SEVENTH EDITION

Handbook of
Nutrition
and the Kidney

SEVENTH EDITION

Handbook of
Nutrition
and the Kidney

Edited by

T. Alp Ikizler, MD

Catherine McLaughlin-Hakim Chair in Vascular Biology
Professor of Medicine
Department of Medicine
Division of Nephrology
Vanderbilt University School of Medicine
Nashville, Tennessee

William E. Mitch, MD

Professor of Medicine and Nephrology
Selzman Institute for Kidney Health
Section of Nephrology
Department of Medicine
Baylor College of Medicine
Houston, Texas

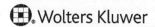 Wolters Kluwer

Philadelphia · Baltimore · New York · London
Buenos Aires · Hong Kong · Sydney · Tokyo

Acquisitions Editor: Kate Heaney
Editorial Coordinator: Annette Ferran
Production Project Manager: Bridgett Dougherty
Manufacturing Coordinator: Beth Welsh
Marketing Manager: Rachel Mante-Leung
Design Coordinator: Steve Druding
Prepress Vendor: S4Carlisle Publishing Services
Seventh Edition

9 8 7 6 5 4

Printed in the United States of America

Library of Congress Cataloging-in-Publication Data

Names: Mitch, William E., editor. | Ikizler, T. Alp., editor.
Title: Handbook of nutrition and the kidney /[edited by] William E. Mitch, MD, Gordon A. Cain Chair in Nephrology, Director, Division of Nephrology, Professor of Medicine, Baylor College of Medicine, Houston, Texas T. Alp Ikizler, MD, Catherine McLaughlin-Hakim Professor of Medicine, Department of Medicine, Division of Nephrology, Vanderbilt University School of Medicine, Nashville, Tennessee.
Description: Seventh edition. | Philadelphia: Wolters Kluwer/Health, [2018] | Includes bibliographical references and index.
Identifiers: LCCN 2017027907 | ISBN 9781496355812
Subjects: LCSH: Kidneys—Diseases—Diet therapy—Handbooks, manuals, etc. | Kidneys—Diseases—Nutritional aspects—Handbooks, manuals, etc.
Classification: LCC RC903.N87 2018 | DDC 616.6/10654—dc23 LC record available at https://lccn.loc.gov/2017027907

LWW.com

We dedicate this book to two outstanding physician-scientists: Joel D. Kopple and Raymond M. Hakim. Each has made seminal contributions to the investigation of mechanisms that underlie nutritional and metabolic abnormalities due to kidney failure. Their contributions to understanding the genesis of complications of kidney disease plus their innovative treatment strategies have become routine practice for patients with kidney disease. They have been recognized through their numerous scientific contributions to practical use of nutritional therapy for patients.

Dr. Kopple was the founding president of the International Society of Renal Nutrition and Metabolism, served as the president of the National Kidney Foundation, and was awarded the Belding H. Scribner Prize by the American Society of Nephrology. Dr. Raymond M. Hakim pioneered clinical studies of mechanisms that cause protein-energy wasting and how to use dialysis for maximum effectiveness. He is widely recognized as a tireless advocate for improving the metabolism and nutritional status of patients receiving renal replacement therapy. His efforts have led to changes in the practice of nephrology and particularly in the area of nutritional support of patients with kidney disease. We are honored to dedicate this book to these giants in our field.

We also dedicate this book to our spouses and children. Without their help, this book devoted to patient care would not have been possible.

CONTRIBUTORS

Naji N. Abumrad, MD
John Sawyers Professor of Surgery and Chairman Emeritus
Vanderbilt University Medical Center
Nashville, Tennessee

Vance L. Albaugh, MD, PhD
Vanderbilt University Medical Center
Nashville, Tennessee

Carla M. Avesani, PhD
Nutrition Institute
Department of Applied Nutrition
Rio de Janeiro State University
Rio de Janeiro, Brazil

Mandeep Bajaj, MD
Department of Medicine
Endocrinology and Diabetes Division
Baylor College of Medicine
Huston, Texas

Melissa B. Bleicher, MD
Assistant Professor of Medicine
Renal, Electrolyte and Hypertension Division
University of Pennsylvania Medical Center
Philadelphia, Pennsylvania

Katrina L. Campbell, PhD AdvAPD
Faculty of Health Sciences and Medicine
Bond University
Department of Nutrition and Dietetics
Princess Alexandra Hospital
Brisbane, Australia

Juan Jesús Carrero, Pharm, PhD
Renal Medicine
Department of Clinical Science
Intervention and Technology
Karolinska Institute
Stockholm, Sweden

Vimal Chadha, MD
Associate Professor of Pediatrics
University of Missouri–Kansas City School of Medicine
Division of Pediatric Nephrology
Children's Mercy Hospital
Kansas City, Missouri

Monica Cortinovis, MD
IRCCS—Istituto di Ricerche Farmacologiche Mario Negri
Clinical Research Center for Rare Diseases Aldo & Cele Daccò
Bergamo, Italy

Lilian Cuppari, MD
Nephrology Division
Federal University of São Paulo
São Paulo, Brazil

Jie Dong, MD, PhD
Professor of Medicine
Renal Division
Peking University First Hospital
Institute of Nephrology
Peking University
Beijing, China

Pieter Evenepoel, MD, PhD
Dienst Nefrologie
Universitair Ziekenhuis Gasthuisberg
Leuven, Belgium

Denis Fouque, MD, PhD
Department Nephrology
Centre Hospitalier Lyon-Sud
University Claude Bernard Lyon 1
Université de Lyon
Pierre-Bénite, France

Simin Goral, MD
Professor of Medicine
Renal, Electrolyte and Hypertension Division
University of Pennsylvania Medical Center
Philadelphia, Pennsylvania

Jane H. Greene, RD, LDN
Vanderbilt University Medical Center
Nashville, Tennessee

Fitsum Guebre-Egziabher, MD
University Grenoble Alpes
Department of Nephrology and Dialysis Transplantation
Centre Hospitalier Universitaire
Grenoble, France

Norio Hanafusa, MD
Associate Professor of Medicine
Department of Blood Purification
Kidney Center
Tokyo Women's Medical University
Tokyo, Japan

Olof Heimbürger, MD, PhD
Renal Medicine
Department of Clinical Science
Intervention and Technology
Karolinska Institutet
Stockholm, Sweden

Adriana M. Hung, MD, MPH
Division of Nephrology and Hypertension
Vanderbilt Center for Kidney Disease
Vanderbilt University Medical Center Nashville Veterans Affairs Hospital
Nashville, Tennessee

T. Alp Ikizler, MD
Catherine McLaughlin-Hakim Chair in Vascular Biology
Professor of Medicine
Department of Medicine
Division of Nephrology
Vanderbilt University School of Medicine
Nashville, Tennessee

Kirsten L. Johansen, MD
Division of Nephrology
University of California
San Francisco, California

Jaimon Kelly, APD, PhD Scholar
Faculty of Health Sciences and Medicine
Bond University
Gold Coast, Australia

Joel D. Kopple, MD
Professor of Medicine and Public Health
Division of Nephrology and Hypertension
Los Angeles Biomedical Research Institute at Harbor-UCLA Medical Center
David Geffen School of Medicine at UCLA
UCLA Fielding School of Public Health
Torrance, California

Maarit Korkeila, MD, PhD
Renal Medicine
Department of Clinical Science
Intervention and Technology
Karolinska Institutet
Stockholm, Sweden

Csaba P. Kovesdy, MD
Division of Nephrology
University of Tennessee Health Science Center
Memphis, Tennessee

John C. Lieske, MD
Professor of Medicine
Department of Internal Medicine
Mayo Clinic Division of Nephrology and Hypertension
Medical Director
Department of Laboratory Medicine and Pathology
Mayo Clinic Renal Testing Laboratory
Rochester, Minnesota

Bengt Lindholm, MD, PhD
Renal Medicine and Baxter Novum
Department of Clinical Science
Intervention and Technology
Karolinska Institutet
Stockholm, Sweden

Michael S. Lipkowitz, MD
Fellowship Program Director
Medstar
Georgetown University Hospital-Division of Nephrology
Washington, D.C.

Kathleen D. Liu, MD, PhD, MAS
Division of Nephrology
University of California
San Francisco, California

Denise Mafra, PhD
Graduate Program in Medical Sciences and Graduate Program in
    Cardiovascular Sciences
Federal Fluminense University, Niterói
Rio de Janeiro, Brazil

Björn Meijers, MD, PhD
Laboratory of Nephrology
Department of Immunology and Microbiology
KU Leuven
Department of Nephrology and Renal Transplantation
University Hospitals Leuven
Leuven, Belgium

William E. Mitch, MD
Professor of Medicine and Nephrology
Selzman Institute for Kidney Health
Section of Nephrology
Department of Medicine
Baylor College of Medicine
Houston, Texas

Miklos Z. Molnar, MD, PhD
Division of Nephrology
University of Tennessee Health Science Center
Memphis, Tennessee

Linda W. Moore, MS, RDN, LD, CCRP
Department of Surgery
Director Clinical Research
Clinical Nutrition Scientist, Outcomes Research
Houston Methodist Hospital Specialty Physician Group
Houston, Texas

Sagar U. Nigwekar, MD, MMSc
Assistant in Medicine
Massachusetts General Hospital
Instructor in Medicine
Harvard Medical School
Boston, Massachusetts

Jose J. Perez, MD
Assistant Professor
Selzman Institute for Kidney Health
Section of Nephrology
Department of Medicine
Baylor College of Medicine
Houston, Texas

Norberto Perico, MD
IRCCS—Istituto di Ricerche Farmacologiche Mario Negri
Clinical Research Center for Rare Diseases Aldo & Cele Daccò
Bergamo, Italy

Giuseppe Remuzzi, MD, FRCP
IRCCS—Istituto di Ricerche Farmacologiche Mario Negri
Centro Anna Maria Astori Science and Technology Park Kilometro Rosso
Bergamo, Italy

Connie M. Rhee, MD
Division of Nephrology and Hypertension
University of California Irvine
Orange, California

Deirdre Sawinski, MD
Assistant Professor of Medicine
Renal, Electrolyte and Hypertension Division
University of Pennsylvania Medical Center
Philadelphia, Pennsylvania

Edward D. Siew, MD, MSCI
Division of Nephrology and Hypertension
Vanderbilt Center for Kidney Disease
Integrated Program for AKI Research
Vanderbilt University Medical Center
Nashville Veterans Affairs Hospital
Tennessee Valley Healthcare Systems
Nashville, Tennessee

Peter Stenvinkel, MD, PhD
Renal Medicine
Department of Clinical Science
Intervention and Technology
Karolinska Institutet
Stockholm, Sweden

Ravi I. Thadhani, MD, MPH
Chief, Division of Nephrology
Massachusetts General Hospital
Professor of Medicine
Harvard Medical School
Boston, Massachusetts

Christoph Wanner, MD
Professor of Medicine
Chief, Division of Nephrology
University Hospital Würzburg
Würzburg, Germany

Bradley A. Warady, MD
Professor of Pediatrics
University of Missouri–Kansas City School of Medicine
Director, Division of Pediatric Nephrology
Director, Dialysis and Transplantation
Children's Mercy Hospital
Kansas City, Missouri

Christopher S. Wilcox, MD, PhD
Chief of Nephrology and Hypertension
Director of Cardiovascular-Kidney Institute
Vice-Chair for Academic Affairs, Department of Medicine
George E. Schreiner Chair of Nephrology
Georgetown University
Washington, D.C.

Rosanne J. Woloschuk, RD
Renal Dietitian
Children's Hospital Colorado
Aurora, Colorado

Biruh Workeneh, MD
Department of Nephrology
The University of Texas MD Anderson Cancer Center
Houston, Texas

In the seventh edition of the *Handbook of Nutrition and the Kidney*, there are important changes and additions. First, there are 28 new authors, including experts from Australia, Brazil, Belgium, China, France, Germany, Italy, Japan, and Sweden. These authors bring new perspectives to the international participation of investigators in this area of patient care. Second, we have added new topics to broaden the scope of the overall goal, namely, how changing the diet influences the course of kidney disease. The new topics include the epidemiology of nutritional metabolic abnormalities in kidney disease, practical approaches to screening and assessment of nutrition status, the influence of gut microbiome in kidney disease, medical nutritional therapy, and a comprehensive but practical chapter detailing nutritional aspects of pediatric patients with kidney disease. Importantly, these new chapters are included without compromising the usefulness of the handbook. Third, we continue to emphasize practical and clinically relevant aspects of manipulating the diet while making the handbook more accessible and useful for physicians, dietitians, nurses, students, and other professionals who provide care for patients with kidney disease. We continue to emphasize the use of figures and tables to demonstrate nutritional principles.

Our goal is to integrate scientific lessons with clinical wisdom to provide readers with clinically useful information plus a rational approach to supplying the nutritional needs of patients with acute and chronic kidney disease, patients undergoing maintenance dialysis (both hemodialysis and peritoneal dialysis) or kidney transplantation, or patients with kidney stones, hypertension, metabolic syndrome, diabetic nephropathy, or nephrotic syndrome. We have made these changes because we believe the role of nutritional principals in the treatment of patients with kidney disease cannot be overestimated and is becoming integrated more completely in the day-to-day management of these individuals. Specifically, the requirements for protein, energy, minerals, and other elements change substantially in patients with advancing kidney disease, and ignoring these changes can contribute to complications that jeopardize the overall well-being of the patient. New advances in understanding the mechanisms behind these derangements, such as the role of the microbiome or systemic inflammation, must be accessible to readers. Besides these new topics, each chapter has been revised and updated by experts in nephrology, metabolism, and clinical nutrition.

We are grateful to the chapter authors for their timely and thoughtful contributions to the handbook.

T. Alp Ikizler
William E. Mitch

CONTENTS

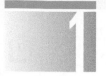

Nutritional Requirements of Healthy Adults

Vance L. Albaugh and Naji N. Abumrad

Over the last few decades, nutritional recommendations have come under intense scrutiny, especially with the increasing prevalence of obesity and other chronic diseases. Through the end of the 20th century, nutritional recommendations in the United States and Canada consisted of the recommended dietary allowance (RDA). Part of the scrutiny of RDAs was that particular nutrients that had been recognized as being important to human health (e.g., dietary fiber, carotenoids) did not necessarily have RDAs, whereas other nutrients that were associated with health or prevention of chronic disease did not have any indication of those benefits reflected by the RDA. To better incorporate nutritional research advances, the Institute of Medicine (IOM) has restructured dietary macro- and micronutrient recommendations, which are currently called dietary reference intakes (DRIs). DRIs for a particular nutrient comprise six components that include the estimated average requirement (EAR), recommended dietary allowance (RDA), tolerable upper intake level (UL), adequate intake (AI), acceptable macronutrient distribution range (AMDR), and estimated energy requirement.

In the following chapter, we review basic biochemistry and digestive physiology of macronutrients and micronutrients as well as the DRIs for healthy adults. Given these requirements change significantly depending on the age and sex of the individual, we discuss these requirements in a general sense and urge the reader to consult the IOM guidelines (www.nam.edu) for specific requirements and up-to-date recommendations.

MACRONUTRIENT REQUIREMENTS FOR HEALTHY ADULTS

Carbohydrates and Fiber

The term carbohydrate, or "carbon hydrates," lends itself directly from the chemical structure (Fig. 1.1). The stoichiometric formula of an unmodified simple carbohydrate molecule or monosaccharide is $(C \cdot H_2O)_n$ or $(CHOH)_n$. The number of carbon atoms per molecule can be as few as three, referred to as triose(s) ($C_3H_6O_3$: e.g., glyceraldehyde and dihydroxyacetone) to as many as nine or nonose(s) ($C_9H_{18}O_9$: like neuraminic acid, also called sialic acid, commonly found in glycoproteins and gangliosides). Although these monosaccharides are naturally occurring, by far the most abundant and commonly used in metabolism are the six-carbon hexoses ($C_6H_{12}O_6$), mainly glucose, galactose, fructose, and mannose. Another important class of monosaccharides is the five-carbon pentoses ($C_5H_{10}O_5$), which includes ribose, a constituent of deoxyribonucleic acid (DNA) and ribonucleic acid (RNA).

Carbohydrates are classified according to the number of saccharide molecules forming the sugar. They are subdivided into mono-, di-, oligo-, and polysaccharides. Monosaccharides have one molecule (e.g., glyceraldehyde, ribose, glucose, galactose, fructose), whereas disaccharides have two molecules linked together (e.g., maltose (glucose-glucose), lactose (glucose-galactose), and sucrose (glucose-fructose)) which is commonly known as "table sugar."

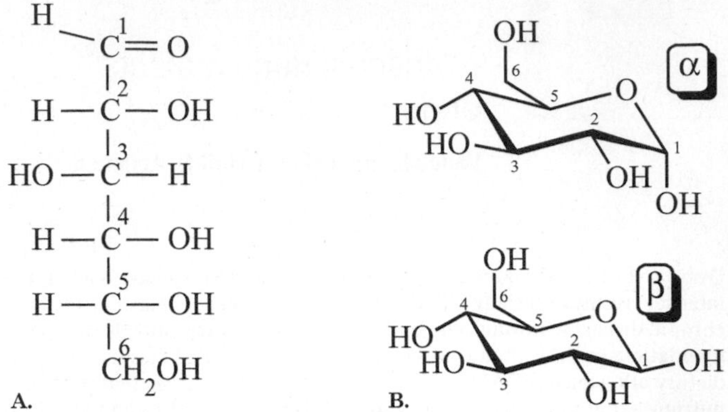

FIGURE 1.1 D-Glucose. **A:** Representation of Dextro-glucose (D-glucose) stereoisomer through Fisher linear projection. **B:** Cyclic representation of D-glucose in a three-dimensional perspective or chain conformation, also called Haworth projection. When the hydroxyl (OH) group on C-1 is on the opposite side of the methyl (CH_2OH) group on C-6 the anomer is called (α) and when both chemical groups are on the same side the anomer is called (β).

Oligosaccharides contain between 3 and 10 monosaccharides; they are often found as components of glycolipids and glycoproteins. Finally, polysaccharides have more than 10 molecules, although usually the number is much higher between 200 and 2,500. The sugar moieties are linked together in a multi-branched structure. Starch is the main plant's polysaccharide whereas glycogen makes its counterpart as the animal's prototype. Both are polymers of glucose, although glycogen has more extensive branching than starch.

The term fiber was coined in 1953, when Hipsley reported a possible association between dietary fibers and the lower occurrence of pregnancy toxemia. Dietary fibers were analytically defined for the first time in 1972 by Trowell et al. as "the skeletal remains of plant cells resistant to digestion by human enzymes." This definition was subsequently modified in 1976 into "all plant polysaccharides and lignins that are resistant to hydrolysis by digestive enzymes of the man." Dietary fibers are complex polysaccharides, and it has been recently recognized that fiber is beneficial to human health. Fiber can be referred to as dietary, functional, and total fiber. Dietary fiber is composed of nondigestible carbohydrates and lignins, which are intrinsic and intact in plants. Functional fiber is isolated, nondigestible carbohydrates that have physiologic effects in humans. Total fiber is the sum of both dietary and functional fibers.

Simple versus Complex Carbohydrates

Cellulose, a typical fiber, is the most abundant natural organic compound on earth. About 33% of all plant matter comprises cellulose, which is the structural component of the cell wall of green plants. Cellulose is a condensation of D-glucose moieties connected through β (1-4) glycosidic bonds (Fig. 1.2). In contrast to α (1-4) present in starch, the β bonds make the linear chain of cellulose less flexible than the amylose chain; accordingly, no coiling occurs, and the molecule adopts an extended and stiff, rod-like conformation (Fig. 1.3). The open chain configuration exposes multiple —OH groups and promotes the formation of hydrogen bonds between the glucose residues. These connections stabilize cellulose, which organizes into microfibrils with high tensile strength.

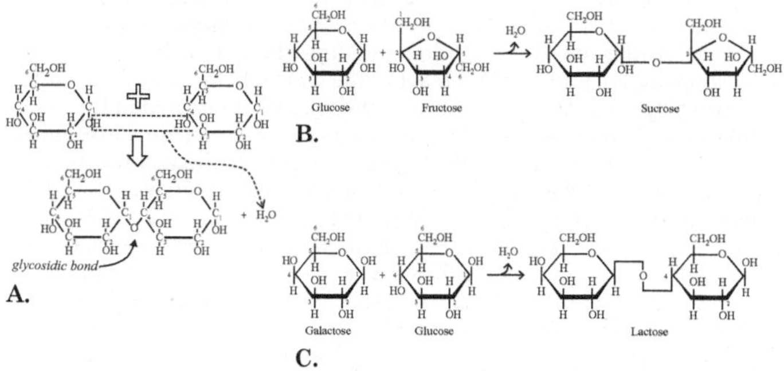

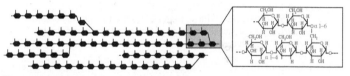

FIGURE 1.2 Glycosidic bond. **A:** Formation of a glycosidic bond between two monosaccharides is a dehydration reaction with liberation of H_2O. **B:** α-glycosidic bond: when the bond is on the opposite side of the substituent group (not H) connected to the carbon (C) flanking the oxygen (O). The O ring is considered as the reference plane (in the case of sucrose the substituent group is CH_2OH C-6 that is connected to C-5 of the glucose ring). **C:** β-glycosidic bond: the substituent group and the bond are on the same side of the ring.

FIGURE 1.3 Starch structure. **A:** Amylose portion of starch showing helical formation because of the bend introduced by the α-glycosidic bonds. The coiling is not interrupted because all the attachments between the glucose moieties are bent in one direction; they are all α (1-4) bonds. This configuration is useful for storage because it relatively occupies less space. At the same time, it gives more resistance to enzymatic access and digestion. **B:** Amylopectin fraction of starch shows a branching structure with less coiling because the bending introduced by α (1-4) bonds is interrupted with the α (1-6) bonds that have different directions.

Physiology of Digestion and Absorption

Cellular metabolic pathways use monosaccharides as their substrates. Monosaccharides are absorbed by the intestinal enterocyte, through the digestive process, which begins in the mouth with salivary amylase that is similar in function to pancreatic amylase. Both amylases are specific for α (1-4) glycosidic bonds present inside the polysaccharide chain but spare other α linkages; that is, α (1-6), terminal α (1-4), and α (1-4) adjacent to a branching point. Amylase digestion of a polysaccharide yields shorter chain polysaccharides, oligosaccharides, and disaccharides. When the mixture of carbohydrates and amylase reaches the stomach, the acidic pH inhibits the hydrolytic activity of the enzyme. This activity is restored in the duodenum by the pancreatic secretions rich in bicarbonate and amylase. Further digestion into monosaccharides occurs just outside the enterocyte in the intestinal lumen by another group of enzymes called oligosaccharidases. These enzymes, secreted locally, break the glycosidic bonds present in the disaccharides and oligosaccharides. The different human oligosaccharidases, the site of their action, their substrates, and the products of their digestive processes are summarized in Table 1.1. Overall, this brush border digestion and subsequent absorption of monosaccharides transforms a mixture of different sugars ingested into glucose, galactose, and fructose that can be taken up by enterocytes by a number of specific transporters.

By definition, fibers are mainly polysaccharides resistant to digestion and absorption. Cellulose (polysaccharide of β (1-4) linear glucose) is indigestible by humans (although it can indirectly be broken down by colonic bacteria and then absorbed by colonocytes). The main reason being that amylase, the only polysaccharidase present in the intestinal tract, is specific for α (1-4) sugars not β (1-4). On the other hand, the table sugar sucrose (disaccharide: α (1-2) glucose–fructose) is completely hydrolyzed by sucrase (Table 1.1) and completely absorbed. Starches from different sources have different contents and complexities. Fiber intake has been associated with improvement in coronary heart disease as well as improved blood glucose homeostasis. High-fiber foods are also satiety-promoting and lower postprandial insulin, which may help preclude development of obesity and type 2 diabetes.

Daily Requirements

Given that carbohydrates are ubiquitous within the diets of most individuals across the world, intake insufficiency is typically not a problem. The current recommended dietary allowance (RDA) and AI values for carbohydrates on average are 130 g per day in both sexes. These RDA/AI values are higher in pregnant or lactating individuals, being 175 and 210 g per day, respectively. Starches and sugars are easily found in grains, vegetables, and fruits. Of note, it is recommended that "added sugars" be limited to no more than 25% of energy intake.

In terms of fiber, the RDIs suggest a range between 20 and 40 g per day depending on the sex and age of the individual, with requirements being slightly higher for males than females. Dietary fiber includes common sources such as grains or those from other plant or animal sources. With regard to the health benefits of naturally occurring fiber, the IOM refers that separation of dietary fiber from other coexisting nutrients that may be having beneficial effects is difficult. Generally speaking, excessive fiber intake is self-limited by the individual.

Amino Acids and Proteins

Proteins are made up of individual amino acids units with the general formula NH_2-CHR-COOH (Fig. 1.4A). Amino acids are organic acids with a central carbon (i.e., the α-carbon) that is bound to a carboxylic acid (COOH) on one side and an amino group (NH_2) on the other side. The remaining two bonds of the α-carbon are linked to a hydrogen atom (H) and an aliphatic side known as the "R group" or the "functional group." One exception to this definition is proline, which is an imino or cyclic amino acid (Fig. 1.4B). The physicochemical properties of amino acids depend on the size, structure, and configuration of the functional groups.

TABLE 1.1

Principle Oligosaccharidases of the Intestinal Lumen

Enzyme	Maltase	Lactase	Sucrase	α-Dextrinase	Trehalase
Action site	α-1,4	β-1,4	α-1,2	α-1,6	α-1,1
Substrate (s)	Maltose	Lactose	Sucrose	α-Dextrins	Trehalose
	α-1,4 Glu*-glu	β-1,4 Glu-galactose	α-1,2 Glu-fructose		α-1,1 Glu-glu
	Maltotriose		Maltose		
	α-1,4 Glu-glu-glu				
	α-Dextrins		Maltotriose		
	α-1,6 Glu-glu-(α-1,4 glu-glu)$_n$				
Product (s)	Glu	Glu	Glu	Glu	Glu
	α-1,6 Glu-glu	Galactose	Fructose	(α-1,4 Glu-glu)$_n$	
Overall result	**Glu, galactose, and fructose**				

*Glu, Glucose.

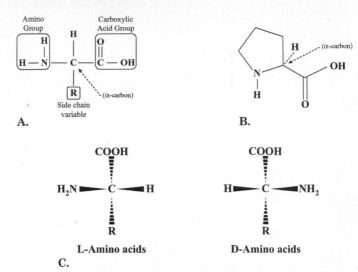

FIGURE 1.4 Structure and configuration of the amino acids. **A:** General formula for an amino acid showing the specificity of each group. The carboxylic acid (COOH) and the amino group (NH₂) are constant, whereas the side chain (R) attached to the main carbon atom (called α-carbon) is variable and it defines the name and structure of each amino acid. **B:** Proline is the only amino acid that does not follow the general rule. Its α-carbon is cyclized within the side chain. **C:** The α-carbon represents a rotational center along which two different configurations can exist; they are called optical Levo- (L) and Dextro- (D) isomers. L and D isomers are mirror images of each other and are not superimposable.

The chiral α-carbon of the amino acid allows for one of two stereoisomers, the "L" or "D" (for "Levo-" and "Dextro-"), respectively (Fig. 1.4C). Glycine is an exception, because the α carbon is bound to two hydrogen atoms and not chiral. In contrast to the carbohydrates in which "D" isomers are utilized for energy production, the human body recognizes "L" amino acids for metabolism and protein synthesis. "D" amino acids, which occur naturally in other organisms are freely filtered at the glomerulus and excreted in the urine.

Proteins are linear polymers of amino acids between the amino group of one amino acid and the carboxy group of another amino acid in an amide linkage, known as the peptide bond. An oligopeptide consists of a protein length between 2 and 12 amino acids (i.e., dipeptide, tripeptide, tetrapeptide, pentapeptide, etc.). Proteins with higher number of amino acids units are called polypeptides and assume a three-dimensional form by changing from the basic linear chain conformation (or primary protein structure) into a secondary and then a tertiary structure depending on chemical properties of the constituent amino acids. Larger protein macromolecules can also be formed by more than one tertiary chain, which is referred to as quaternary structure.

A large number of molecules can follow the general formula of an amino acid; however, only 20 are normally incorporated during protein synthesis in humans directly from the ribosome. Amino acid synthesis can occur through breakdown and recycling of cellular protein or de novo endogenous synthesis from metabolic intermediates that are structurally related to amino acids. For example, D-pyruvate and L-alanine are distinguished by the absence or presence of an amino group, respectively. Many metabolic intermediates share this structural similarity with amino acids and are interconvertible. Thus, this is why the human body has a preference for D-sugars and L-amino acids.

Essential versus Nonessential Amino Acids

Amino acids can be divided into essential and nonessential. Essential amino acids must be derived from the diet because the body cannot synthesize these amino acids endogenously. On the other hand, nonessential amino acids can be synthesized endogenously from other metabolic intermediates (as mentioned earlier). In addition to essential and nonessential, some amino acids can also be referred to as being "conditionally essential," meaning the body cannot produce sufficient quantities in times of stress or rapid growth—situations like trauma, infection, catabolic diseases, or neonatal/infant growth. Eleven amino acids are considered nonessential: alanine, arginine, aspartic acid, asparagine, cysteine, glutamic acid, glutamine, glycine, proline, serine, and tyrosine. Of these nonessential amino acids, arginine, cysteine, glutamine, and serine are conditionally essential. The remaining nine essential amino acids are isoleucine, leucine, lysine, methionine, phenylalanine, threonine, tryptophan, valine, and histidine.

Physiology of Digestion and Absorption

In a typical Western diet, 70 to 100 g of protein is ingested daily, and an additional 35 to 200 g of protein joins this pool from endogenous sources (i.e., gastrointestinal [GI] secretions, desquamated intestinal cells, and plasma proteins). More than 95% of total protein delivered to the intestines is normally digested and absorbed. Protein digestion begins in the stomach where the acidic milieu denatures proteins and promotes proteolytic enzyme function. The acidic milieu converts protein-degrading pepsinogens (inactive) into pepsins (active), which are the proteolytic enzymes of the stomach and work best in an acidic pH. The amount of proteins digested in the stomach is minimal; however, even people with a previous total gastrectomy digest and absorb protein normally.

Following the initiation of protein digestion in the stomach, further digestion involves a number of peptidases and other enzymes that degrade complex proteins to individual amino acids or short peptides. In the duodenum, the protein load is digested by proteolytic enzymes of the pancreas to approximately 60% by the time it reaches the proximal jejunum. These duodenal enzymes include trypsinogen, chymotrypsinogen, proelastase, and procarboxypeptidases A and B. All these enzymes are secreted as inactive zymogens in the pancreatic juice. An enteropeptidase originating from the brush border of the duodenal epithelial cells activates trypsinogen to trypsin and then trypsin is available to activate these other pancreatic proenzymes. In contrast to pepsin in the stomach, pancreatic enzymes require an optimum pH of 8. Except for the carboxypeptidases, which are exopeptidases (cleaving amino acids at the terminal end of a peptide), all pancreatic enzymes mentioned are endopeptidases (cleave amino acids within a polypeptide chain). Trypsin cleaves at peptide bonds with lysine or arginine at one end, but it refrains when the other end is occupied by proline. Chymotrypsin has similar specificity to pepsin (neutral amino acids or aromatic ones). Elastase has a relatively broader specificity attacking peptide bonds adjacent to small amino acids with aliphatic (linear) chains such as alanine, glycine, serine, and valine. Carboxypeptidase A splits aromatic amino acids from the terminal end of a peptide chain, and carboxypeptidase B cleaves terminal arginine residues at the carboxyl end also. After the combined action of pancreatic enzymes, approximately 70% of proteins are transformed into oligopeptides and 30% into free amino acids.

At the mucosal brush border, cell surface peptidases produced by the enterocytes cleave amino acids from the oligopeptide pool present at their contact, releasing free amino acids and smaller peptides. The outcome of the intraluminal and brush border digestive processes culminates in the release of free amino acids, dipeptides, and tripeptides that are absorbed across the apical cell membrane of enterocytes by specific transporters. Further hydrolysis of dipeptides and tripeptides into amino acids occurs inside the cell by several cytosolic peptidases. From a load of proteins entering the digestive lumen, only simple amino acids are transferred to the basolateral space of the enterocyte. As a rule, proteins are successfully broken down into smaller size entities as they progress along the digestive tract, releasing amino acids and small peptides (di- and tripeptides) into the portal circulation.

Daily Requirements

The requirements for daily protein intake are generally weight based (i.e., 1.5 g/kg/d for infants, 1.1 g/kg/d for ages 1 to 3 years, 0.95 g/kg/d for 4 to 13 years, 0.85 g/kg/d for 14 to 18 years, 0.8 g/kg/d for adults, and 1.1 g/kg/d for pregnant individuals [i.e., based on prepregnancy weight] and lactating women). The AMDR for protein and amino acids is from 10 to 35 g per day for healthy adults, with the lower limit at the RDA for protein and the upper limit intended to complement the dietary intake when considering carbohydrates and lipids collectively. The large majority of individuals have no difficulties sustaining adequate protein intake, with high-protein foods being mostly meat, poultry, eggs, cheese, and other dairy products. Even individuals consuming a vegan diet can maintain adequate protein intake by consuming high-protein foods like legumes, grains, nuts, seeds, and other vegetables.

Lipids

Lipids can exert a wide array of biologic functions, although their high energy density (9 kcal per g) makes them a preferred fuel for storage. Dietary lipids consist mostly of triglycerides (>95%), whereas the remainder is cholesterol, fatty acids, phospholipids, and plant sterols. A triglyceride, also known as triacylglycerol, is formed from a single molecule of glycerol, combined through ester bonds on each of the three –OH groups of glycerol with a fatty acid. A monoglyceride (monoacylglycerol) or diglyceride (diacylglycerol) has one glycerol connected to one or two fatty acids, respectively (Fig. 1.5).

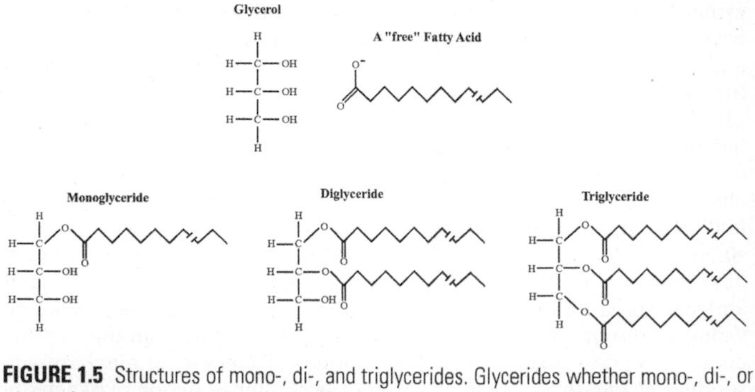

FIGURE 1.5 Structures of mono-, di-, and triglycerides. Glycerides whether mono-, di-, or triglycerides are formed through esterification of the carboxyl group (COOH) on a fatty acid to the hydroxyl group (OH) on the glycerol molecule with the release of a molecule of water (H_2O) for every esterification reaction.

In contrast to triglycerides, fatty acids are carboxylic acids with long, generally unbranched hydrocarbon tails (chain) that are either unsaturated (i.e., with a double bond) or saturated without any doubly bonded carbons. Fatty acids can be esterified to glycerol to synthesize triglyceride molecules for fuel storage in times of surplus or can be hydrolyzed from the glycerol backbone of triglycerides and then oxidized to acetyl CoA molecules via β-oxidation during times of high energy demand. The net flux of lipids is highly dependent on the energy status of the individual. It is important to note that glucose metabolized via glycolysis can be converted to acetyl CoA through the action of pyruvate dehydrogenase, which catalyzes an irreversible reaction (Fig. 1.6). Thus, glucose can be used to synthesize fatty acids, but fatty acids cannot be converted back into glucose for use by the body. This is especially important during periods of prolonged fasting when tissues selectively switch to using predominately fatty acids and ketone bodies for metabolic fuels to preserve glucose for organs that are dependent on it (e.g., red blood cells, brain). During these periods, the liver is the source of ketone body formation (e.g., acetoacetate and β-hydroxybutyrate), which are synthesized from acetyl CoA.

Essential versus Nonessential Fatty Acids

The double bond, characteristic of the unsaturated fatty acids, induces two conformations of the linear chain, *cis* and *trans*. The "*cis*" form, with adjacent hydrogens on the same side, causes the chain to bend and restricts the conformational freedom of the fatty acid. This decreased flexibility of the *cis* conformation hinders the ability of the fatty acids to be closely packed, for example, in lipid droplets. It also favors a lower melting temperature compared to the *trans* conformation. In contrast, in "*trans*" fatty acids (or trans fats), adjacent hydrogen atoms are bound to opposite sides of the double bond and enable them to be more closely packed. This does not cause much bending, and the chain will look similar to straight saturated fatty acids (Fig. 1.7A). The higher melting point and the higher conformational flexibility of the trans fatty acids have major biologic effects. Consumption of trans fatty acids by humans has been positively associated with harmful changes in serum lipids, systemic inflammation, and risk of heart disease. All naturally

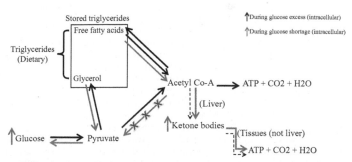

FIGURE 1.6 Diagram showing energy pathways during different metabolic states. In postprandial periods, the supply of glucose and free fatty acids provides enough ATP for energy consumption, and the excess is driven toward storing this energy in the form of triglycerides with very little formation of ketone bodies. During fasting, especially prolonged ones, mobilization of triglycerides toward glucose is limited (no reverse reaction forming glucose from acetyl CoA), with accumulation of more ketone bodies to be used as a source of alternative energy.

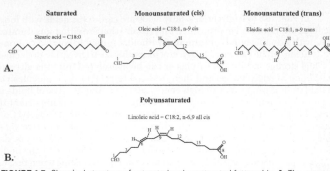

FIGURE 1.7 Chemical structure of saturated and unsaturated fatty acids. **A:** The presence of a double bond in a fatty acid chain characterizes the unsaturated state. In a "cis" configuration, both hydrogen (H) atoms are present on one side of the double bond giving the chain a bent shape. In the "trans" configuration, each H is on one side of the double bond and this keeps the chain in nearly a linear form. Metabolic consequences of these two forms are explained in the text. **B:** Example of a polyunsaturated fatty acid structure illustrating the "$n - x$" (or "$\omega - x$") nomenclature style. Linoleic acid is an example for polyunsaturated fatty acid; in the $n - x$ nomenclature, it is written as C18:2, n-6-9 all cis, meaning that this is an 18 carbon (C) chain length with 2 double bonds, one located at C-6 (between C-6 and C-7) and the second one at C-9 (between C-9 and C-10), all in the cis configuration. Numbering of C atoms starts from the methyl end (CH_3).

occurring unsaturated fatty acids are cis, and most trans fatty acids are the result of human processing.

Polyunsaturated fatty acids are another type of fatty acid, with double bonds almost invariably occurring at three carbon atoms further along the chain from the preceding one. Different systems of nomenclature for unsaturated fatty acids are described. The more commonly used in popular literature is "$n - x$" (n minus x; also "$\omega - x$" or omega minus x) nomenclature. It starts by designating the total number of carbon atoms and double bonds in a fatty acid by C:D called the code (C is the number of carbons, and D is the number of double bonds). Then, it identifies the placement of the double bond "x" relative to the methyl end (CH3) of the carbon chain and the conformation cis/trans. For example, linoleic acid is described as "C18:2, $n - 6{,}9$ all cis" or "C18:2, $\omega - 6{,}9$ all cis." It indicates that the chain has 18 carbons and 2 double bonds where the first one is located between the sixth and seventh carbon atoms from the methyl end. The second double bond is definitely located at the ninth carbon. All double bonds are cis (Fig. 1.7B).

Similar to amino acids, the terminology essential and nonessential indicates those fatty acids that can be produced de novo or must be obtained from the diet, respectively. During de novo formation, the human enzymes are capable of inserting double bonds at n-9 or higher. Meanwhile, mammalian tissues contain four families of polyunsaturated fatty acids (n-3, n-6, n-7, and n-9). Thus, polyunsaturated fatty acids that have their first double bond below n-9 are essential and must be obtained in the diet. In humans, there are two major short chain polyunsaturated fatty acids that are essential, linolenic acid and linoleic acid, which can be used to make longer length n-3 and n-6.

Physiology of Digestion and Absorption

The digestive process of dietary lipids begins with the lingual lipase secreted in the oral cavity. A gastric lipase has a similar function in the stomach. These enzymes act on ester bonds present on the third carbon of the glycerol, releasing diacylglycerol and free fatty acids. Further digestion by the gastric lipase produces free fatty acids and glycerol. The majority of lipid digestion, however, begins in the duodenum where pancreatic lipases work in concert with other digestive enzymes (e.g., co-lipase) to reduce lipid surface tension and allow for efficient hydrolysis and absorption. Other lipases also hydrolyze cholesterol esters into cholesterol and fatty acids as well as fat-soluble vitamins and phospholipids.

The overall impact of the digestive process on ingested lipids is the formation of a mixture of substances made up of monoglycerides, free fatty acids, and cholesterol. Monoglycerides are relatively water soluble whereas free fatty acids and cholesterol are more hydrophobic molecules. The transport of the water insoluble products into the mucosal cells requires passage through an unstirred hydrophilic water layer at the mucosal brush border. This is accomplished by the formation of micelles mainly by bile salts and phospholipids. Through an amphipathic interaction between the bile salts and the phospholipids, free fatty acids and cholesterol are incorporated in a spherical shape. Thus, the polar (water soluble) extremities of the bile salts are exposed to the water milieu, whereas the nonpolar groups (i.e., hydrocarbon tails of the free fatty acids and cholesterol) are imbedded inside the sphere. Incorporation of monoglycerides in a micelle increases its ability to solubilize free fatty acids and cholesterol. On contact with the mucosal cell membrane, the polar heads in the micelles and the hydrophilic side (external) of the cell membrane interact and open the way for the more lipophilic substances to pass through the lipid part of the membrane and into the cell.

Daily Requirements

Given that excess carbohydrates and amino acids can be converted to fatty acids and stored as triglycerides, there are no specific RDA/AI for total fat intake for adults; however, the AMDR values are generally between 25 and 35 g per day for both adult sexes. Because high-dietary intake of fat has been linked to chronic disease, this is the rationale for determining the upper limit of the AMRD, whereas the lower limit is recommended to ensure AI of fat-soluble nutrients. Cholesterol, as well as trans and saturated fats have no determined RDAs or AMDR. With respect to n-3 polyunsaturated fatty acids, the RDA/AI values are generally 1.1 to 1.6 g per day depending on the sex and age of the individual, whereas the RDA/AI values for n-6 polyunsaturated fatty acid (linoleic acid) are much higher than those of n-3, with values of 10 to 17 g per day. Excellent sources of n-3 (linolenic acid) and n-6 (linoleic acid) polyunsaturated fats are soybean, flax seed, safflower, corn and canola oils, fish, nuts, as well as some meats and eggs.

MICRONUTRIENT REQUIREMENTS FOR HEALTHY ADULTS

Dietary Vitamins and Minerals

Micronutrients are vitally important for human health, and a number of classic deficiencies have been described over the last 100 years. With the availability diverse foods as well as dietary supplementation, micronutrient deficiencies are rare but their effects can be devastating if not identified and treated. As a brief review for this text, we describe the basic functions (if known) for the various micronutrients. Where applicable, the RDA/AI and other information from the nutrient's DRIs has been included. For more information on the age-dependent dietary recommendations as well as other information on the potential deficiencies or consequences of overconsumption, we encourage the reader to review the DRI information from the IOM.

Fat-Soluble Vitamins

Vitamin A, also known as **retinol**, is necessary for vision, embryologic development, normal immune function as well as gene transcription in a number of cases. The RDA/AI ranges between 600 and 900 μg per day with slightly higher requirements for males and increases to 750 to 770 μg per day or 1,200 to 1,300 μg per day in pregnancy or lactation. Foods high in Vitamin A include liver, dark leafy green vegetables, fruits, and fish products. The upper limit of recommended intake is below 3,000 μg per day in most individuals because of hepatic toxicity or teratogenic effects.

Vitamin D, also known as **calciferol**, is used biologically to maintain calcium and phosphorous homeostasis and is important in maintenance of bone health. The RDA/AI values are 600 IU per day across all individuals including those pregnant or lactating. Liver, fish, eggs, and fortified dairy and cereal products are all excellent sources of vitamin D. Excessive consumption can lead to hypercalcemia and altered cardiovascular or kidney function in certain cases, which is why the upper limit intake is not greater than 4,000 IU per day.

Vitamin E, also known as α-**tocopherol**, functions as an antioxidant and may have various roles in gene transcription or cellular signaling processes. The RDA/AI is 15 mg per day in adults with increased requirements in those lactating, requiring 19 mg per day. Vitamin E deficiency can lead to myopathies, neuropathies, and immune impairment. The upper limit of normal intake is not greater than 1,000 mg per day for most individuals. Sufficient vitamin E can be found in vegetables and their oils, fruits, nuts, and meat.

Vitamin K, also known as **phylloquinone**, is a coenzyme important in the synthesis of factors involved in the blood-clotting cascade. The RDA/AI values range from 60 to 90 μg per day in most individuals, with the higher recommendations in those older, pregnant, or lactating. Vitamin K is found in excellent quantities in green leafy vegetables as well as plant oils. There are no known adverse effects with excess vitamin K supplementation.

Water-Soluble Vitamins

Vitamin B$_1$, also known as **thiamin**, is a coenzyme that is necessary for a number of chemical processes in the body, including adequate function of pyruvate dehydrogenase as well as branched-chain α-keto acid dehydrogenase. The dietary requirements range from 0.9 to 1.1 mg per day across both sexes, and 1.4 mg per day is recommended for pregnant and lactating individuals. Thiamin can be found in enriched whole grains and grain-containing foods like cereals. There are no known effects of excess thiamin intake, but a number of conditions associated with its deficiency including Beriberi, optic neuropathy, and Wernicke-Korsakoff syndrome.

Vitamin B$_2$, also known as **riboflavin**, is a coenzyme in a number of redox reactions within the body. The RDA/AI values range from 0.9 to 1.1 mg per day for both sexes, with increased requirements of 1.4 and 1.6 mg per day for pregnant and lactating individuals, respectively. Dietary sources of riboflavin include fortified cereals, organ meats, milk, and other bread products. There have been no described adverse effects of excess riboflavin intake.

Vitamin B$_3$, also known as **niacin** (or nicotinic acid), is a coenzyme in redox reactions within the body. The RDA/AI ranges from 12 to 14 mg per day for both sexes, with increased requirements of 17 to 18 mg per day in lactating or pregnant individuals. High-niacin foods include meats, fish, poultry, and fortified bread products. There are no known adverse effects of excess niacin consumption, although acute intake can lead to flushing or GI upset. In particular, individuals on hemodialysis or peritoneal dialysis may require supplemental niacin.

Vitamin B₅, also known as **pantothenic acid** is a coenzyme that is used in the synthesis of Coenzyme A, which is involved in a wide range of biochemical processes. These include acylation and acetylation as well as synthesis of fatty acids, cholesterol, and acetylcholine. The RDA/AI ranges from 4 to 5 mg per day in both sexes, with 6 to 7 mg per day recommended for pregnant and lactating individuals, respectively. Excellent sources of pantothenic acid include chicken, beef, potatoes, oats, kidney, yeast, egg yolks, and whole grains.

Vitamin B₆, also called **pyridoxine**, is used as part of a number of pyridoxine-containing compounds that function as coenzymes in amino acid, glycogen, and neurotransmitter synthesis. The RDA/AI is 1.0 to 1.7 mg per day, with slightly increased requirements for males. Similar to other nutrients, 1.9 and 2.0 mg per day are recommended for pregnant and lactating individuals. Pyridoxine is found in a number of foods that include cereals, organ meats, and soy-based meat substitutes. No adverse effects have been described with excessive pyridoxine consumption.

Vitamin B₇, also known as **biotin**, is a coenzyme in fatty acid, glycogen, and amino acid synthesis. It is naturally found in many foods including the liver and other meat products. The RDA/AI is similar for both sexes at 20 to 330 μg per day, with increased requirements for lactating women. There has not been an established upper limit of intake because there are no known adverse effects of excess intake.

Vitamin B₉, also known as **folate** (folic acid), is an important cofactor in nucleic acid and amino acid synthesis, and maternal deficiency has been linked to neural tube defects in newborns. The RDA/AI ranges from 300 to 400 μg per day, with increased requirements for pregnant or lactating women. Folate is particularly enriched in dark leafy green vegetables as well as whole grains and fortified cereals. Of particular clinical significance, excess folate intake can mask neurologic deficiencies in vitamin B₁₂-deficient individuals; however, there are no other known adverse effects of excess of excessive folate intake.

Vitamin B₁₂, also known as **cobalamin**, is a coenzyme involved in nucleic acid synthesis and is linked to the clinical condition of megaloblastic anemia. The RDA/AI ranges from 1.8 to 2.4 μg per day in both sexes depending on age of the individual, with increased requirements of 2.6 and 2.8 μg per day in pregnant and lactating individuals. Vitamin B₁₂ can be found in fortified cereals as well as meat, fish, and poultry. There are no adverse effects that have been described by excessive intake.

Vitamin C, also known as **ascorbic acid**, is an antioxidant and cofactor in chemical reactions that involved the reduced form of copper or other metalloenzymes. The RDA/AI values range from 45 to 90 mg per day in both sexes, with slightly increased requirements in males as well as increased requirements in pregnancy and lactation of 80 to 85 mg per day and 115 to 120 mg per day, respectively. Citrus foods as well as potatoes, green vegetables like broccoli, brussels sprouts, and spinach are all excellent sources of vitamin C.

Choline is a molecule involved in the biosynthesis and other metabolic reactions as a precursor to acetylcholine and phospholipids. The RDA/AI differs among the sexes but ranges from 375 to 550 mg per day with increased requirements suggested for pregnant and lactating individuals. Choline is commonly found in milk, eggs, liver, and peanuts.

Minerals

Minerals play a number of key biochemical roles in human metabolism as well as a plethora of other physiologic processes within the body. Several minerals are known to have multiple recognized functions. **Calcium** and **phosphorous** are intimately involved in bone health. **Phosphorus** is also involved in pH regulation as well as ATP and nucleic acid synthesis. Other minerals including **calcium, sodium, potassium,** and **chloride** are involved in signal transduction and neural function. Many minerals including **magnesium, copper,** and **manganese**, the predominate known functions include acting as a cofactor in various biochemical reactions of metabolism or, like **molybdenum**, are involved in amino acid or nucleic catabolism. **Iron** is well known as an integral component of hemoglobin and other proteins that make up the electron transport chain which is vital to oxidative metabolism. **Iodine** is necessary for thyroid hormone synthesis. **Selenium** is involved in redox reactions and is an antioxidant. It is well accepted that **chromium** is necessary for maintenance of normal blood glucose concentrations. Furthermore, **zinc** is a key structural component of proteins controlling gene expression. There are even a number of minerals that are present in humans with no suggested RDA/AI values because these minerals have unknown functions in human metabolism; these include **boron, nickel, silicon,** and **vanadium**. These minerals do have UL values, but data on excessive intake are scarce in these situations. For brevity, we have not presented all the RDA/AI data for minerals, but consuming a balanced diet of a variety of foods typically allows AI of all micronutrients. Regardless, these deficiencies may manifest in some clinical situations, and the clinician should be aware of these rare situations.

Suggested Readings

Bray GA, Smith SR, de Jonge L, et al. Effect of dietary protein content on weight gain, energy expenditure, and body composition during overeating: a Randomized Controlled Trial. *JAMA* 2012;307(1):47–55. doi:10.1001/jama.2011.1918.

Buchholz AC, Schoeller DA. Is a calorie a calorie? *Am J Clin Nutr* 2004;79(5):899S–906S.

Galgani J, Ravussin E. Energy metabolism, fuel selection and body weight regulation. *Int J Obes Relat Metab Disord* 2008;32:S109-S119. doi:10.1038/ijo.2008.246.

Intakes SCOTSEODR, Intakes SOURLONAIAUODR, Macronutrients AROTPO, Board FAN, Institute of Medicine. *Dietary Reference Intakes for Energy, Carbohydrate, Fiber, Fat, Fatty Acids, Cholesterol, Protein, and Amino Acids (Macronutrients)*. National Academies Press; 2005. doi:10.17226/10490.

Joint FAO. *WHO Expert Consultation on Fats and Fatty Acids in Human Nutrition (10-14 November 2008, WHO, Geneva)*. Geneva: World Health Organization; 2008.

Joint FAO. *WHO Expert Consultation on Human Vitamin and Mineral Requirements. Vitamin and Mineral Requirements in Human Nutrition*. Geneva: World Health Organization and Food and Agriculture; 2004.

Joint WHO/FAO/UNU Expert Consultation. *Protein and Amino Acid Requirements in Human Nutrition*. 2007:1–265, backcover.

Paddon-Jones D, Westman E, Mattes RD, et al. Protein, weight management, and satiety. *Am J Clin Nutr* 2008;87(5):1558S–1561S.

Prentice AM. Macronutrients as sources of food energy. *Public Health Nutr.* 2005;8(7A):932–939. doi:10.1079/PHN2005779.

World Health Organization. *Iodine I. Trace Elements in Human Nutrition and Health*. Geneva: World Health Organization.

World Health Organization. *Human Energy Requirements: Report of a Joint FAO/WHO/UNU Expert Consultation, Rome 17–24 October 2001*. Rome: Food Agric Organ United Nations; 2004.

World Health Organization. *WHO Guideline: Sodium Intake for Adults and Children*. Geneva: World Health Organization; 2012.

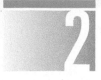

Nutrition Screening and Assessment in Kidney Disease

Katrina L. Campbell, Carla M. Avesani, and Lilian Cuppari

THE IMPORTANCE OF NUTRITION IN KIDNEY DISEASE

The loss of renal function and the dialysis procedure result in multiple consequences that adversely affect the patient's nutritional condition. The nutritional disturbances in chronic kidney disease (CKD) include not only protein-energy wasting (PEW) but also obesity (including visceral obesity and sarcopenic obesity), nutrient deficiencies (vitamin D, zinc, folic acid, and other B vitamins), and undesirable accumulation of nutrients (potassium and phosphorus). Therefore, nutrition assessment and dietary management are complex and involve a number of tools and strategies to identify and to successfully prevent and treat the various nutrition-related aspects of CKD.

Overview of Nutrition-Related Problems in Kidney Disease
Protein-Energy Wasting in Kidney Disease
Protein-energy wasting (PEW) is a term proposed by the International Society of Renal Nutrition and Metabolism (ISRNM) that refers to a state of nutritional and catabolic derangements that occur in CKD characterized by depletion of body protein (muscle mass) and energy stores and is associated with hospitalization and death risk. There are many contributing causes of PEW in CKD, including not only inadequate dietary intake due to poor appetite but also several other CKD-related alterations such as persistent inflammation, metabolic acidosis, increased energy expenditure, endocrine disorders, and the dialysis procedure itself. Associated comorbidities, sedentary lifestyle, and aging are also important risk factors for PEW in CKD patients. Further details on the consequences are provided in Chapter 3.

Given the multifactorial nature of PEW in CKD patients, screening and assessment of nutritional status must be made using various complementary measures, in particular, assessment of recent change. The ISRNM proposed a list of four criteria affected by PEW in CKD patients detailed in Figure 2.1. To classify a patient as having PEW, at least one of the following four criteria should be met: serum biochemistry, body mass, muscle mass, and dietary intake. Furthermore, assessment of nutritional status may be established through the use of comprehensive screening and assessment tools, formulating a score or classification based on several criteria detailed later in this chapter.

Sarcopenia and Functional Decline in Kidney Disease
Sarcopenia, like PEW, is characterized by a state of progressive muscle wasting. Although sarcopenia and PEW share common etiologic factors and diagnostic criteria, they have distinct definitions. Sarcopenia was first defined by Irwin Rosemberg as "an age-related condition of decrease in muscle mass." Of importance, however, is that sarcopenia is not a condition present exclusively in older people.

The *European Working Group on Sarcopenia in Older People* proposed two categories of sarcopenia according to its etiology: *primary* sarcopenia, concerning the age-related causes, and *secondary* sarcopenia, encompassing

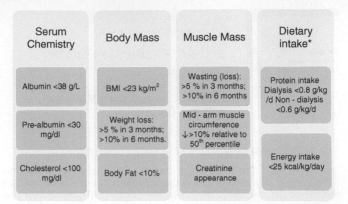

Serum Chemistry	Body Mass	Muscle Mass	Dietary intake*
Albumin <38 g/L	BMI <23 kg/m²	Wasting (loss): >5 % in 3 months; >10% in 6 months	Protein intake Dialysis <0.8 g/kg /d Non - dialysis <0.6 g/kg/d
Pre-albumin <30 mg/dl	Weight loss: >5 % in 3 months; >10% in 6 months.	Mid - arm muscle circumference ↓>10% relative to 50th percentile	
Cholesterol <100 mg/dl	Body Fat <10%	Creatinine appearance	Energy intake <25 kcal/kg/day

FIGURE 2.1 Summary of the protein-energy wasting (PEW) criteria of the International Society of Renal Nutrition and Metabolism (ISRNM).

other causes not related to aging (related to disease, activity, and nutrition). These conditions lead not only to decreased muscle mass but also to diminished muscle strength and muscle functionality, representative of the concept of sarcopenia. Moreover, the catabolic conditions present in kidney disease, coupled with the dialysis procedure and in addition to aging (Fig. 2.2), make individuals with kidney disease a group with high susceptibility to develop sarcopenia.

Progressive functional decline, one criterion of sarcopenia, also deserves attention in the setting of CKD. Muscle weakness is an important potential contributor to poor physical performance, which connects sarcopenia to frailty (syndrome resulting from cumulative declines in multiple physiologic

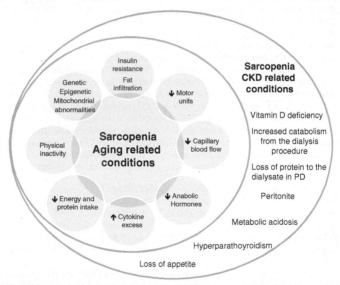

FIGURE 2.2 Chronic kidney disease (CKD)-related conditions leading to sarcopenia and the overlapping with aging-related conditions.

TABLE 2.1   Criteria for the Assessment of PEW, Sarcopenia, and Frailty Phenotype

Criteria	PEW*	Sarcopenia[†]	Frailty Phenotype[‡]
Low body mass (body weight, BMI, body fat)	x		x
Low muscle mass (lean body mass)	x	x	x
Serum chemistry (low albumin, prealbumin, cholesterol)	x		
Diminished food intake (24-h food recall, food records/diaries, food frequency questionnaire)	x		
Physical function, including:		x	x
Low muscle strength (handgrip strength and knee flexion/extension)			
Low physical performance (short physical performance battery, gait speed, get-up-and-go test, stair climb power test)			
Low activity			x

*International Society of Renal Nutrition and Metabolism (Fouque et al., 2007).
[†]European Working Group on Sarcopenia in Older People (Cruz-Jentoff et al., 2010).
[‡]Fried et al., 2001.
BMI, body mass index; PEW, protein-energy wasting.

systems) and disability (difficulty in walking, climbing stairs, and rising from a chair). Altogether, it is clear that PEW, sarcopenia, and frailty share common causes, criteria, and diagnostic methods (Table 2.1), but refer to different clinical conditions that require attention for the correct diagnosis and distinct treatments.

Obesity
Obesity is a well-documented risk factor for diabetes and hypertension, the two primary causes of CKD. Moreover, obesity has been shown to be an independent risk factor for the development and progression of CKD. The potential mechanisms involved in the direct effect of obesity in the kidney include glomerular hyperfiltration, systemic and local inflammation, and alterations in production of adipokines and growth factors. Conversely, when CKD is established, obesity determined by body mass index (BMI, weight/height^2) has been paradoxically associated with improved survival, particularly in patients receiving maintenance dialysis.

Of the several hypotheses have been proposed to explain this paradoxical association, the most likely one is that the short-term benefits of excess of body fat may outweigh its long-term risks. However, in moderate CKD (Stages 3 and 4), obesity assessed by BMI seems not to offer protection and in the earlier stages of CKD (Stages 1 and 2), seems to be a risk factor for mortality. The limited ability of BMI to distinguish between fat mass and muscle mass and to differentiate the distribution of body fat (visceral vs. subcutaneous fat) is a cause for concern when reflecting on the heterogeneous association between obesity and outcomes in CKD patients. Indeed, it appears that the harmful impact of obesity in CKD is due to the proportion of body fat, in particular, abdominal obesity. Therefore, in the assessment of nutritional status in CKD, it is essential to implement the assessment of total body fat as well as central fat in clinical practice. For further discussion on obesity in kidney disease, please refer to Chapter 20.

Challenges of Measuring Nutritional Status in Kidney Disease

There is no single measurement that is able to provide a complete assessment of nutritional status. Some disturbances related to kidney disease and/or to the dialysis treatment, such as fluid retention, inflammation, and residual renal function, can interfere in the interpretation of markers of nutritional status and methods of body composition.

The choice of method applied to the assessment of both nutritional status and body composition will depend on the time, the cost, and ease of measurement, in addition to the purpose of its use (clinical or research setting). In practice, utilizing a range of measures and monitoring change over time is advised as best practice. This approach requires frequent and well-documented consecutive patient measurements, and therefore overcomes the need to focus on definitive cutoffs to define nutritional status in CKD patients, which can be problematic for several measures.

Body Composition Assessment in Practice

Key measures and considerations for undertaking body composition measurement in practice to inform the assessment of obesity, PEW, and low muscle mass are detailed in Table 2.2. The assessments should be performed after the dialysis session for hemodialysis patients or with an empty cavity for peritoneal dialysis patients, in order to diminish errors coming from fluid retention. In addition, good training is of importance to standardize the method of assessment and diminish the intra- and interobserver error. This is of particular importance for anthropometric measurements that rely on the skills of the observer.

Biochemical Parameters and Relationship to Nutritional Status and Nutrition Assessment

Biochemical parameters can be routinely used to complement the assessment of nutritional status in kidney disease patients. Biochemical parameters have the potential to be useful biomarkers that can be objectively measured and evaluated as indicators of normal biologic processes, pathogenic processes, or pharmacologic responses to therapeutic interventions. An ideal biochemical marker for clinical practice should be inexpensive, directly linked to the pathophysiologic process that it represents, closely correlated with symptom severity, and be sensitive and specific. It is clear that it will be highly difficult to reach such standards for any biomarker. In the uremic milieu, this is challenging because the currently favored biomarkers have significant limitations for assessing nutritional status in CKD, being influenced by systemic inflammation and by the important role of the kidney in metabolizing circulating peptides, as well as by fluid status and losses of the biomarker in urine or dialysate.

Albumin is an acute-phase reactant, and inflammatory stimuli are important factors affecting its production. Because the disease itself and dialysis treatment trigger the production of proinflammatory cytokines in response to inflammatory stimuli, the utility of serum albumin as a marker of poor nutritional status in dialysis patients has been questioned. Despite this limitation, measurement of serum albumin is a simple test, which is readily available in most clinical settings monthly or quarterly. Because the PEW syndrome represents not only malnutrition but also inflammation, serum albumin remains an outcome marker that reflects the severity of disease. Moreover, lower concentration of albumin is strongly associated with increased death risk. Considering the above, serum albumin is an accessible

TABLE
22

Methods to Assess Body Composition in Kidney Disease Populations with High Utility in Clinical Practice

Modality	Method	Body Compartment	Advantages	Limitation
Anthropometry	MAMC, calf circumference, APMT	Muscle mass	Widely available, low cost, quick, portable, predictor of mortality in CKD.	Low precision, high inter- and intraobserver variation, subject to hydration status.*
	Sum of skinfold thicknesses	Total body fat		
	Waist circumference	Central body fat		
Impedance	BIA	Body water, FFM, and body fat	Widely available, medium cost, low inter- and intraobserver variation, quick, portable.	Indirect measurement, equations not validated to CKD patients, pacemaker precludes its use (common in older adults), subject to hydration status.*
	BIS	Body water, FFM, and body fat	Medium cost, low interobserver variation, quick, portable, validated for patients on dialysis.	Indirect measurement, pacemaker precludes its use (common in older adults), subject to hydration status.*
Creatinine kinetics	Urinary creatinine excretion	Muscle mass	Low cost, allows assessment in routine appointments in outpatient clinic.	Subject to the quality of 24-h urine collection. Influenced by creatine intake (typically from cooked meat). Not applicable for patients on dialysis.
	Serum creatinine	Muscle mass	Low cost, allows assessment in routine appointments	Influenced by creatine intake (typically from cooked meat).

*In order to diminish the influence of fluid retention on the interpretation, the assessment should be performed after the dialysis session for hemodialysis or with an empty cavity for peritoneal dialysis patients.
APMT, adductor pollicis muscle thickness; BIA, bioelectrical impedance analysis; BIS, bioelectrical impedance spectrometry; CKD, chronic kidney disease; FFM, fat-free mass; MAMC, midarm muscle circumference.

biomarker, but its use as a marker of PEW should be interpreted with caution, taking into account the patient's inflammatory and hydration status, in order to avoid a misinterpretation of a low serum albumin concentration.

Prealbumin (transthyretin, which is a preferred term) is also affected by systemic inflammation, and a reduced renal catabolism can influence its serum concentration. Even with these limitations, low concentration of serum transthyretin and negative changes over 6 months were both associated with increased mortality risk. Also of interest is that transthyretin was able to evaluate the effect of oral energy and protein supplementation. These data underline the utility of serum transthyretin as a nutritional marker in the CKD setting.

In predialysis kidney disease patients, serum creatinine is used to evaluate kidney function. In maintenance dialysis patients who have minimal or no residual renal function and who undergo a stable dialysis treatment regimen, time-averaged serum creatinine concentration (assessed before the dialysis session) can be used as a surrogate of muscle mass, and its changes over time may represent parallel changes in skeletal muscle mass. Low serum creatinine in this setting is a powerful risk factor for death, both in cross-sectional and longitudinal studies. However, as mentioned in Table 2.2, limitations of serum creatinine as a marker of nutritional status include the fact that the amount of creatine (typically from cooked meat) and protein intake can influence the concentration of serum creatinine and it is reflective of kidney function in patients who are not maintenance dialysis yet.

Considerations for Dietary Assessment in Kidney Disease

Examining the food intake of patients with CKD in terms of quality and quantity is of great importance because of the extensive diet modifications considered in the management of these patients. The most frequently used methods for dietary assessment in the general population and in patients with CKD include dietary recalls (e.g., 24-hour recall), food records (3 to 7 days), and food frequency questionnaires. The choice of method to be used depends on the purpose of the investigation and the type of dietary information to be obtained (nutrients, food and food groups, dietary patterns, etc.). In addition, the accuracy of dietary information depends on the ability of the investigator and on the cooperation of the patient. Table 2.3 describes briefly the characteristics of each method, the strengths and limitations, and the considerations for applicability in patients on dialysis. More recently, the assessment of food patterns and dietary quality has emerged as a way to assess food intake. This approach is complementary to the traditional evaluation of energy, nutrients, and micronutrients (mostly protein, potassium, sodium, and phosphorous), because it allows a broad assessment of the food intake. Recent studies have demonstrated that adherence to a healthier dietary pattern was associated with a decreased risk of developing end-stage renal disease, and improved survival. Therefore, understanding the pattern of nutrient insufficiencies from the diet may be the first step toward building nutritional interventions focusing not on isolated nutrients, but on healthier patterns.

Nutrition Screening and Assessment Tools in Practice

Nutrition screening and assessment are distinct yet complementary processes. Nutrition screening is the initial evaluation to detect patients who have or are at high risk of poor nutritional status and warrant further investigation from formal nutrition assessment.

Distinguishing features between nutrition screening and nutrition assessment relate to skills, information, and time required to undertake each process. Administration of screening requires minimal training, is designed for any health care professional to complete, and is recommended to occur

Strengths and Limitations of Methods Used to Assess Dietary Intake in Kidney Disease Populations

Method	Strengths	Limitations
24-h recall: During a face-to-face or telephone interview, patient is questioned about food intake during the day before.	• Convenient • Quick • Low cost • Does not change the usual diet • Estimation of usual diet can be obtained with repeated application.	• Open to recall bias • Reliance on interviewer's training • Atypical food intake on the previous day • Application of two 24-h recalls is necessary to capture food intake of dialysis and nondialysis days.
Food records/diaries: Patients are instructed to record in detail the type and amount of foods ingested during 3 to 7 d.	• Low cost • Increases the possibility of capturing usual food intake. • Capture differences in food intake between dialysis days and nondialysis days.	• Reliance on patient's ability and compliance to complete. • Potential for modifying usual food intake. • There is a need to review the records to obtain additional relevant information.
Food frequency questionnaire: A large list of commonly eaten food items (with specified serving sizes) with multiple choices for the frequency of ingested food and is self- or interviewer administrated.	• Capture long-term dietary intake • Dietary patterns can be captured. • Convenient for use in large-scale population studies.	• Open to recall bias • Does not capture current food intake • May be time consuming • Of limited value for evaluating individual intake and informing nutrition interventions

routinely (i.e., every month or on admission to acute care) to indicate risk for poor nutritional status or PEW. Nutrition assessment, however, is more comprehensive, requiring specific training and skill development to provide a definitive diagnosis. The recommended frequency for routine assessment is every 3 to 6 months or upon screening at risk.

Nutrition Screening Tools in Kidney Disease

Nutrition screening tools identify characteristics known to be associated with nutritional risk and therefore identify individuals likely to have poor nutritional status; however, this is not a definitive diagnosis. Nutrition screening tools previously applied to the patients with kidney disease cover appetite, recent weight change, body mass index, and, less frequently, laboratory values or disease severity. Each tool has a different scoring process to identify high nutritional risk.

Nutrition Assessment Tools in Kidney Disease

Subjective Global Assessment (SGA) is the most widely adopted comprehensive nutrition assessment tool and has been established as a diagnostic standard for assessing malnutrition in end-stage kidney disease since the National

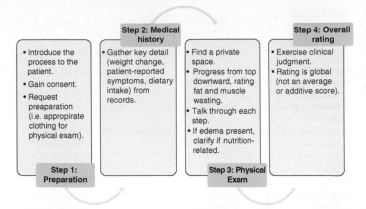

FIGURE 2.3 Steps for undertaking a subjective global assessment.

Kidney Foundation Kidney Disease Outcomes Quality Initiative (NKF K/DOQI) recommendation in 2001. This assessment formalizes information generally collected in the patients' medical history and by undertaking a physical exam. The assessment components of the SGA include changes in weight, dietary intake, persistent (>2 weeks) gastrointestinal symptoms, and functional capacity. The physical examination should include an evaluation of subcutaneous fat, muscle wasting, ankle and sacral edema, and ascites. The steps for preparing and undertaking an SGA are detailed in Figure 2.3. After reviewing each parameter, patients are assigned a rating, on a 3-point or 7-point scale: SGA A or 6 to 7 is well nourished; SGA B or 3 to 5 is at risk of malnutrition, or is suspected to be malnourished; and SGA C or 1 to 2 means the patient is severely malnourished.

A modification of the SGA, the Malnutrition Inflammation Score (MIS), is designed as an additive score incorporating the characteristics of PEW. This score contains the seven components of the SGA together with three additional components: BMI, serum albumin, and transferrin (or total iron-binding capacity). Each MIS component is scored from 0 (*normal*) to 3 (*severely abnormal*). The sum of all 10 components, therefore, ranges from 0 (*normal*) to 30 (*severely malnourished*); a higher score reflects more severe malnutrition and inflammation. Although the applicability of the MIS may be limited by the availability of albumin and transferrin measurements in the clinical setting, it can be used without transferrin and provides a scored tool for components across the PEW categories.

Validation and Considerations of Nutrition Screening and Assessment Tools in Kidney Disease

When evaluating the range of comprehensive tools specifically designed for nutrition screening and assessment, it is important to identify their validity for use in kidney disease populations. Having validity indicates that the tools can accurately identify risk of malnutrition or PEW (criterion validity), are associated with other measures of nutritional status (clinical or concurrent validity), and are also associated with poor outcome (predictive validity). The following section will cover the range of tools applied in CKD populations and validation summarized in Table 2.4.

Most validation studies to date have covered criterion validity, ability to detect poor nutritional state according to the SGA or the MIS as the

Validity of Nutrition Screening and Assessment Tools
Applied to the Kidney Disease Population

Tool	Components and Scoring	Scoring	Validated Against
Nutrition screening tools			
Malnutrition Screening Tool (MST)	Weight loss, poor intake or appetite	0–5; Risk > 3	SGA, MIS
Malnutrition Universal Screening Tool (MUST)	Body mass index (BMI), weight loss, acute disease	0–6; Risk > 2	SGA, MIS, hospitalization
Nutrition Risk Screening (NRS)	BMI, weight loss, appetite, intake, severity of disease	0–15; At risk > 4	MIS, mortality
Geriatric Nutrition Risk Index (GNRI)	$GNRI = [1.489 \times albumin (g/dL)] + 41.7 \times (body\ weight/ideal\ body\ weight)]$	At risk < 91	SGA, MIS, mortality, hospitalization
Mini-Nutrition Assessment	Intake, weight loss, mobility, acute disease; BMI	0–14; At risk < 11	MIS
Nutrition assessment tools			
Subjective Global Assessment (SGA)	Medical history and physical examination	ABC or 1–7	Body composition, biochemistry, mortality, hospitalization
Malnutrition Inflammation Score (MIS)	Scored SGA with: Total iron-binding capacity, albumin, BMI	0–30	Biochemistry, body composition, mortality, hospitalization
Mini-Nutrition Assessment (MNA)	Intake, weight loss, mobility, stress or acute disease, BMI	0–14	Mortality
Objective Score of Nutrition on Dialysis (OSND)	Weight, BMI, SFT, MAC, albumin, transferrin, cholesterol	5–32	Biochemistry, body composition, hospitalization

reference method, in addition to prospective validity, with hospitalization or all-cause mortality. Of note, the Geriatric Nutrition Risk Index demonstrated the greatest potential; however, it is validated for use only in maintenance dialysis patients. This tool was consistently predictive of mortality, likely to be related to the feature of serum albumin in the equation.

Numerous studies have been dedicated to the evaluation of nutrition assessment tools in the maintenance dialysis population, with only a few in the nondialysis CKD population. The SGA has been identified in large-scale studies to be an independent and significant predictor of morbidity and mortality, with established validity and reliability, in both dialysis and nondialysis populations. The MIS has primarily undergone validation in the maintenance dialysis population and presents a strong prognostic indicator. However, various cutoff points for determining nutritional status have been presented in the literature, making a definition of PEW based on the MIS score alone difficult in practice.

Implementation of Nutrition Screening and Assessment in Practice

A protocol for the routine implementation of screening and assessment practices is recommended in all dialysis and kidney disease care settings. Scheduling of nutrition screening and assessment should be routine with screening practices adopted into routine practice (at minimum monthly), and comprehensive assessments (e.g., the use of assessment tools such as SGA) every 3 to 6 months (or more frequently if identified at risk). Parameters with the highest ease of measurement and clinical effectiveness (see Table 2.5) should be implemented as tools for routine nutrition screening and assessment.

Summary of the Utility of Parameters Assessing Nutrition Status in Dialysis

Nutrition Assessment Parameters	Ease of Measurement*	Clinical Applicability†
Anthropometry and body composition		
Weight and weight change, including BMI	+ + + +	+ +
Anthropometry: skinfold thickness and midarm muscle circumference	+ + +	+ + +
Impedance: bioimpedance analysis or spectroscopy	+ +	+ + +
Lean muscle mass (and/or fat mass) using gold-standard body composition instruments (Dual-Energy X-ray Absorptiometry, BodPod, etc.)	+	+ + + +
Handgrip strength	+ + + +	+ + +
Biochemistry		
Serum proteins	+ + + +	+ +
Inflammation markers	+ + +	+ +
Adequacy of intake		
Protein and energy intake (diet recall or record)	+ +	+ + + +
Protein nitrogen appearance (PNA)	+ + +	+ +
Comprehensive tools		
Screening tools (e.g., Malnutrition Screening Tool)	+ + + +	+ +
Assessment tools (e.g., Subjective Global Assessment, Malnutrition Inflammation Score)	+ + +	+ + + +

Scale reflects the ease of measurement or applicability: highest + + + + to lowest +.
*Considers availability in clinical practice, cost, time, and degree of training required.
†Considers validity and reliability; influence of nonnutritional factors.

Suggested Readings

Carrero JJ, Johansen KL, Lindholm B, et al. Screening for muscle wasting and dysfunction in patients with chronic kidney disease. *Kidney Int* 2016;90:53–66.

Carrero JJ, Stenvinkel P, Cuppari L, et al. Etiology of the protein-energy wasting syndrome in chronic kidney disease: a consensus statement from the International Society of Renal Nutrition and Metabolism (ISRNM). *J Ren Nutr* 2013;23:77–90.

Cruz-Jentoft AJ, Baeyens JP, Bauer JM, et al. Sarcopenia: European consensus on definition and diagnosis: Report of the European Working Group on Sarcopenia in Older People. *Age Ageing* 2010;39:412–423.

Fouque D, Vennegoor M, ter Wee P, et al. EBPG guideline on nutrition. *Nephrol Dial Transplant* 2007;22(Suppl 2):ii45–ii87.

Fried LP, Tangen CM, Walston J, et al. Frailty in older adults: evidence for a phenotype. *J Gerontol A Biol Sci Med Sci* 2001;56:M146–M156.

Harmon BE, Boushey CJ, Shvetsov YB, et al. Associations of key diet-quality indexes with mortality in the Multiethnic Cohort: the Dietary Patterns Methods Project. *Am J Clin Nutr* 2015;101:587–597.

Huang X, Jiménez-Moleón JJ, Lindholm B. Mediterranean diet, kidney function, and mortality in men with CKD. *Clin J Am Soc Nephrol* 2013;8:1548–1555.

Rhee CM, Ahmadi S-F, Kalantar-Zadeh K. The dual roles of obesity in chronic kidney disease: a review of the current literature. *Curr Opin Nephrol Hypertens* 2016;25:208–216.

3

Epidemiology of Protein-Energy Wasting in Chronic Kidney Disease

Connie M. Rhee, Miklos Z. Molnar, and Csaba P. Kovesdy

Protein-energy wasting (PEW) is a highly prevalent condition and a major risk factor for adverse outcomes including higher risk of hospitalization, impaired health-related quality of life, and mortality in advanced chronic kidney disease (CKD) and end-stage renal disease (ESRD) patients receiving dialysis. Indeed, various markers of PEW such as hypoalbuminemia, lower body mass index (BMI), and reduced muscle mass are among the most potent predictors of death risk in this population. In order to better characterize the syndrome of malnutrition, muscle wasting, and inflammation commonly observed in CKD and ESRD patients, the International Society of Renal Nutrition and Metabolism convened an expert panel in 2007 to operationalize the concept and definition of PEW. Although there has been substantial research advancing our understanding of the risk factors and sequelae of wasting in kidney disease over the past 9 years, there are many remaining knowledge gaps. In this chapter, we review the epidemiology of PEW, including its diagnostic criteria, incidence and prevalence, and associated clinical outcomes in the CKD and ESRD population.

NOMENCLATURE

PEW is defined as a condition of reduced body stores of protein and energy and is ascertained by the presence of biochemical abnormalities, low body weight, reduced muscle mass, and decreased protein and energy intake. Although PEW is characterized by mild degrees of depleted protein and energy mass, cachexia has also been used to describe a severe form of PEW that portends very poor outcomes and for which there are limited therapeutic options. PEW is also considered to be a distinct entity from malnutrition. Although malnutrition is precipitated by insufficient dietary intake, it has been suggested that PEW, which is characterized by heightened catabolism of body protein stores, cannot be corrected by increased dietary intake alone. However, some evidence suggests that nutritional supplementation can indeed improve nutritional status in CKD and ESRD patients with PEW.

DIAGNOSIS

The International Society of Renal Nutrition and Metabolism has established four broad categories in the diagnosis of PEW, including: (1) at least one or more biochemical abnormalities; (2) low body weight, low total body fat, and/or weight loss; (3) reduced muscle mass; and (4) low protein or energy intake (Fig. 3.1). In order to make a diagnosis of PEW, abnormalities should be present in at least three out of four categories, with each criterion documented on at least three occasions, preferably about 2 to 4 weeks apart.

With respect to the *biochemical criteria*, serum albumin has been the most widely used marker of mortality in observational studies of CKD and ESRD patients and it is also widely measured in routine clinical practice, thus making it a feasible tool for widespread clinical utilization. The important

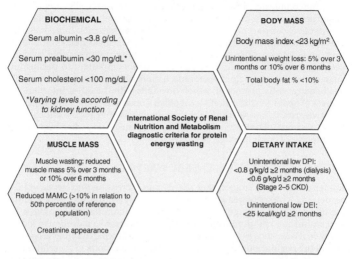

FIGURE 3.1 International Society of Renal Nutrition and Metabolism diagnostic criteria for protein-energy wasting. CKD, chronic kidney disease; DEI, dietary energy intake; DPI, dietary protein intake; MAMC, mid-arm muscle circumference.

conclusion is that a decrease in serum albumin is principally associated with the presence and severity of inflammation rather than with a low serum albumin and inadequacies of dietary factors. Serum prealbumin (i.e., transthyretin), percentage of lymphocytes, and total cholesterol may also be used as potential biochemical markers.

Regarding the diagnosis of inadequate *body mass criteria*, BMI is the most practical marker of body mass, although there can be fluctuations with increases or decreases in intra- and extracellular volume status. Notably, the BMI threshold for PEW of <23 kg per m^2 may not be appropriate for certain racial/ethnic groups (e.g., Asians), and it should not be applied to the general population in whom BMIs of 18.5 to 25.0 kg per m^2 are recommended by the World Health Organization. Unintentional weight loss (≥5% or ≥10% loss of nonedematous weight over 3 months vs. 6 months, respectively) may also be used in assessing PEW. Given the inability to determine fat versus muscle mass when BMI alone is used, a low total body fat percentage (<10%) may identify the presence of PEW.

Although ascertainment of *loss of muscle mass* may be challenging owing to a lack of robust clinical metrics, mid-arm muscle circumference (MAMC) area or assessment of predialysis serum creatinine or creatinine appearance in hemodialysis patients may serve as convenient measures. If at all possible, this measurement should be made serially by the same examiner to reduce the likelihood of relying on erroneous perceived changes in body compartments.

Lastly, given the role of diminished appetite in PEW, identification of unintentional *low dietary protein intake* or unintentional *low dietary energy intake* for at least 2 months (<0.80 g/kg/d or <0.6 g/kg/d in dialysis vs. Stages 2 to 5 CKD patients, respectively) and estimated from urea kinetics and the nonurea nitrogen excretion may be used to ascertain PEW. This biochemical estimate provides results that are superior to the diagnosis of PEW obtained from results of dietary diaries and interviews.

The complexity of diagnosing PEW necessitates an equally complex diagnostic approach, but many of the above criteria are only available if collected prospectively, as part of dedicated nutritional assessments. This conclusion prevents making a formal diagnosis of PEW based on measurements obtained from large retrospective registries difficult or at times impossible. In short, gathering nutritional information is a critical component to performing large-scale epidemiologic assessments. A more simplified assessment of PEW has been recently promoted, which dovetails with the latest International Society of Renal Nutrition and Metabolism Consensus Statement suggesting that two criteria may be sufficient for a diagnosis of PEW. The critical issue is that accuracy of nutritional measurements is necessary when maximizing the analysis of epidemiologic results.

PREVALENCE OF PROTEIN-ENERGY WASTING

Epidemiologic data suggest that there in an increasing prevalence of PEW associated with a greater severity of kidney dysfunction, and both findings are likely caused by augmented activation of inflammatory cytokines, hypercatabolism, and diminished appetite in response to a decline in kidney function. Prevalence estimates vary across studies, owing to the heterogeneity of patient populations, diagnostic criteria, and methods of ascertainment; results from the United States, Canada, South America, and Europe suggest that the prevalence of PEW increases as patients progress from predialysis CKD to dialysis (Table 3.1).

Predialysis Chronic Kidney Disease

Among predialysis CKD patients, few studies have examined the prevalence of PEW using diagnostic criteria from the International Society of Renal Nutrition and Metabolism. The diagnosis of PEW has mainly relied upon laboratory markers or nutritional scoring tools as a proxy for careful measurements of nutritional status. For example, larger population-based studies ($N > 100$ patients) using the Subjective Global Assessment tool have estimated the prevalence of PEW to be 11% to 31% across countries in Europe and South America.

In one of the largest studies of predialysis CKD patients, the prevalence of PEW was estimated among 1,220 US veterans with Stage 1 to 5 CKD using biochemical criteria (i.e., presence of ≥ 2 out of 3 of the following biochemical abnormalities: (1) serum albumin < 3.7 g per dL, (2) percentage of lymphocytes in white blood cell [WBC] count $< 22\%$, and (3) WBC count $> 7,500$ per mm^3). Using this definition, 33% of patients were found to have PEW, and an increasing probability of PEW was observed with progressive impairment of the estimated glomerular filtration rate.

Hemodialysis

Most studies in the hemodialysis population have also utilized the Subjective Global Assessment nutritional scoring tool to ascertain PEW. Across these studies, the prevalence has widely ranged from 20% to 62% in South American regions to 14% to 94% in Europe. In a study of 11,422 hemodialysis patients from the Euro-DOPPS cohort, the prevalence of PEW based upon Subjective Global Assessment was compared across various countries (e.g., France, Germany, Italy, Spain, and United Kingdom) and found to have the lowest prevalence in Spain (i.e., 14%) and the highest prevalence in France (i.e., 23%); the overall prevalence was 19%.

Given that longitudinal studies have shown that ESRD patients undergoing hemodialysis develop worsening body anthropometry measures (declining weight, muscle mass, and fat mass) plus inflammatory status (increased C-reactive protein) with increasing vintage, it has been suggested the PEW

TABLE
3.1

Selected Studies of the Prevalence of PEW among CKD, HD, PD, and Tx

Author (Year)	Study Population	Definition of PEW	Prevalence (%)
CKD			
Kovesdy et al. (2009, AJCN)	1,220 Stages 1–5 CKD patients (United States)	≥2 out of 3 biochemical markers of PEW: (1) Serum albumin < 3.7 g/dL (2) Percent of lymphocytes < 22 (3) WBC count > 7,500/mm^3	33
Sanches et al. (2008, AJKD)	122 CKD patients (Brazil)	SGA	18 (mild to moderate)
Cuppari et al. (2014, JREN)	922 Stages 2–5 CKD patients (Brazil)	SGA	11
Gama-Axelsson et al. (2012, JREN)	280 Stage 5 CKD patients (Sweden)	SGA	31
Westland et al. (2014, JREN)	376 CKD patients attending predialysis clinics (Netherlands)	SGA	11
HD (*Notes HD + PD Combined)			
Nascimento et al. (2004, NDT)	180 HD patients (Brazil)	SGA	62
Sanabria et al. (2008, KI Supp)	923 dialysis patients (Colombia)*	SGA	44 (mild to severe)
Gracia-Iguacel et al. (2013, Nefrologia)	122 HD patients (Spain)	ISRNM definition	Baseline: 37.0 12 mo: 40.5 24 mo: 41.1
Oliveira et al. (2012, Rev Assoc Med Bras)	575 HD patients (Brazil)	SGA	19.5
Hecking et al. (2004, NDT)	11,422 HD patients (Euro-DOPPS)	SGA	France: 23 Germany: 17 Italy: 18 Spain: 14 United Kingdom: 22 All Euro-DOPPS: 19

(continued)

29

TABLE 3.1 Selected Studies of the Prevalence of PEW among CKD, HD, PD, and Tx (*continued*)

Author (Year)	Study Population	Definition of PEW	Prevalence (%)
Carrero et al. (2007, AJCN)	223 HD patients (Sweden)	SGA	43
Gurreebun et al. (2007, JREN)	141 HD patients (United Kingdom)	SGA	32 (mild to moderate malnutrition)
Elliott et al. (2009, Dial Transp)	122 HD patients (Scotland)	SGA	33 ("at-risk" of malnutrition)
Gama-Axelsson et al. (2012, CJASN)	458 incident dialysis patients*	SGA	Incident: 31
	383 prevalent dialysis patients (Sweden)*		Prevalent: 42
Huang et al. (2012, JIM)	222 HD patients (Sweden)	SGA	20
Laegreid et al. (2014, Renal Failure)	233 dialysis patients (Norway)*	SGA	49
Isoyama et al. (2014, CJASN)	330 dialysis patients (Sweden)*	SGA	~19–21
De Mutsert et al. (2009, AJCN)	1,601 dialysis patients (Netherlands)*	SGA	28 (moderate to severe)
Mazairac et al. (2011, NDT)	560 HD patients (Netherlands, Norway, Canada)	SGA	17
Sclauzeo et al. (2013, J Renal Care)	203 HD patients (Italy)	SGA	34
Moreira et al. (2013, Nutr Hosp)	103 HD patients (Portugal)	SGA	94
Segal et al. (2009, NDT)	149 HD patients (Romania)	SGA	27
Garneata et al. (2014, JREN)	263 HD patients (Romania)	SGA	15
PD			
Leinig et al. (2011, JREN)	109 PD patients (Brazil)	ISRNM definition	18
Vavruk et al. (2012, J Bras Nefrol)	110 PD patients (Brazil)	SGA	37
Davies et al. (2000, KI)	153 PD patients (United Kingdom)	SGA or >5% below desirable body weight	31
Tx			
Molnar et al. (2010, AJKD)	993 Tx recipients (Hungary)	MIS > 5	19

CKD, chronic kidney disease; HD, hemodialysis; ISRNM, International Society of Renal Nutrition and Metabolism; MIS, Malnutrition-Inflammation Score; PD, peritoneal dialysis; PEW, protein-energy wasting; SGA, subjective global assessment; Tx, kidney transplant patients.

may progress during the course of ESRD. In one study of 122 Spanish hemodialysis patients that examined PEW using the International Society of Renal Nutrition and Metabolism diagnostic criteria, a gradual rise in the prevalence was observed over time: 37.0% at baseline measurement, 40.5% at 12 months, and 41.1% at 24 months. In one Swedish study of 458 incident dialysis patients and 383 prevalent dialysis patients (hemodialysis and peritoneal dialysis combined), the prevalence of PEW based on the Subjective Global Assessment was found to be 31% in the incident cohort and 42% in the prevalent cohort.

Peritoneal Dialysis
Among larger studies of patients solely receiving peritoneal dialysis ($N >$ 100 patients), prevalence estimates of PEW using Subjective Global Assessment criteria have ranged from 31% to 37%. In the only study of peritoneal dialysis patients that has used International Society of Renal Nutrition and Metabolism diagnostic criteria, 18% of the cohort was found to have PEW. Clearly, additional, large population-based studies examining the prevalence of PEW and its longitudinal trends across the spectrum of predialysis CKD to ESRD using formal diagnostic criteria (i.e., International Society of Renal Nutrition and Metabolism definitions) are needed.

Kidney Transplantation
There is only one published study ($N >$ 100 patients) of prevalent kidney transplant recipients that estimates PEW using the Malnutrition-Inflammation Score. The prevalence of PEW was 19% in that Hungarian cohort.

OUTCOMES ASSOCIATED WITH PROTEIN-ENERGY WASTING

Multiple studies have shown that markers of PEW (biochemical metrics, BMI, body composition, and nutritional scoring tools) are strong predictors of mortality in predialysis CKD and ESRD patients (Table 3.2).

Biochemical Markers
Aberrant levels of PEW biomarkers, including lower serum albumin, prealbumin, creatinine, and normalized protein nitrogen appearance levels, have also been associated with higher death risk in patients with kidney disease. For example, in a study of 58,058 hemodialysis patients from a large US dialysis organization, it was shown that both baseline and time-dependent values of serum albumin (as a proxy of long- and short-term albumin—mortality associations, respectively) <3.8 g per dL were independently associated with higher death risk. In a subcohort of 30,827 patients who had survived the first 6 months, mild increases in serum albumin of ≥0.2 g per dL over that time period were associated with improved survival, whereas a mild decrease of ≥0.1 g per dL was associated with higher death risk in the ensuing 18-month period. Given that serum prealbumin bears a relatively short half-life (i.e., 1.8 to 8 days), it has sometimes been used in lieu of serum albumin in studies of markers of change in nutritional status. In a study of 798 hemodialysis patients who underwent serum prealbumin levels at study entry, levels <20 mg per dL were associated with higher mortality risk, although prealbumin was not found to be superior to albumin in predicting survival.

Among dialysis patients who no longer have residual kidney function, serum creatinine has also been used as a proxy of muscle protein content and nutritional status. Although muscle mass varies across race/ethnicity, in a study of two nationally representative cohorts of Korean hemodialysis patients ($N = 20,818$) and matched US hemodialysis patients comprised of whites and blacks ($N = 20,000$), higher serum creatinine was found to be associated with better survival across all three racial groups.

TABLE 3.2 Selected Studies of Various Protein-Energy Wasting Markers and Mortality in Predialysis CKD and ESRD Patients

Author (Year)	Study Population	PEW Marker	Outcome
Biochemical Metrics			
Kalantar-Zadeh et al. (2005, NDT)	58,058 HD patients (United States)	Serum albumin (baseline and time-dependent)	Albumin levels <3.8 g/dL associated with ↑ all-cause death risk.
Rambod et al. (2008, AJCN)	798 HD patients (United States)	Serum prealbumin (baseline)	Prealbumin <20 mg/dL associated with ↑ all-cause death risk.
Park et al. (2013, Mayo Clinic Proceedings)	20,818 HD patients (Korea) and 20,000 matched HD patients (United States)	Serum creatinine	Linear association between higher creatinine and lower all-cause mortality. Creatinine ≤6.0 mg/dL with 76% higher mortality risk vs. >12.0 mg/dL.
Ravel et al. (2013, J Nutrition)	98,489 HD patients (United States)	Normalized protein nitrogen appearance (g/kg/d) Protein nitrogen appearance (g/d)	Normalized protein nitrogen appearance <1.0 and ≥1.3 associated with ↑ all-cause death risk. Linear association between lower protein nitrogen appearance <60 g/d and ↑ all-cause death risk.
Kovesdy et al. (2009, AJCN)	1,220 Stages 1–5 CKD patients (United States)	Biochemical markers of PEW: (1) Serum albumin <3.7 g/dL (2) Percent of lymphocytes <22% (3) WBC count >7,500/mm³	Incrementally ↑ all-cause death risk with increasing number of markers: 1 marker: 1.7-fold ↑ risk. 2 markers: 2.4-fold ↑ risk. 3 markers: 3.6-fold ↑ risk.

BMI

Kovesdy et al. (2007, AJKD)	521 Stages 1–5 CKD patients (United States)	BMI (baseline and time-dependent): <10, 10–50, 50–90, >90 percentiles of observed values	Inverse association between lower BMI and ↑ all-cause death risk.
Lu et al. (2014, JASN)	453,946 Stages 3–5 CKD patients (United States)	BMI (baseline): (<20, 20–<25, 25–<30, 30–<35, 35–<40, 40–<45, 45–<50, and ≥50 kg/m²)	BMI levels <25 kg/m² associated with ↑ all-cause death risk in all patients. BMI levels ≥35 kg/m² associated with ↑ all-cause death risk in Stages 4 and 5 CKD only.
Lu et al. (2015, Lancet Diab Endo)	3,376,187 patients with eGFR >60 mL/min/1.73 m² stratified by age	BMI (baseline): <20, 20–<25, 25–<30, 30–<35, 35–<40, and ≥40 kg/m²	BMI <20 kg/m² and BMI >35 kg/m² were associated with higher mortality across all ages.
Kalantar-Zadeh et al. (2010, Mayo Clin Proc)	21,762 HD patients (United States)	BMI (3-mo averaged)	BMI <23.0 kg/m² associated with ↑ all-cause death risk.
Doshi et al. (2016, NDT)	123,624 HD patients (United States)	BMI (time-dependent) using marginal structural model	Inverse association between lower BMI and ↑ all-cause death risk. Lowest BMI category (BMI < 18.0 kg/m²) associated with a 3.2-fold higher death risk (ref: BMI 25.0–27.5 kg/m²).
Molnar et al. (2011, AJT)	14,632 wait-listed HD patients (United States)	BMI (13-wk averaged)	BMI <22.0 kg/m² associated with ↑ all-cause death risk.
Stenvinkel et al. (2016, JASN)	5,904 HD patients (Europe) stratified by inflammatory status (defined by C-reactive protein levels)	BMI (time-dependent) divided into quintiles: <21.5, 21.5–24.0, >24.0–26.4, >26.4–29.8, and >29.8 kg/m²	In inflamed patients, there was an inverse association between lower BMI levels and ↑ death risk. In noninflamed patients, only BMI levels < 21.5 kg/m² associated with ↑ death risk.

(continued)

TABLE 3.2 Selected Studies of Various Protein-Energy Wasting Markers and Mortality in Predialysis CKD and ESRD Patients *(continued)*

Body Weight and Composition

Molnar et al. (2011, AJT)	14,632 wait-listed HD patients (United States)	Weight change over 6 mo	Compared to minimal (<±1 kg) weight change over 6 mo, 3–<5 kg and ≥5 kg weight loss associated with ↑ all-cause death risk.
Noori et al. (2010, CJASN)	792 HD patients (United States)	Mid-arm muscle circumference divided into quartiles	Highest mid-arm muscle circumference quartile with 36% ↓ death risk vs. lowest quartile.
Kalantar-Zadeh et al. (2006, AJCN)	535 HD patients (United States)	Near-infrared interactance (total body fat)	Total body fat <12% associated with four-fold ↑ all-cause death risk among patients with body fat 24%–36%.

Nutritional Scoring Tools

Lawson et al. (2001, JREN)	50 CKD patients (United States)	Subjective Global Assessment	Malnourished patients determined by Subjective Global Assessment with ↑ death risk.
Chung et al. (2000, PDI)	91 PD patients (Korea)	Subjective Global Assessment	Malnourished patients determined by Subjective Global Assessment with ↑ death risk.
Rambod et al. (2009, AJKD)	809 HD patients (United States)	Malnutrition Inflammatory Score divided into quartiles: 0–2, 3–4, 5–7, ≥8	Patients in the second, third, and fourth quartiles with ↑ death risk vs. patients in the first quartile.

CKD, chronic kidney disease; BMI, body mass index; eGFR, estimated glomerular filtration rate; ESRD, end-stage renal disease; HD, hemodialysis; PD, peritoneal dialysis; PEW, protein-energy wasting.

Normalized protein nitrogen appearance is derived from the urea nitrogen appearance rate and is used as a proxy of dietary nitrogen and protein intake. In one study of 98,489 hemodialysis patients, both lower and higher normalized protein nitrogen appearance levels (i.e., <1.0 and ≥1.3 g/kg/d) were associated with higher risk of all-cause deaths. It may be speculated that the relationship between higher normalized protein nitrogen appearance levels and death is because of confounding factors such as low body weights of patients (i.e., total protein nitrogen appearance is scaled to patient's body weight in the denominator) and increased catabolism is associated with illness or directly because of toxicities associated with high-protein intakes. In analyses of protein nitrogen appearance (i.e., studies not scaled to body weight), there was a linear association between lower protein nitrogen appearance levels (<60 g per day and a higher death risk).

Considering the complex pathophysiology of PEW, the presence of various wasting markers (serum albumin <3.7 g per dL, percentage of lymphocytes in WBC count <22%, and WBC count >7,500 per mm^3) were examined separately and in combination with mortality among 1,220 Stages 1 to 5 CKD patients. Patients with a greater number of markers were found to have an increasingly higher death risk: 1.7-, 2.4-, and 3.6-fold higher death risks with the presence of 1, 2, and 3 markers, respectively.

Low Body Mass Index

Among studies of BMI and mortality in the predialysis CKD population, various patterns of association have been observed. In a single-center study of 521 US veterans with Stages 1 to 5 CKD, there was an inverse association between baseline and time-dependent BMI levels with all-cause mortality. However, in a subsequent study of 453,946 nationwide US veterans with Stages 3 to 5 CKD, differential associations were observed across varying levels of kidney dysfunction. In patients with Stages 3A and 3B CKD, a U-shaped association between BMI and death risk was observed (i.e., both lower and higher BMI levels were associated with higher mortality). But, among patients with Stages 4 and 5 CKD, there was an inverse linear association between lower BMI levels and higher death (i.e., lower BMI levels only were associated with higher mortality). More recently, associations between BMI and mortality across strata of age were examined among >3 million U.S. veterans who had normal baseline kidney function (>60 mL/min/1.73 m^2). Although this was an evaluation of patients with normal kidney function at baseline, both those with lower and higher BMI levels (<20 and >35 kg per m^2, respectively) were associated with increased mortality in these patients without CKD.

In contrast, a rather consistent association between obesity and either a greater survival or reduced mortality rates have been observed in the hemodialysis population. A number of large national and international hemodialysis cohort studies have uncovered robust associations between a higher BMI and a lower mortality risk. For example, in a large population-based study of 21,762 US hemodialysis patients from a large dialysis organization, BMI levels <23.0 kg per m^2 were independently associated with higher death risk. Although these prior studies have largely examined BMI at a single point in time (i.e., baseline BMI ascertained at study entry), hemodialysis patients experience fluctuations in BMI. This finding may result from changes in dietary intake, dialysis prescriptions, and/or comorbidity over time. In a study of 14,632 wait-listed hemodialysis patients were examined for changes in weight over 6 months, patients who experienced a 3 to <5 kg and ≥5 kg weight loss had higher death risks compared to the risk of hemodialysis patients who had minimal (<±1 kg) weight change. In an analysis of dynamic BMI changes over time, the association between BMI as a time-dependent exposure with all-cause mortality was examined among 123,625 US hemodialysis patients using a marginal structural modeling approach. Similar to baseline BMI studies, an inverse association between lower BMI and higher mortality was observed, such that the lowest BMI category (BMI < 18.0 kg per m^2) was associated with a 3.2-fold higher death risk versus the BMI reference of 25.0 to 27.5 kg per m^2.

Underlying inflammatory status may be a key modifier of the relationship between BMI and outcomes in dialysis patients. In a study of 5,904 incident hemodialysis patients across 312 European facilities, inflammatory status (determined by C-reactive protein levels) was found to modify the BMI–mortality association. Among inflamed patients, incrementally lower BMI categories across the spectrum of high and low BMI were associated with increasingly higher death risk, whereas in noninflamed patients only BMI levels <21.5 kg per m^2 were associated with higher mortality.

Body Composition

Studies of body composition have suggested that having both a higher muscle and fat mass are protective for dialysis patients. As a proxy of muscle mass, quartiles of MAMC, estimated as MAMC (cm) = mid-arm circumference (cm) − 3.142 × triceps skinfold, and mortality were examined among 792 hemodialysis patients. Incrementally higher quartiles of MAMC were associated with lower mortality: the highest quartile was associated with a 36% lower death risk versus results from the lowest quartile.

As an estimate of body fat percentage and fat-free body mass, near-infrared interactance body fat (%) has been measured using a portable sensor evaluating the nonvascular access upper arms of dialysis patients. The body fat is highly correlated with other body fat and nutritional metrics in this population. Among 535 hemodialysis patients who underwent near-infrared interactance testing, those with total body fat <12% had a four-fold higher death risk compared to patients with body fat of 24% to 36%.

Nutritional Scoring Systems

The Kidney Disease Outcomes Quality Initiative expert panel for nutrition and the European Best Practice Guidelines Wave II have recommended serial assessments by Subjective Global Assessment of Nutrition in hemodialysis patients. Indeed, studies of both predialysis CKD and dialysis patients reveal that malnutrition determined from the Subjective Global Assessment tool is associated with higher death risk. Efforts have been made to improve upon this tool because it is a semi-quantitative grading system and objective measures of nutrition such as laboratory tests and body mass are not included. To address this limitation, the Malnutrition-Inflammation Score was developed from the Subjective Global Assessment tool, and the change includes values of BMI, serum albumin, and prealbumin. It is scored 0 to 30 for the examination of the presence of PEW (i.e., higher levels indicate worse PEW). In a study of 809 US hemodialysis patients who underwent Malnutrition-Inflammation Score testing, patients with scores in the second, third, and fourth quartiles had a higher death risk compared to patients in the lowest quartile. Similar results were found in prevalent kidney transplant recipients.

PRACTICAL IMPLICATIONS

Given the high burden of PEW that is present in predialysis CKD and ESRD patients, plus its potent relationship with mortality, additional studies are needed to more accurately assess the incidence and prevalence of PEW. What is needed is a system that defines robust and practical methods of assessing the nutritional status of the vast numbers of patients suffering from kidney disease worldwide. In the aforementioned study of 1,220 US veterans with CKD, the population attributable fraction (i.e., proportion of outcomes attributed to the exposure of a disease or condition within the population) was estimated to be as high as 38% and 40% for low serum albumin and low lymphocyte percentage, respectively. The observational studies we have presented in the chapter cannot prove causality, but there are data suggesting that the amelioration of mortality linked to various PEW parameters (i.e., increases in serum albumin or body fat) over time suggests that the deleterious complications of PEW can be modified. Consequently, interventional therapeutic trials testing this hypothesis are needed. This need is highlighted by the report that mathematical simulations of the influence of a 0.2 g per dL therapeutic increase in serum albumin indicate that as many as 1,400 lives could be saved, 6,000 hospitalizations could be averted, and $36 million in Medicare costs are saved. Finally, there are the paradoxical associations that have been uncovered in subjects with nonkidney disease but with heart failure or malignancies. These reports show that BMI or other estimates of PEW can be related to an increase in mortality. Consequently, investigations of the outcomes of patients with PEW are likely to advance our understanding of the causes and treatment of wasting in other populations with chronic diseases.

Suggested Readings

Fouque D, Kalantar-Zadeh K, Kopple J, et al. A proposed nomenclature and diagnostic criteria for protein-energy wasting in acute and chronic kidney disease. *Kidney Int* 2008;73(4):391–398.

Ikizler TA, Cano NJ, Franch H, et al. Prevention and treatment of protein energy wasting in chronic kidney disease patients: a consensus statement by the International Society of Renal Nutrition and Metabolism. *Kidney Int* 2013;84(6):1096–1107.

Kalantar-Zadeh K, Kilpatrick RD, Kuwae N, et al. Revisiting mortality predictability of serum albumin in the dialysis population: time dependency, longitudinal changes and population-attributable fraction. *Nephrol Dial Transplant* 2005;20(9):1880–1888.

Kovesdy CP, George SM, Anderson JE, et al. Outcome predictability of biomarkers of protein-energy wasting and inflammation in moderate and advanced chronic kidney disease. *Am J Clin Nutr* 2009;90(2):407–414.

Kovesdy CP, Kopple JD, Kalantar-Zadeh K. Management of protein-energy wasting in non-dialysis-dependent chronic kidney disease: reconciling low protein intake with nutritional therapy. *Am J Clin Nutr* 2013;97(6):1163–1177.

Lacson E Jr, Ikizler TA, Lazarus JM, et al. Potential impact of nutritional intervention on end-stage renal disease hospitalization, death, and treatment costs. *J Ren Nutr* 2007;17(6):363–371.

Lu JL, Kalantar-Zadeh K, Ma JZ, et al. Association of body mass index with outcomes in patients with CKD. *J Am Soc Nephrol* 2014;25(9):2088–2096.

Lu JL, Molnar MZ, Naseer A, et al. Association of age and BMI with kidney function and mortality: a cohort study. *Lancet Diabetes Endocrinol* 2015;3(9):704–714.

Molnar MZ, Streja E, Kovesdy CP, et al. Associations of body mass index and weight loss with mortality in transplant-waitlisted maintenance hemodialysis patients. *Am J Transplant* 2011;11(4):725–736.

Rambod M, Bross R, Zitterkoph J, et al. Association of Malnutrition-Inflammation Score with quality of life and mortality in hemodialysis patients: a 5-year prospective cohort study. *Am J Kidney Dis* 2009;53(2):298–309.

4 Effects of Chronic Kidney Disease on Metabolism and Hormonal Function

Adriana M. Hung

The primary function of the kidney is to maintain a near complete homeostasis of the internal *milieu*, the blood is filtered continuously by the kidneys, resulting in a stable chemical composition of the blood compartment over a wide range of nutrient and fluid intakes. Kidney function thus plays a critical role in maintaining circulatory and organ system functional homeostasis, and the loss of kidney function in chronic kidney disease (CKD) and especially end-stage renal disease (ESRD) leads to dysregulation of many metabolic pathways. This results clinically in the uremic syndrome in ESRD, and metabolic disturbances characterized by subtle dysfunction of many organ systems that are present in variable degree since early stages of the disease.

The kidney also regulates body homeostasis not only by excretory function also but by a number of synthetic and degradative properties dependent on glomerular and tubular epithelial cell function. These properties include synthesis of hormones, degradation of peptides and low–molecular-mass proteins (less than 50 kDa), and metabolic events aimed at conserving energy and regulating the composition of body fluids. The kidney is the site of synthesis of a number of hormones (i.e., erythropoietin [EPO], 1,25-dihydroxyvitamin D_3 [1,25-dihydroxycholecalciferol], and rennin) and is an important catabolic site for several polypeptide hormones (e.g., insulin, glucagon, and parathyroid hormone [PTH]) and glycoproteins. Furthermore, the kidney has important metabolic functions such as neoglucogenesis (Table 4.1).

SOLUTE ACCUMULATION

In CKD, as glomerular filtration rate (GFR) decreases, solutes that are excreted by the kidney (such as creatinine and urea) accumulate in body fluids, and the plasma concentration of these solutes increases. Other solutes, including phosphates, sulfates, uric acid, and hydrogen ions, also can accumulate in body fluids. Accumulation of hydrogen ions is caused by impairment of both amoniagenesis and hydrogen ion secretion in tubular cells, resulting in the development of metabolic acidosis. Although the most profound changes occur with severe impairment of GFR, many of these abnormalities with associated adaptive or maladaptive responses begin around a GFR of 60 mL/min/1.73 m^2 or even higher. As CKD progresses, other compounds that are retained in body fluids include phenols, guanidines, organic acids, indols, myoinositol and other polyols, polyamines, β_2-microglobulin, certain peptides, urofuremic acids, and trace elements, such as aluminum, zinc, copper, and iron. The accumulation of these toxic substances can lead to hormonal deficiencies (testosterone, fetuin, growth hormone, etc.), inability to appropriately respond to stimuli (insulin resistance, EPO resistance, etc.), or overproduction (prolactin). As kidney function declines, patients' abilities to adapt to changes in dietary intake, particularly those involving sodium, potassium, phosphorus, and water, becomes more restricted. Solute and water excretion per nephron increases as kidney function decreases; however, this is counterbalanced by

Components of Kidney Function

Excretion of metabolic waste products (urea, creatinine, and uric acid)
Elimination and detoxification of drugs and toxins
Maintenance of volume and ionic composition of body fluids
Acid–base regulation
Regulation of systemic blood pressure (renin, angiotensin, prostaglandins, nitric
    oxide, and sodium homeostasis)
Production of erythropoietin
Control of mineral metabolism through endocrine synthesis
    (1,25-dihydroxycholecalciferol and 24,25-dihydroxycholecalciferol)
Degradation and catabolism of peptide hormones (insulin, glucagon, and
    parathyroid hormone) and clearance of low–molecular-weight proteins
    (β_2-microglobulin and light chains)
Regulation of metabolic processes (gluconeogenesis and lipid metabolism)

the fewer number of functional nephrons. As kidney disease progresses, the capacity to respond to changes in the intake of sodium, other solutes, and water becomes less flexible, and eventually, this loss of capacity can result in changes in the volume and composition of the extracellular fluid. Thus, dietary intake in patients with CKD needs to be adjusted.

METABOLIC PATHWAYS FREQUENTLY ALTERED IN CHRONIC KIDNEY DISEASE

CKD is known to be associated with alterations in multiple metabolic pathways. Recent studies indicate that these alterations might lead to a milieu highly conducive to the development of atherosclerosis and might explain, at least to some extent, the exaggerated cardiovascular disease risk in this patient population (Fig. 4.1).

Inflammation

Chronic noninfectious inflammation is a common feature of CKD and ESRD. It has been demonstrated that 30% to 50% of patients with advanced CKD have serologic evidence of an activated inflammatory response in cross-sectional studies. In longitudinal studies, virtually, all dialysis patients have evidence of intermittent inflammation. Elevated plasma levels of the pro-inflammatory cytokine interleukin 6 (IL-6) and the prototypical acute-phase protein C-reactive protein (CRP) have emerged as powerful independent predictors of cardiovascular events and mortality, often exceeding the prognostic value of traditional cardiovascular risk factors such as low-density lipoprotein (LDL) cholesterol in the CKD population. Moreover, plasma IL-6 and CRP levels do not change significantly over the course of time after initiation of dialysis therapy, suggesting that dialysis only partially improves the inflammatory metabolic alterations associated with loss of kidney function. A plethora of additional inflammatory markers have been studied in kidney disease, including sICAM-1, serum amyloid A, IL-8, IL-18, myeloperoxidase (MPO), sCD40 ligand, and matrix metalloproteinase-9. Fibrinogen is also an important acute-phase reactant, and fibrinogen levels significantly predict cardiovascular events in patients with CKD undergoing peritoneal and hemodialysis.

The underlying etiology of the augmented inflammatory response in kidney disease remains poorly understood, and it is most likely multifactorial. The hemodialysis procedure itself contributes to a pro-inflammatory milieu by increasing the synthesis of fibrinogen, IL-6, and other pro-inflammatory

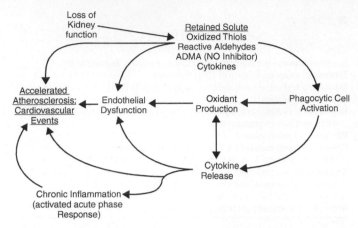

FIGURE 4.1 A proposed mechanism for uremia-induced cardiovascular disease risk.

peptides. This is primarily because of exposure to the dialysate and the plastic tubing during the extracorporeal procedure. Subclinical vascular access infections may also contribute to augmented inflammation in many dialysis patients. However, although multiple dialysis-related factors can contribute to maintenance of a chronic inflammatory response, studies have demonstrated that plasma IL-6 and CRP levels are elevated in earlier stages of CKD, suggesting a more proximate relationship to loss of kidney function and chronic inflammation. Loss of kidney function is directly associated with reduced renal clearance of cytokines, complement peptides, oxidants, and other pro-inflammatory solutes. Biologic priming of inflammatory cells may also be an important contributor to increased inflammation in CKD. Inflammation is exacerbated by comorbid conditions such as diabetes mellitus, cardiovascular disease, gout, and inflammatory renal disease (glomerulonephritis).

Recent data have demonstrated a key role of the NLRP3 inflammasome, a cytosolic protein structure that activates caspase 1, and IL-1β and leads to chronic inflammation. A study demonstrated in kidney biopsies the activation of NLRP3 and caspase 1, regardless of the CKD etiology, suggesting its role in CKD progression. The inflammasome is also activated in other chronic inflammatory conditions, particularly in gout and diabetes, which are highly prevalent in patients with CKD.

Oxidative Stress

Increased oxidative stress is known to contribute to the pathogenesis of atherosclerosis. According to the widely accepted oxidized LDL hypothesis, atherogenicity of LDL is greatly increased by oxidative modification. Oxidatively modified LDL is taken up into monocyte/macrophages via scavenger receptors, leading foam cell formation in the subendothelial space, an early step in the atherosclerotic process. Reactive oxygen species directly oxidize LDL, stimulate vascular smooth muscle cell proliferation and migration, and potentiate the production of pro-inflammatory cytokines. Reactive oxygen species activate matrix metalloproteinases, which can lead to atherosclerotic plaque instability and rupture, as a precipitant of cardiovascular events. Reactive oxygen species also increase production of pro-inflammatory cytokines and acute-phase proteins via activation of the transcription factor nuclear factor-κB (NF-κB). NF-κB activation is controlled by the oxidation–reduction (redox) status of the cell, and generation of intracellular reactive oxygen species may be a common step in all of the signaling pathways that lead to activation of NF-κB.

Uremia is now well recognized as an increased oxidative stress state. Increased oxidative stress in CKD and ESRD is characterized by excess formation and retention of lipid peroxidation products, α-, β-unsaturated reactive aldehydes, and oxidized thiols. Levels of plasma F_2-isoprostanes, a lipid peroxidation end product, are 2 to 4 times higher in hemodialysis patients than in age- and gender-matched healthy subjects. Levels of minimally oxidatively modified LDL are also higher in dialysis patients than healthy subjects. Several recent studies demonstrate that plasma levels of individual plasma-oxidized solutes or antioxidants can predict subsequent cardiovascular mortality in dialysis patients. A linkage between increased oxidative stress and acute-phase inflammation in severely hypoalbuminemic dialysis patients has been described. Kidney transplantation, dialysis therapy, and antioxidant and anti-inflammatory therapy may each have limited but beneficial effects on oxidative stress-related metabolic abnormalities.

Although the dialysis population is better studied, data now convincingly demonstrates that patients with less severe degrees of CKD are also subject to high levels of oxidative stress. Multiple biomarkers of oxidative stress (and inflammation) are elevated in patients with moderate CKD compared to healthy subjects. Increased lipid peroxidation end products, protein carbonyls, advanced oxidation protein products, and changes in glutathione content have all been observed. Thus, there is a surprisingly high prevalence of inflammation and oxidative stress associated with the development of mild to moderate CKD.

The pathogenesis of uremic oxidative stress is not well understood. However, leukocyte activation clearly is an important contributor. Stimulated neutrophils and monocytes generate superoxide and hydrogen peroxide (after dismutation) and release the heme enzyme MPO during degranulation. MPO is one of the most abundant proteins in phagocytes, constituting approximately 5% neutrophil protein and 1% monocyte protein. MPO has the unique property of converting chloride in the presence of hydrogen peroxide to hypochlorous acid. A substantial body of evidence suggests that MPO is involved in uremic inflammation and oxidative stress. Catalytically, active MPO can be released during the hemodialysis procedure, and 3-chlorotyrosine, an oxidative stress biomarker specific for MPO-catalyzed oxidation through hypochlorous acid, has been demonstrated in the plasma proteins of dialysis patients. Other factors that contribute to increased oxidative stress in patients with CKD include dietary deficiency of antioxidants and scavenging systems, diabetes, inflammation, and age-related changes in antioxidant defenses.

Insulin Resistance

Glucose metabolism can be impaired by defects in insulin secretion from pancreatic β-cells and/or from defects in cellular sensitivity to insulin. Frank hyperglycemia may ensue (diabetes) or impair fasting glucose may happen depending on the balance between these two parameters. There are a number of diagnostic techniques available for the assessment of insulin resistance. Fasting glucose measurements and oral glucose tolerance tests are routinely used to clinically identify disease, such as prediabetes (impaired fasting glucose or impaired glucose tolerance) or type 2 diabetes. More invasive diagnostic tests can be used to define underlying pathophysiology. These tests include glucose clamp studies and the intravenous glucose tolerance test (IVGTT). During the IVGTT, glucose and insulin concentrations are measured after a standard IV glucose bolus. The insulin response to the glycemic load reflects insulin secretion, while modeling relates glucose disappearance to insulin concentrations to calculate insulin sensitivity. Fasting insulin concentrations or practical indices of insulin sensitivity are calculated from fasting insulin and fasting glucose (e.g., the Homeostasis Model Assessment) and are also frequently used to estimate insulin sensitivity under basal conditions, particularly in large epidemiologic studies. The hyperinsulinemic euglycemic clamp procedure is the gold standard for quantifying peripheral insulin sensitivity in a stimulated state. During administration of exogenous supraphysiologic doses of insulin, an infusion of glucose is titrated to a rate which maintains peripheral glucose concentration at a normal fasting level. The glucose infusion rate equals the rate of glucose utilization by the body, providing a global measure of insulin sensitivity.

Glucose metabolism is frequently impaired in CKD (Fig. 4.2). In ESRD, the predominant disturbance is insulin resistance, as demonstrated by euglycemic and hyperglycemic clamp techniques. The main defect resides in a reduced insulin-mediated glucose uptake in skeletal muscle. Some patients with ESRD are able to compensate for insulin resistance by increasing insulin secretion, although defects in insulin secretion are also common in ESRD. It is not clear whether impaired glucose metabolism contributes to the pathogenesis of CKD and its progression (in the absence of overt diabetes), whether impaired kidney function causes impaired glucose metabolism, or both. In mild to moderate CKD, there is a high prevalence of insulin resistance, which is strongly associated with the degree of adiposity. A synergistic effect of increase adiposity and decreased kidney clearance of adipokines with CKD may also exacerbate these disturbances.

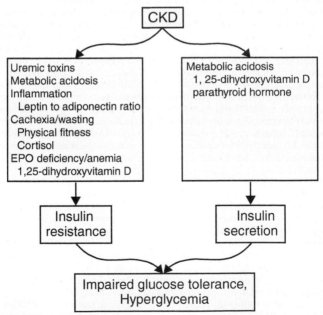

FIGURE 4.2 Potential CKD-related alterations leading to insulin resistance. CKD, chronic kidney disease.

Impaired glucose metabolism is an established risk factor for cardiovascular events and mortality, and thus represents an important potential therapeutic target in CKD to decrease incidence and progression of CKD and to reduce CV risk. In the Modification of Diet in Renal Disease Study, participants with CKD Stages 3 and 4 without diabetes who had higher hemoglobin A1C levels had increased mortality over long-term follow-up. Other smaller observational studies have correlated the extent of insulin resistance in mild to moderate CKD with cardiovascular and all-cause mortality risk. Among patients with ESRD with diabetes, several studies have observed that higher hemoglobin A1c levels are associated with increased mortality, although this association was apparent only for very high levels. Insulin resistance and frank hyperglycemia may lead to cardiovascular risk and mortality risk through endothelial dysfunction, activation of the renin–angiotensin–aldosterone system, increasing dyslipidemia, and by amplifying oxidative stress and inflammatory pathways.

Endothelial Dysfunction

The endothelium plays a key role in the maintenance of vascular tone, structure, and hemostasis. This occurs primarily through the secretion of several vasodilating factors, among which the most important is nitric oxide (NO). Endothelium-derived NO has potent antiatherogenic properties which are mediated through inhibition of platelet aggregation, prevention of smooth muscle cell proliferation, and reduction of endothelial adhesion molecule expression. Low production of NO has been found in patients with CKD and could contribute to the development of hypertension, atherosclerosis, and the progression of kidney disease. NO abnormalities might also contribute to intradialytic hypotension in patients receiving hemodialysis therapy. Several endogenous inhibitors of NO synthesis which accumulate in CKD have been identified, of which asymmetric dimethylarginine (ADMA) and symmetric dimethylarginine (SDMA) and homocysteine have received the most attention. ADMA is a naturally occurring methylated form of the amino acid arginine that competes with arginine as a substrate for all three isoforms of NO synthase. SDMA competitively inhibits uptake of arginine by endothelial cells, thereby decreasing substrate availability for NO synthesis. Patients with CKD and ESRD have high plasma levels of ADMA and SDMA, which have been closely associated with cardiovascular risk. Hyperhomocysteinemia is also highly prevalent in patients with CKD. Homocysteine circulates predominantly as an oxidized dimer (e.g., as homocysteine or a mixed disulfide), and considerable experimental data suggests that plasma homocysteine levels are an independent risk factor for cardiovascular disease. Homocysteine has proatherogenic effects by inhibiting endothelial cell growth and promoting vascular smooth muscle cell proliferation. On the other hand, a recent randomized clinical trial failed to show any benefit of folic acid supplementation to reduce cardiovascular and overall mortality in patients with CKD Stages 4 and 5. Oxidative stress is also closely linked with endothelial dysfunction in CKD. In increased oxidative stress states, superoxide anion produced via nicotinamide adenine dinucleotide phosphate-oxidase (NADPH) oxidase reacts extremely rapidly with NO, resulting in loss of NO bioactivity. The end product of this reaction is peroxynitrite, itself a highly reactive and toxic reactive nitrogen species. A recent study showed that treatment of vascular inflammation in patients with CKD with IL-1 blockade improved both endothelial function (measured as endothelium-dependent vasodilation) and decreases markers of oxidative stress.

ALTERATIONS IN RENAL METABOLISM OF PEPTIDE HORMONES

The kidney is a major site for the catabolism of plasma proteins with a molecular mass less than 50 kDa but not for proteins with a molecular mass

| TABLE 4.2 | Circulating Levels of Hormones and Related Peptides in Advanced CKD |

Increased	Decreased
Insulin, proinsulin, C-peptide	Erythropoietin
Glucagon	1,25-Dihydroxycholecalciferol
Growth hormone	Progesterone
Parathyroid hormone	Testosterone
Calcitonin	Thyroxine
Gastrin	Triiodothyronine
FGF-23	Renalase
Prolactin (particularly in women)	
Vasopressin	
Adipocytokines: leptin, adiponectin, and resistin	
Luteinizing hormone	
Follicle-stimulating hormone	
Luteinizing hormone–releasing hormone	
Secretin	
Cholecystokinin	
Vasoactive intestinal peptide	
Gastric inhibitory peptide	

CKD, chronic kidney disease; FGF-23, fibroblast growth factor-23.

greater than 68 kDa (e.g., albumin and immunoglobulins). Because most polypeptide hormones have molecular masses greater than 30 kDa, they are metabolized by the kidney to a variable extent. Renal metabolism of polypeptide hormones often involves the binding of the hormone to specific receptors in the basolateral membrane of tubular epithelia or alternatively glomerular filtration and tubular reabsorption. Degradation results in the generation of amino acids, which are reabsorbed and returned to the circulation. Removal of peptide hormones by filtration depends on the molecular mass, shape, and charge of the molecule; for example, growth hormone, with a molecular mass of 21.5 kDa, has a filtration coefficient of 0.7, whereas insulin, with a molecular mass of 6 kDa, is freely filtered. Binding of a hormone to large proteins prevents its filtration. Other factors, including impaired renal and extrarenal degradation of a hormone or abnormal secretion, are also operative in kidney disease. Most filtered peptides are reabsorbed in the proximal tubule so that less than 2% of filtered polypeptides appear in the urine. In experimental animals, nephrectomy prolongs the plasma half-life of insulin, proinsulin, glucagon, PTH, and growth hormone. Consequently, the circulating levels of numerous peptide hormones are elevated in advanced CKD (Table 4.2). In most instances, successful kidney transplantation rapidly restores the circulating levels of many peptide hormones to normal levels.

Insulin, Proinsulin, and C-Peptide
The major sites of insulin degradation are the kidney and the liver. In humans, less than 1% of the filtered insulin is excreted in the urine, and catabolism of insulin in the kidney involves both filtration reabsorption and peritubular uptake. The kidney also catabolizes proinsulin and C-peptide. The kidney accounts for most of the catabolism of the insulin precursor, proinsulin. Conversely, the kidney accounts for only one-third of the metabolic clearance rate of insulin; the liver and muscle account for two-thirds of the disappearance of this peptide. In patients with advanced CKD, the high plasma

levels of immunoreactive insulin probably represent a greater contribution of proinsulin and C-peptide rather than of the active insulin. Consequently, when kidney function is decreased, dissociation can occur between the insulin level indicated by radioimmunoassay and the amount of biologically active insulin actually present.

Glucagon

The kidney accounts for about one-third of the metabolic clearance of glucagon. Glomerular filtration is the major route of glucagon removal. Plasma glucagon levels are increased in patients with advanced CKD, and the metabolic clearance rate of injected glucagon is markedly prolonged. Glucagon secretion in response to stimulants is exaggerated in these patients, but the high plasma glucagon levels in uremia are apparently caused by decreased metabolic clearance, rather than hypersecretion of the hormone.

Growth Hormone and Insulin-like Growth Factor I

The kidney accounts for approximately 40% to 70% of the metabolic clearance rate of growth hormone in experimental animals. It is reabsorbed along the nephron, and less than 1% of filtered hormone is excreted in the urine. In advanced renal insufficiency, the metabolic clearance of growth hormone is markedly decreased, and plasma levels of the immunoreactive hormone are increased; but excess growth hormone production also contributes to the high growth hormone levels observed in subjects with uremia. Some of the biologic effects of growth hormone are mediated by insulin-like growth factors I and II (IGF-I and IGF-II). Growth hormone stimulates the synthesis and release of IGFs, and circulating IGFs exert a negative effect on growth hormone secretion, thereby forming a hormonal axis.

Recent evidence indicates that IGF-I plays a role in compensatory renal hypertrophy. Administering IGF-I increases GFR and kidney weight in intact animals. After uninephrectomy, IGF-I levels increase in the contralateral kidney, although IGF-I receptor levels remain unchanged. In patients with ESRD, the plasma levels of IGF-I are normal, but the levels of IGF-II are elevated. Interestingly, the biologic effects of IGF-I and IGF-II are blunted when assayed in the presence of uremic serum, suggesting that a uremic factor (or factors) interferes with the biologic activity of IGF-I and perhaps IGF-II. However, long-term administration of supraphysiologic amounts of growth hormone to humans increases plasma IGF-I, improves nitrogen balance, and can have an anabolic effect. Clinical trials, mainly in children with kidney disease, have shown that administering growth hormone improves both the rate of growth and the amount of growth. For this reason, growth hormone is routinely administered to children with CKD or after kidney transplantation. The use of growth hormone in adults with CKD as a therapeutic for protein energy wasting is under active investigation.

Gastrin

The plasma concentration of gastrin in humans is increased after nephrectomy. The hypergastrinemia seen in patients with CKD is most likely caused by reduced degradation of this hormone by the kidney.

Catecholamines

Plasma levels of norepinephrine are within normal limits in patients with mild to moderate CKD, but high levels are found in patients with CKD Stages 4 and 5. In these patients, a threefold increase in plasma norepinephrine levels occurs when patients assume an upright position, and this response exceeds that measured in healthy subjects. Patients with CKD metabolize norepinephrine abnormally because the activity of tyrosine hydroxylase, the critical enzyme involved in the synthesis of norepinephrine in certain organs (e.g., heart and brain), is reduced. However, the norepinephrine level in patients with CKD does not appear to be caused by increased synthesis but rather by decreased degradation.

Prolactin

Approximately 16% of circulating prolactin is extracted during passage through the kidney. This hormone, which has a molecular mass of 23 kDa, is filtered to a modest extent and then is reabsorbed by the proximal tubules (less than 1% appears in the urine). Elevated plasma prolactin levels occur in approximately 80% of women, but in only 30% of men with CKD. Notably, the increase in prolactin is not modified by the administration of dopamine or bromocriptine. Patients with CKD experience a prolonged increase in prolactin levels after administration of thyroid-releasing factor, indicating that a pituitary gland disorder, plus a defect in the peripheral metabolism of the hormone, is present. The metabolic clearance of prolactin is diminished to about one-third in patients with moderate to severe CKD. Apart from galactorrhea and amenorrhea, other biologic effects of prolactin in patients with CKD are not clearly established.

Antidiuretic Hormone (Vasopressin)

Antidiuretic hormone (ADH) is metabolized in the liver and kidney. ADH is filtered at the glomerular level, and the kidney accounts for approximately 60% of the total metabolic clearance of ADH. Whether vasopressin is filtered and reabsorbed in the proximal tubule with intracellular degradation, or is degraded at the brush-border membrane of proximal tubular cells, remains unclear. In patients with CKD and especially with long-term hemodialysis, removal of ADH is decreased, resulting in high circulating levels of vasopressin.

Glucocorticoids

Plasma levels of cortisol are normal or high in patients with advanced CKD, especially in dialysis patients. The response of the adrenal gland to adreno-corticotropin (ACTH) is decreased, but the response of ACTH to stimulatory agents such as hypoglycemia is nearly normal. Thus, the normal or high cortisol level found might be the consequence of reduced clearance by the diseased kidney or in response to increased physiologic stress. The net effect is that adrenal function remains normal, and the expected diurnal variation remains unaltered in patients with CKD. Metabolic acidosis has been reported to increase glucocorticoid production.

Aldosterone

Aldosterone is the major mineral corticoid produced by the adrenal gland and, to a lesser extent, by endothelial and vascular smooth muscle cells. As a result, systemic and local production of aldosterone can each produce target organ effects. Aldosterone levels are elevated in most patients with CKD and in most animal models of CKD. Increasing evidence suggests that aldosterone partici-pates in the development of fibrosis, proteinuria, and cardiomyopathy. These conditions may, therefore, respond therapeutically to aldosterone blockade.

Thyroid Hormones

Abnormalities of thyroid function are present in patients with CKD, because kidney disease affects the metabolism of thyroid hormones at different steps. Levels of both serum total thyroxine (TT_4) and free thyroxine index (FT_4I), measured as the product of TT_4 and the triiodothyronine (T_3) resin uptake, are frequently low. Plasma iodide levels are usually high, and the plasma level of TSH is in general within normal limits, but the response to thyroid-releasing factor is blunted, especially when metabolic acidosis is present. The prevalence of goiter in patients with CKD is high compared to that in the general population. Individuals with CKD are subject to easy fatigability, lethargy, and cold intolerance; however, these changes are not accompanied by alterations in the basal metabolic rate or in the relaxation time for tendon reflexes (indicators of the biologic function of thyroid hormone). Low circulating levels of thyroid hormones in patients with ESRD may have a protective action on protein catabolism. Recent data have associated low levels of triiodothyronine with a poor outcome in patients with CKD and ESRD, which may be because of an inverse association with levels of inflammation. Thyroid supplementation is not advisable unless firm evidence of hypothyroidism exists.

Leptin

Leptin is a 16-kDa protein that is synthesized predominately in adipocytes under the control of the *ob* gene. Leptin's main target is the hypothalamus, where binding to the leptin receptor induces satiety, decreased food intake, increased energy expenditure, and weight loss. Leptin is mainly cleared by the kidney in the setting of normal kidney function, although nonrenal clearance is also evident and may increase in importance in CKD. Levels of free leptin are generally increased (when corrected for body mass) in patients with CKD and also correlate with low EPO levels and insulin resistance. Leptin may play a role in the cachexia and anorexia associated with uremia, but this remains controversial.

Other Adipocytokines

Adiponectin is exclusively secreted from adipose tissue (and also from the placenta during pregnancy) into the bloodstream and is very abundant in plasma relative to many hormones. It is one of the most potent molecules in the human body with respect to its insulin-sensitizing activity, along with its well-established anti-inflammatory, antioxidant and antiatherogenic properties. Reduction in adiponectin secretion has been associated with insulin resistance, dyslipidemia, and atherosclerosis in humans and animal models. These metabolic actions are closely associated with activation of 5' adenosine monophosphate-activated protein kinase (AMPK) and modulation of NF-κB through the activation of adiponectin receptors (AdipoR) 1 and 2, mostly in the liver and muscle. In CKD, adiponectin levels are in the overall increased because adiponectin is cleared by the kidney; however, the production of adiponectin is suppressed by inflammation which is common in CKD and which alters the ratio of adiponectin and other adipokines. For example, leptin to adiponectin ratio has been shown to be one of the main biomarkers (or determinants) of insulin sensitivity in ESRD.

Resistin is a 12.5-kDa adipokine that is predominantly produced by macrophages, with lower levels released from adipocytes with increasing levels associated with adiposity. Resistin circulates in the blood in two forms (minor and major), the minor form and the major active form. Elevated resistin levels are associated with an enhanced inflammatory response. In CKD, the levels of resistin are increased. High resistin levels correlate with increased endothelin (ET)-1 expression. ET-1 is a potent vasoactive factor that causes endothelial dysfunction in cardiovascular disease and has also been linked to obesity-related hypertension.

Sex Hormones

The kidney is a major site for the removal of glycoprotein hormones and their metabolites, including luteinizing hormone (LH), follicle-stimulating hormone (FSH), and human chorionic gonadotropin. Studies in animals suggest that the kidney accounts for 95% and 78% of the metabolic clearance rate of LH and FSH, respectively. Sexual dysfunction is a bothersome disorder for patients with advanced CKD. Sexual dysfunction is manifested clinically by impotence, decreased libido, testicular atrophy, and reduced sperm count in men and amenorrhea, irregular cycles, dysmenorrhea, and decreased libido in women. Its cause is frequently related to dysfunction of the hypothalamic–pituitary–adrenal axis, characterized by elevated circulating levels of LH, FSH, prolactin, and LH–releasing hormone. These changes lead to lower levels of progesterone or testosterone in women and men, respectively. Contributory roles have been suggested for PTH, anemia, decreased levels of NO, and zinc deficiency in the pathogenesis of these abnormalities. Androgen therapy was used as an adjunctive therapy for anemia in CKD for many years, but androgen therapy for anabolic indications in patients with CKD remains controversial. Increased levels of prolactin can cause galactorrhea and am-menorrhea, whereas high levels of LH can cause gynecomastia. Many of these abnormalities are reversed or markedly improved after successful kidney transplantation, and thus the patients regain their reproductive function.

HORMONAL DEFICIENCIES IN CHRONIC KIDNEY DISEASE

Erythropoietin (EPO)

Although resistance of the bone marrow to EPO can occur, decreased synthesis of EPO by the diseased kidney is the major cause of anemia in patients with CKD. Patients with CKD have lower EPO levels than anemic persons who have normal renal function when adjusted for the hemoglobin concentration. Uncomplicated anemia of kidney disease is classified into normocytic and normochromic. Administering pharmacologic doses of recombinant human EPO to patients with CKD can correct the anemia, reduce the need for blood transfusions, and improve quality of life.

Renalase

Renalase is a novel Flavin-adenine-dinucleotide–dependent amine oxidase that circulates after synthesis and secretion in the kidney. Under basal conditions, circulating renalase lacks amine oxidase activity (prorenalase), and conver-sion from prorenalase to renalase occurs after exposure to norepinepherine. Active renalase metabolizes and degrades circulating catecholamines, and renalase activity has been demonstrated to be altered in animal models and human CKD. It has been hypothesized that abnormal renalase activity may contribute to hypertension, increased sympathetic activity, and increased cardiac risk in CKD by reducing catecholamine clearance.

25-Hydroxycholecalciferol and 1,25-Dihydroxycholecalciferol (Calcitriol)

In healthy individuals, cutaneous synthesis is the predominant source of vitamin D, with smaller quantities coming from diet. Cholecalciferol and ergo-calciferol from these sources are converted to 25-hydroxyvitamin D (25-OHD) in the liver, and circulating 25-OHD reflects cutaneous and dietary vitamin D intake. 25-OHD is filtered at the glomerulus and actively reabsorbed into renal tubular cells via megalin and cubulin, where it is converted to the potent hormone 1,25-dihydroxyvitamin D (calcitriol) by the enzyme 1-α hydroxylase.

Vitamin D metabolism is profoundly disordered in CKD. Abnormalities begin during early CKD stages (i.e., Stage 3 or sooner) and progress as kidney function declines. The central feature of this process is a decline in circulating calcitriol, which occurs early and is because of diminished and suppresses 1-α hydroxylase activity and contribution of low substrate (Fig. 4.3). While CKD is not an independent risk factor for 25-OHD insufficiency, it is clear that low 25-OHD concentrations are common in all CKD stages. Contribut-ing factors may include decreased cutaneous synthesis (owing to older age,

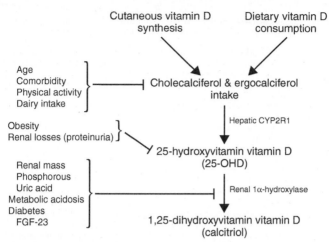

FIGURE 4.3 Vitamin D metabolism and factors that influence its homeostasis in CKD. CKD, chronic kidney disease.

comorbidities, and decreased physical activity), decreased dietary intake of fortified dairy products, obesity, and renal 25-OHD losses, which are most severe with heavy proteinuria. Diminished 1-α hydroxylase activity is probably the most important cause of declining calcitriol levels in CKD. Hyperphosphatemia, hyperuricemia, metabolic acidosis, and diabetes are associated with decreased 1-α hydroxylase activity. Elevated levels of fibroblast growth factor-23, which act to maintain serum phosphorous concentration as GFR falls, potently suppress 1-α hydroxylase activity.

The main function of calcitriol is maintenance of calcium and bone homeostasis, which is accomplished through regulation of dietary calcium absorption, PTH secretion, and osteoclast activity. However, vitamin D receptors are present throughout the body in diverse tissues, and hundreds of human genes contain vitamin D response elements. Thus, potential pleiotropic or nonclassic actions of vitamin D have recently attracted increasing interest. These actions may include suppression of the renin–angiotensin–aldosterone system, blood pressure reduction, modulation of immune function and cellular proliferation, prevention of myocyte hypertrophy, albuminuria reduction, prevention of glomerulosclerosis, β-cell function in the pancreas, and preservation of cognition.

Suggested Readings

Annuk M, Zilmer M, Lind L, et al. Oxidative stress and endothelial function in chronic renal failure. *J Am Soc Nephrol* 2001;12:2747–2752.

DeFronzo RA, Tobin JD, Rowe JW, et al. Glucose intolerance in uremia. Quantification of pancreatic beta cell sensitivity to glucose and tissue sensitivity to insulin. *J Clin Invest* 1978;62:425–435.

Dusso AS, Brown AJ, Slatopolsky E. Vitamin D. *Am J Physiol Renal Physiol* 2005;289:F8–F28.

Himmelfarb J, Stenvinkel P, Ikizler TA, et al. The elephant in uremia: oxidant stress as a unifying concept of cardiovascular disease in uremia. *Kidney Int* 2002;62:1524–1538.

Hung AM, Sundell MB, Egbert P, et al. A comparison of novel and commonly-used indices of insulin sensitivity in African American chronic hemodialysis patients. *Clin J Am Soc Nephrol* 2011;6(4):767–774.

Kalantar-Zadeh K, Ikizler TA, Block G, et al. Malnutrition-inflammation complex syndrome in dialysis patients: causes and consequences. *Am J Kidney Dis* 2003;42:864–881.

Levin A, Bakris GL, Molitch M, et al. Prevalence of abnormal serum vitamin D, PTH, calcium, and phosphorus in patients with chronic kidney disease: results of the study to evaluate early kidney disease. *Kidney Int* 2007;71:31–38.

Liu S, Quarles LD. How fibroblast growth factor 23 works. *J Am Soc Nephrol* 2007;18:1637–1647.

Mak RH. Intravenous 1,25-dihydroxycholecalciferol corrects glucose intolerance in hemodialysis patients. *Kidney Int* 1992;41:1049–1054.

Oberg BP, McMenamin E, Lucas FL, et al. Increased prevalence of oxidant stress and inflammation in patients with moderate to severe chronic kidney disease. *Kidney Int* 2004;65:1009–1016.

Siew ED, Ikizler TA. Determinants of insulin resistance and its effects on protein metabolism in patients with advanced chronic kidney disease. *Contrib Nephrol* 2008;161:138–144.

Stenvinkel P. Inflammation in end-stage renal disease: the hidden enemy. *Nephrology (Carlton)* 2006;11:36–41.

Teng M, Wolf M, Ofsthun MN, et al. Activated injectable vitamin D and hemodialysis survival: a historical cohort study. *J Am Soc Nephrol* 2005;16:1115–1125.

Vallance P, Leone A, Calver A, et al. Accumulation of an endogenous inhibitor of nitric oxide synthesis in chronic renal failure. *Lancet* 1992;339:572–575.

Zimmermann J, Herrlinger S, Pruy A, et al. Inflammation enhances cardiovascular risk and mortality in hemodialysis patients. *Kidney Int* 1999;55:648–658.

Zoccali C, Tripepi G, Cutrupi S, et al. Low triiodothyronine: a new facet of inflammation in end-stage renal disease. *J Am Soc Nephrol* 2005;16:2789–2795.

Calcium, Phosphorus, and Vitamin D in Kidney Disease

Sagar U. Nigwekar and Ravi I. Thadhani

CALCIUM, PHOSPHOROUS, AND VITAMIN D METABOLISM IN CHRONIC KIDNEY DISEASE

As chronic kidney disease (CKD) develops and progresses, a host of changes in mineral metabolism take place. One of the earliest changes is increased levels of fibroblast growth factor-23 (FGF-23) in response to reduced phosphorous excretion. As glomerular filtration rate declines, it is also accompanied by a fall in the activity of the renal vitamin D 1α-hydroxylase enzyme. FGF-23 also suppresses 1α-hydroxylase, limiting the production of 1,25-dihydroxyvitamin D. As a result, conversion of vitamin D from its inactive form (25-hydroxyvitamin D) to the active form (1,25-dihydroxyvitamin D) is impaired. With reduced 1,25-dihydroxyvitamin D activity, the vitamin D-dependent calcium absorption from the gastrointestinal tract is limited and patients develop hypocalcemia. Phosphorous excretion, in contrast, becomes restricted in the setting of advanced CKD because of decreased tubular function. In addition to the effects of declining kidney function and FGF-23 on production of 1,25-dihydroxyvitamin D, its synthesis may also be limited by a reduction in substrate, that is, 25-hydroxyvitamin D for 1α-hydroxylase. Reduction in 25-hydroxyvitamin D results at least in part from the urinary loss of the vitamin D-binding protein (DBP) and 25-hydroxyvitamin D bound to DBP in individuals with proteinuria. In addition, the ability of the skin to produce vitamin D in response to ultraviolet radiation appears to be impaired in CKD. Reduced dietary intake and overall limited sun exposure may also play a role in promoting 25-hydroxyvitamin D deficiency in this population.

One of the roles of 1,25-dihydroxyvitamin D is to suppress the production of parathyroid hormone (PTH) gene transcription. Not only is 1,25-dihydroxyvitamin D synthesis impaired in CKD, but the amount of vitamin D receptor (VDR) in the parathyroid gland is also reduced. Furthermore, in advanced CKD, the binding of 1,25-dihydroxyvitamin D to VDR and of the VDR complex to vitamin D response elements (VDRE) in DNA is also decreased. As a result of decreased vitamin D action, including reduced serum calcium from decreased gastrointestinal absorption, PTH production increases in a counterregulatory attempt to release calcium from bone stores. Unfortunately, the accompanying phosphate release further exacerbates the hyperphosphatemia of CKD and promotes further production of PTH.

The net result of these metabolic changes is a progressive and persistent increase in PTH levels (secondary hyperparathyroidism). Although extremely high levels of PTH have been associated with worsened survival in patients with end-stage renal disease (ESRD) on hemodialysis, PTH and mineral parameters are not established surrogates of ESRD-related mortality. The principal association of hyperparathyroidism has been an increased risk of CKD-related bone disease. It is noteworthy that extremely low levels of PTH and phosphorous in the patients with ESRD are also associated with poor outcomes.

BONE DISEASE AND CHRONIC KIDNEY DISEASE

The hyperparathyroidism of CKD has been most closely linked to the form of bone disease known as osteitis fibrosa cystica, characterized by markedly increased rates of bone turnover. Mineralization is preserved and bone volume is variable. The disease is often accompanied by bone marrow fibrosis. The persistently high turnover seen in this disease is associated with a replacement of lamellar bone by woven bone, which is less resilient to stress. As a result, individuals with osteitis fibrosa cystica may be predisposed to fractures out of proportion to their bone density. While hyperparathyroidism is felt to be the strongest contributor to the development of osteitis fibrosa cystica, there may also be a contribution from 1,25-dihydroxyvitamin D deficiency itself.

The use of vitamin D replacement in CKD has been largely driven by the goal of preventing osteitis fibrosa cystica. Early studies demonstrated improvement in bone histology after treatment with 25-hydroxyvitamin D. Further studies have noted the ability of intravenous calcitriol to increase osteoblastic osteoid while reducing marrow fibrosis in patients on hemodialysis. Because of these findings, along with the physiology supporting suppression of PTH, vitamin D is considered to be well-established standard therapy, particularly in patients on maintenance dialysis.

Increased use of vitamin D analogs may not come without risk, particularly with respect to bone disease. Adynamic bone disease, characterized by markedly reduced bone turnover, is the other major form of bone disease seen in CKD. Although mineralization is preserved, bone volume is usually low. As with osteitis fibrosa cystica, this disease has been linked to increased skeletal fragility. The prevalence of adynamic bone disease appears to be increasing over time, especially in patients on peritoneal dialysis. This may be, at least in part, the result of excessive use of active vitamin D analogs, because the development of adynamic bone disease has been reported in patients treated with these agents.

The osteomalacia of CKD, characterized by a reduction in bone turnover and low to normal bone volume, is a third form of bone disease. Unlike adynamic bone disease, bone mineralization is markedly abnormal in osteomalacia. The distinguishing characteristic is an abundance of unmineralized osteoid, which is not typically seen in either adynamic bone disease or osteitis fibrosa cystica. The primary cause of osteomalacia is thought to be accumulation of aluminum and other heavy metals in bone, which can disrupt normal mineralization of the bone matrix. Because aluminum-based phosphate binders have greatly declined in use, the prevalence of osteomalacia in CKD has reduced over time.

TREATMENT OF MINERAL METABOLISM ABNORMALITIES IN CHRONIC KIDNEY DISEASE

The changes in calcium, phosphorous, and PTH that accompany CKD can be modified through the use of several therapeutic strategies, including an increasingly broad range of medications. However, it is important to note that although these medications achieve correction of biochemical abnormalities, their effects on "hard outcomes" remain unknown.

Phosphate Restriction and Binders

Phosphate control is a critical component in the management of CKD because of the protean effects of phosphate retention and hyperphosphatemia on a range of metabolic processes. Because PTH promotes phosphate wasting, hyperphosphatemia can drive the development of hyperparathyroidism and osteitis fibrosa cystica. Phosphate retention promotes the production of FGF-23, leading to suppression of 1α-hydroxylase and reduced production

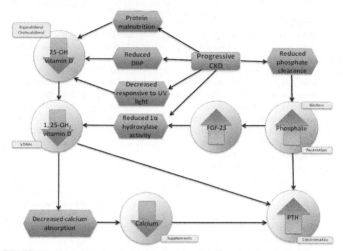

FIGURE 5.1 Changes in vitamin D and mineral metabolism associated with progressive chronic kidney disease. CKD, chronic kidney disease; DBP, vitamin D-binding protein; FGF-23, fibroblast growth factor 23; PTH, parathyroid hormone; VDRA, vitamin D receptor antagonists.

of 1,25-dihydroxyvitamin D (Fig. 5.1). Chronic elevation in serum phosphate, at least in patients with ESRD, also contributes to calcium phosphate deposition in tissues and vessel walls. In maintenance hemodialysis patients, elevated serum phosphate levels have been linked to an increased risk of early mortality and importance of hyperphosphatemia has also been recognized in early-stage CKD mortality.

Given the wide-ranging deleterious effects of hyperphosphatemia, control of phosphate levels is an important focus of CKD management. Kidney Disease: Improving Global Outcomes (KDIGO) guidelines recommend maintaining serum phosphate within or close to normal range. Dietary phosphate restriction is a reasonable initial approach with mild hyperphosphatemia, although it may have limited efficacy and practicability in some patients. Phosphate intake of 800 to 1,000 mg daily for patients with CKD exceeding the target range for serum phosphate is recommended. Dairy products, beans, and meats are not only common sources of dietary phosphate but also important sources of protein. Thus, excessive focus on reducing dietary phosphorous could lead to inadvertent and excessive reduction in dietary protein. This may be particularly important in the dialysis population, where nutritional status has been linked to patient outcomes. There are few studies directly evaluating the effects of dietary phosphate restriction alone on either serum phosphate or PTH levels.

Given the limitations of dietary phosphate restriction, the addition of oral phosphate binders is often necessary to achieve adequate control of serum phosphate. These agents are taken with food to reduce absorption of food-derived phosphate from the gastrointestinal tract.

Calcium-based phosphate binders include calcium acetate and calcium carbonate. Calcium citrate, a calcium supplement used in the non-CKD population, can increase absorption of aluminum and is not recommended for use as a phosphate binder. These agents are popular because of their low cost and providers' familiarity with them. Although the calcium content of these drugs may seem beneficial in balancing the hypocalcemia of CKD, there has been concern about the propensity of excessive calcium exposure to promoting vascular calcification. Additional side effects of these binders include gastrointestinal effects such as constipation.

Sevelamer hydrochloride is a nonabsorbed polymer that avoids the risk of excess calcium load of the calcium-based binders. A concern with the use of sevelamer hydrochloride is the potential for worsening metabolic acidosis, particularly in the nondialysis population; an updated formulation of this agent, sevelamer carbonate, has been developed to attenuate this risk.

Lanthanum is an element with the ability to bind phosphate and has been used in its carbonate form as a phosphate binder in CKD. This newer agent has the potential advantage of both sevelamer (lower calcium load) without the increase in metabolic acidosis risk. Despite the potential appeal of this agent, as with sevelamer, the higher cost of lanthanum compared to the calcium-based binders is a potential downside.

In a recent meta-analysis that pooled data from 11 randomized controlled trials comparing calcium-containing versus calcium-free phosphate binders in the patients with CKD, 22% mortality risk reduction was associated with the use of the non–calcium-based binders. A recent KDIGO workgroup suggested that the choice of phosphate binder in patients with CKD should take into account the CKD stage, the presence of other components of mineral bone disease including vascular calcification, concomitant therapies, and side effect profile.

Additional novel calcium-free phosphate binders including sucroferric oxyhydroxide, ferric citrate, and nicotinamide are now available. However, data on their effects on cardiovascular outcomes (similar to other binders) are not available. Aluminum-based phosphate binders such as aluminum hydroxide were first-line agents for hyperphosphatemia in the past because of their high efficacy. However, they have fallen out of favor because of the long-term risks of aluminum toxicity, particularly osteomalacia and neurotoxicity. Short-term use of aluminum compounds (e.g., a 4-week course) is still considered reasonable for individuals with persistent severe hyperphosphatemia.

Vitamin D Receptor Agonists for Hyperparathyroidism

Considering the risk of hyperparathyroidism and consequent osteitis fibrosa cystica as well as the underlying deficiency of 1,25-dihydroxyvitamin D that accompanies progressive CKD, treatment with active vitamin D and its analogs plays a central role in patients with ESRD and, to a lesser extent, in predialysis CKD. These analogs generally referred to as vitamin D receptor agonists (VDRAs), include the native calcitriol as well as agents such as 22-oxacalcitriol, paricalcitol, doxercalciferol, falecalcitriol, and alfacalcidol (1-hydroxyvitamin D, converted to 1,25-dihydroxyvitamin D in the liver).

A recent KDIGO workgroup concluded that for patients with CKD Stages 3 to 5 not on dialysis, the optimal PTH level is unknown. However, the workgroup suggested that patients with elevated PTH should be first evaluated for hyperphosphatemia, hypocalcemia, and vitamin D deficiency and that these abnormalities be corrected with approaches such as dietary phosphate restriction, phosphate binders, calcium supplements, and/or nutritional vitamin D. For patients with CKD Stages 3 to 5 not on dialysis, in whom PTH remains persistently elevated despite these approaches, the group suggested treatment with calcitriol or vitamin D analogs.

PTH goals are higher in the more advanced stages of CKD because of the development of PTH resistance in bone. Because of the inability to directly measure bone PTH activity and the impracticality of routine bone biopsy, PTH levels have remained the primary, albeit imperfect, guide to VDRA treatment. There has been much interest in the potential of newer VDRAs to suppress PTH while minimizing promotion of calcium and phosphate absorption from the gastrointestinal tract. This is supported by animal data and limited human studies. Use of one VDRA over another cannot be strongly recommended at this time.

Nutritional Vitamin D

Nutritional forms of vitamin D include the fungal-derived ergocalciferol and the animal-based cholecalciferol. These must be hydroxylated by both the hepatic 25-hydroxylase and the renal 1α-hydroxylase; the utility of these agents in CKD has, therefore, been thought to be limited. However, recent data suggest that treatment of 25-hydroxyvitamin D deficiency with ergocalciferol is effective at reducing PTH in Stage 3 CKD. The presence of extrarenal 1α-hydroxylase also points to the potential importance of these nutritional forms. However, effects of nutritional vitamin D compounds beyond mineral bone metabolism have not been confirmed in recent randomized clinical trials.

Calcimimetics

The advent of calcimimetic drugs added a more direct pathway for the suppression of PTH. This class of drugs binds to the calcium-sensing receptor (CaSR) on the parathyroid gland, thus simulating a hypercalcemic state in the setting of normal serum calcium levels. Consequently, PTH production is decreased. In addition, increased stimulation of the CaSR may be helpful in minimizing parathyroid gland hyperplasia. Only one calcimimetic, cinacalcet, is currently available in the United States. Cinacalcet offers the potential to control PTH without the risk of hypercalcemia or hyperphosphatemia associated with VDRAs. Because of the underlying mechanism of action, cinacalcet should be avoided in patients with a serum calcium level below 7.5 mg per dL.

Cinacalcet is approved for use in the maintenance dialysis population. Use in predialysis CKD is not Food and Drug Administration approved for management of hyperparathyroidism and remains controversial given the potential for severe hypocalcemia and seizures.

In the EVOLVE trial, maintenance hemodialysis patients with moderate-to-severe secondary hyperparathyroidism were randomized to cinacalcet or placebo. This trial found that the primary composite end point (time until death, myocardial infarction, hospitalization for unstable angina, heart failure, or a peripheral vascular event) was not different between the cinacalcet and placebo groups. However, after adjustment for baseline characteristics, there was a significant 12% reduction in risk ($p = 0.008$). Also, >20% of cinacalcet group patients discontinued the study medication, and censored analysis of these patients showed significant reductions in the primary composition end point and mortality.

PARATHYROIDECTOMY

Surgical parathyroidectomy in the setting of ESRD is reserved for hyperparathyroidism that is refractory to medical therapies. However, threshold PTH for parathyroidectomy is not clearly established, and most patients who undergo parathyroidectomy in this setting have PTH levels >1,000 pg per mL.

VITAMIN D AND SURVIVAL

Although much of the focus on VDRA use has centered on management of PTH, calcium, and phosphorus, there has been increasing attention on potential effects of VDRAs on improved outcomes in CKD. A retrospective study in over 60,000 maintenance hemodialysis patients demonstrated a 16% reduction in all-cause mortality associated with paricalcitol over calcitriol. This reduction persisted despite adjustment for a wide range of clinical characteristics, including levels of calcium, phosphorous, and PTH, suggesting that any mortality benefits may result from actions beyond the traditional axis of mineral metabolism. In a later study, the same group found a 26% reduction in 2-year mortality in patients who received any form of active vitamin D compared with those who did not receive the therapy.

Intriguingly, one study suggests that the dialysis survival benefit associated with the black race may be explained by increased use of VDRAs in this population. However, retrospective cohort studies such as these cannot prove a causative link, and unfortunately adequately powered randomized placebo-controlled trials to address this question have not been conducted and are challenging considering widespread utilization of these agents and challenges involved in randomizing to placebo arm.

In the CKD population, the PRIMO trial evaluated the effect of paricalcitol on the left ventricular mass index and diastolic function. Despite reduction in PTH with paricalcitol, the change in the left ventricular mass index and standard measures of diastolic dysfunction did not differ between treatment groups. Interestingly, treated patients had fewer cardiovascular-related hospitalizations, and left atrial size appeared to decrease in treated patients as well.

Potential Mechanisms of a Survival Benefit of Vitamin D Receptor Agonists

Because cardiovascular mortality is the leading cause of death in CKD and the risk of cardiovascular disease is dramatically increased in this population, the potential actions of vitamin D on the cardiovascular system have been a topic of great interest. These mechanisms have largely been explored through animal models. VDRAs appear to suppress renin production, thus potentially mitigating the risk of heart failure. An animal model at high risk of developing left ventricular hypertrophy and heart failure demonstrated improved cardiac function following treatment with paricalcitol, and observational data have suggested that similar benefits may exist in humans. Although high doses of vitamin D have been implicated in vascular calcification in animals, newly elucidated pathways suggest that vitamin D has the potential to reduce this calcification at lower doses. Although cardiovascular disease has been the focus of research on the link between VDRAs and improved patient outcomes, recent research tying vitamin D to expression of antimicrobial peptides raises the possibility of an effect on infectious disease as well, which represents the second-leading cause of death in dialysis. At this time, these actions in humans remain speculative and are active areas of investigation.

It should be noted that in the absence of data from randomized controlled trials, routine use of VDRAs other than for reduction of PTH, such as for improving patient outcomes, cannot be definitively substantiated by existing research. Observational studies such as those described above are helpful for generating testable hypothesis and guiding further research. Despite the fact that these studies adjusted for potential confounding from mineral levels and patient health, there is always the potential for residual confounding from unmeasured factors.

CALCIPHYLAXIS

Calciphylaxis is a rare vascular calcification disorder that affects patients with advanced CKD/ESRD. Calciphylaxis primarily involves dermal vasculature and is associated with a heavy burden of morbidity and mortality. The current understanding of its pathogenesis is limited; however, experts recommend the following practical considerations: (1) calciphylaxis patients should be evaluated by specialists from nephrology, dermatology, wound care, surgery, pathology, and pain/palliative medicine; (2) a punch biopsy has an overall low complication rate and should be considered for diagnostic confirmation; (3)

serum calcium and phosphorous levels should be maintained in the normal range, and serum PTH level should be maintained between 150 and 300 ng per mL. Calcium supplements, high dialysate calcium bath, and vitamin D preparations should be avoided; (4) dialysis prescription should be optimized to achieve dialysis adequacy. Evidence to support routine intensification of dialysis is limited; (5) intravenous sodium thiosulfate at doses ranging from 12.5 to 25 g in the last 30 minutes of each hemodialysis session has been shown to improve outcomes in small retrospective studies; (6) hyperbaric oxygen therapy can be considered a second-line treatment if wounds not improving; (7) nutrition consult to address protein energy malnutrition should be obtained; and (8) risk versus benefit discussion is needed to decide whether to continue potential calciphylaxis triggers such as warfarin and iron compounds.

CONCLUSION

A cascade of changes in the metabolism of calcium, phosphorous, and vitamin D leads to a disordered state of mineral metabolism that accompanies the progression of CKD. Given the risk of metabolic bone disease associated with hyperparathyroidism, attempts to normalize levels of calcium and phosphorous and regulate the level of PTH have been central to the management of CKD. This may be achieved through modification of diet or use of phosphate binders, calcimimetics, VDRAs, or parathyroidectomy. The choice of agents is dictated in part by levels of minerals and PTH. Importantly, calcium, phosphorous, and PTH have not been established as surrogate outcomes of survival. Despite initial enthusiasm for VDRAs in the observational studies, data from randomized trials are either limited or negative to support positive effects of these agents beyond mineral metabolism abnormalities. Similarly, cinacalcet did not improve mortality in a large randomized trial. Studies focused on personalizing these treatments for an individual patient will guide future recommendations.

Suggested Readings

Andress D, Norris KC, Coburn JW, et al. Intravenous calcitriol in the treatment of refractory osteitis fibrosa of chronic renal failure. *N Engl J Med* 1989;321:274–279.

Bhan I, Dobens D, Tamez H, et al. Nutritional vitamin D supplementation in dialysis: a randomized trial. *Clin J Am Soc Nephrol* 2015;10(4):611–619.

Block GA, Klassen PS, Lazarus JM, et al. Mineral metabolism, mortality, and morbidity in maintenance hemodialysis. *J Am Soc Nephrol* 2004;15:2208–2218.

EVOLVE Trial Investigators, Chertow GM, Block GA, et al. Effect of cinacalcet on cardiovascular disease in patients undergoing dialysis. *N Engl J Med* 2012;367(26):2482–2494.

Goodman WG, Ramirez JA, Belin TR, et al. Development of adynamic bone in patients with secondary hyperparathyroidism after intermittent calcitriol therapy. *Kidney Int* 1994;46:1160–1166.

Jamal SA, Vandermeer B, Raggi P, et al. Effect of calcium-based versus non-calcium-based phosphate binders on mortality in patients with chronic kidney disease: an updated systematic review and meta-analysis. *Lancet* 2013;382(9900):1268–1277.

Ketteler M, Elder GJ, Evenepoel P, et al. Revisiting KDIGO clinical practice guideline on chronic kidney disease—mineral and bone disorder: a commentary from a Kidney Disease: Improving Global Outcomes controversies conference. *Kidney Int* 2015;87(3):502–528.

LaClair RE, Hellman RN, Karp SL, et al. Prevalence of calcidiol deficiency in CKD: a cross-sectional study across latitudes in the United States. *Am J Kidney Dis* 2005;45:1026–1033.

Moe S, Drücke T, Cunningham J, et al.; Kidney Disease: Improving Global Outcomes (KDIGO). Definition, evaluation, and classification of renal osteodystrophy: a position statement from Kidney Disease: Improving Global Outcomes (KDIGO). *Kidney Int* 2006;69(11):1945–1953.

Nigwekar SU, Bhan I, Thadhani R. Ergocalciferol and cholecalciferol in CKD. *Am J Kidney Dis* 2012;60(1):139–156.

Nigwekar SU, Kroshinsky D, Nazarian RM, et al. Calciphylaxis: risk factors, diagnosis, and treatment. *Am J Kidney Dis* 2015;66(1):133–146. doi:10.1053/j.ajkd.2015.01.034.

Qunibi W, Moustafa M, Muenz LR, et al. A 1-year randomized trial of calcium acetate versus sevelamer on progression of coronary artery calcification in hemodialysis patients with comparable lipid control: the Calcium Acetate Renagel Evaluation-2 (CARE-2) study. *Am J Kidney Dis* 2008;51:952–965.

Teng M, Wolf M, Lowrie E, et al. Survival of patients undergoing hemodialysis with paricalcitol or calcitriol therapy. *N Engl J Med* 2003;349:446–456.

Thadhani R, Appelbaum E, Pritchett Y, et al. Vitamin D therapy and cardiac structure and function in patients with chronic kidney disease: the PRIMO randomized controlled trial. *JAMA* 2012;307(7):674–684.

Wolf M. Forging forward with 10 burning questions on FGF23 in kidney disease. *J Am Soc Nephrol* 2010;21(9):1427–1435.

Zisman AL, Hristova M, Ho LT, et al. Impact of ergocalciferol treatment of vitamin D deficiency on serum parathyroid hormone concentrations in chronic kidney disease. *Am J Nephrol* 2007;27:36–43.

6

Management of Lipid Abnormalities in the Patient with Kidney Disease

Christoph Wanner

Dyslipidemia is associated with adverse cardiovascular (CV) outcomes in the general population and in patients with chronic kidney disease (CKD). The absolute risk of CV events in individuals with CKD is similar to that of patients with established coronary artery disease in the general population, or exceeds in individuals with end-stage kidney disease (ESKD) on dialysis, but the increase in risk is associated with multifactorial conditions: a higher prevalence of insulin resistance, high blood pressure, vascular calcification, inflammation, and protein-energy wasting. Kidney failure is associated with a range of metabolic abnormalities, the so-called milieu of uremic toxicity, activation of the neurohormonal axis, vitamin D receptors, and increased fibroblast growth factor-23 that may all contribute to accelerated aging of the vasculature and damage to the heart. The hemodialysis procedure itself may have a direct negative effect on the heart, the so-called myocardial stunning.

Owing to the risk from multiple causes and confounding factors, it has been a challenge to explore the impact of dyslipidemia on CV outcomes in cohort studies and observational databases. Intervention studies are necessary to dissect a causal role of lipoproteins and lipids in that respect. Few intervention studies have been conducted and focused on lipid lowering through statins rather than on a dietary intervention. Certainly, diet and lifestyle modification are the basis of every hyperlipidemia treatment in the general population, but the complexity of the overall situation in later stages of CKD makes specific dietary interventions for dyslipidemias clinically implausible and less feasible. For example, a dietary approach which has changed or corrected the fundamental abnormality of lipoprotein composition in CKD and kidney failure, namely the enrichment of lipoproteins by apolipoprotein C, has not been done in patients with CKD especially not with hard CV outcomes.

To date, four large randomized controlled trials (RCTs) have been conducted to form a relatively solid basis of evidence for treatment of dyslipidemia in patients with CKD. These RCTs are represented by the ALERT study (Assessment of LEscol in Renal Transplantation Study), the 4D study (Die Deutsche Diabetes Dialyse Studie), AURORA (A Study to Evaluate the Use of Rosuvastatin in Subjects on Regular Hemodialysis: An Assessment of Survival and Cardiovascular Events), and SHARP (Study of Heart and Renal Protection). The results of these studies are also supported by post hoc analyses from these RCTs of statin versus placebo from the general population that focus on the subset of participants with CKD at baseline. In general, these analyses suggest that statins reduce the relative risk of CV events to a similar extent among patients with and without CKD, but that the absolute benefit of treatment is larger in patients with CKD because of their higher baseline CV risk.

ASSESSMENT OF LIPID STATUS IN ADULTS WITH CHRONIC KIDNEY DISEASE

Initial evaluation of the lipid profile (total cholesterol, low-density lipoprotein [LDL] cholesterol, high-density lipoprotein [HDL] cholesterol, and triglycerides) is intended to diagnose severe hypertriglyceridemia and/or hypercholesterolemia while ruling out any underlying secondary causes. Medical conditions that cause secondary dyslipidemias include hypothyroidism, excessive alcohol consumption, nephrotic syndrome, diabetes mellitus, and liver disease. Medications that may lead to dyslipidemias include immunosuppressants (corticosteroids, cyclosporine, and sirolimus), diuretics, and oral contraceptives. A fasting lipid profile should ideally be obtained, but nonfasting values provide useful information as well. Other major factors predisposing to dyslipidemia in people with CKD are lower *glomerular filtration rate* (GFR), modality of renal replacement with heparin use or protein loss across the peritoneal membrane, presence of comorbidities, and nutritional status.

TREATMENT OF DYSLIPIDEMIAS IN KIDNEY DISEASE

Statins in *Glomerular Filtration Rate* Categories G3a to G5

The SHARP trial is the largest study of lipid-lowering agents in patients with CKD, involving more than 9,000 patients, randomized to placebo or a combination of low-dose simvastatin and ezetimibe, with a median follow-up of 4.9 years. Overall, the study found that statin–ezetimibe therapy reduced the risk of major CV events by 17% (95% confidence interval [CI], 6% to 26%, $p = 0.0021$). Roughly, two-thirds ($n = 6,247$) of the participants in the study were not receiving maintenance dialysis at entry. In this population, statin therapy reduced the risk of major CV events by 22% (95% CI, 9% to 33%), with no increase in the risk of adverse events.

Based on these results, KDIGO (Kidney Disease Improving Global Outcomes) issued lipid-lowering guidelines with the following recommendations: (1) in adults aged ≥50 years with estimated GFR (eGFR) < 60 mL/min/1.73 m^2 but not treated with chronic dialysis or kidney transplantation (GFR categories G3a to G5), treatment with a statin or statin–ezetimibe combination is recommended (highest level of evidence; Grade 1A). A slightly lower, but still strong grading (1B) is recommended for statin treatment in adults aged ≥50 years with CKD and eGFR >60 mL/min/1.73 m^2 (GFR categories G1 and G2). Similarly (Grade 2A), in adults aged 18 to 49 years with CKD but not treated with chronic dialysis or kidney transplantation, treatment with a statin is suggested in people with one or more of the following: (a) known coronary disease (myocardial infarction [MI] or coronary revascularization), (b) diabetes mellitus, (c) prior ischemic stroke, (d) estimated 10-year incidence of coronary death or nonfatal MI >10%.

Statin Treatment in Dialysis Patients

Along with the subgroup of maintenance dialysis patients in SHARP, two other large trials have failed to show a conclusive benefit of statin treatment among prevalent maintenance dialysis patients. The 4D study investigated 1,255 subjects with type 2 diabetes mellitus receiving maintenance hemodialysis who were randomly assigned to receive 20 mg of atorvastatin or matching placebo daily. During a median follow-up period of 4 years, atorvastatin had no significant effect on the primary endpoint, defined as composite of death from cardiac causes, fatal stroke, nonfatal MI, or nonfatal stroke (relative risk [RR], 0.92; 95% CI, 0.77% to 1.10%), except that there was an increase in the risk of fatal stroke (RR, 2.03, 95% CI, 1.05 to 3.93) among those receiving atorvastatin. Atorvastatin reduced the rate of all cardiac events combined

(RR, 0.82, 95% CI, 0.68 to 0.99; $p = 0.03$, nominally significant) but not all cerebrovascular events or combined or total mortality.

In the AURORA study, 2,776 participants on hemodialysis were randomized to receive rosuvastatin 10 mg or matching placebo daily and 804 patients developed major CV events during the follow-up period, of which 396 were in the rosuvastatin group and 408 were in the placebo group (9.2 and 9.5 events per 100 person-years of follow-up, respectively). There was no significant effect of treatment with rosuvastiatin on the primary combined endpoint (hazard ratio [HR], 0.96; 95% CI, 0.84 to 1.11). The lack of efficacy of rosuvastatin on the primary endpoint was consistent among all subgroups, including diabetes mellitus, high LDL cholesterol levels, elevated C-reactive protein, hypertension, and preexisting CV disease. There was a small but statistically significant increase in the incidence of hemorrhagic stroke in the patients with diabetes mellitus who received rosuvastatin—an observation also reported in the 4D study. A post hoc analysis of the 731 patients with diabetes mellitus reported a 32% risk reduction of composite primary endpoint the treatment arm (HR, 0.68; 95% CI, 0.51 to 0.90).

A recent meta-analysis of more than 180,000 individual participant data from 28 randomized trials by the Cholesterol Treatment Trialists' (CTT) collaboration found that even after allowing for the smaller reductions in LDL cholesterol achieved by patients with more advanced CKD, and for differences in outcome definitions between dialysis trials, the relative reductions in major vascular events observed with statin-based treatment became smaller as eGFR declined, with little evidence of benefit in patients on dialysis. The CTT collaborators recommended for patients with earlier stages of CKD, statin-based regimens should be chosen to maximize the absolute reduction in LDL cholesterol to achieve the largest treatment benefits. For maintenance dialysis patients, the KDIGO guideline work group used a different wording and speculated that these patients might elect to receive statin treatment if they are interested in a relatively uncertain and small reduction in CV events. Because very high LDL cholesterol might increase the likelihood of benefit from statin in a dialysis patient, patients who meet this criterion may be more interested in receiving statin treatment, recognizing that the benefit remains speculative. Other factors that might influence a patient's decision to receive statin treatment could include a recent CV event (MI or stroke). On the other hand, if these patients are already receiving statins or statin–ezetimibe combination at the time of dialysis initiation, the treatment ought to be continued.

Studies of Statin Therapy in Kidney Transplant Recipients

The risk of future CV events in kidney transplant recipients is substantially elevated compared with people without CKD: the rate of CV death or nonfatal MI is approximately 21.5 per 1,000 patient-years. The ALERT study showed that fluvastatin (40 to 80 mg per day) nonsignificantly reduced the risk of coronary death or nonfatal MI, compared with placebo (RR, 0.83; 95% CI, 0.64 to 1.06). However, fluvastatin led to a significant 35% relative reduction in the risk of cardiac death or definite nonfatal MI (HR, 0.65; 95% CI, 0.48 to 0.88) in an unblinded extension study. A significant reduction in the original primary outcome was found after 6.7 years of follow-up.

It appeared that fluvastatin produces a safe and effective reduction of LDL cholesterol and CV risk in kidney transplant recipient, compared to those of statins in general population. However, the lack of statistical significance in the primary analysis and the fact that only one randomized trial was available both favored a relatively weak recommendation by KDIGO (Grade 2B).

SHOULD THE USE OF CHOLESTEROL LOWERING AGENTS IN CHRONIC KIDNEY DISEASE BE BASED ON LIPID LEVELS?

Although LDL cholesterol is widely used in estimating future CV risk in the general population, kidney function is not incorporated in current risk calculators despite the fact that reduced GFR confers increased CV risk. The prescription of statins using standard absolute risk algorithms may, therefore, result in many patients with renal impairment who would benefit from statins not receiving this therapy.

Among patients with advanced-stage CKD, the magnitude of risk associated with LDL cholesterol levels decreases with progression of the stage of CKD. For dialysis patients with the lowest level of LDL cholesterol and total cholesterol, the all-cause and CV mortality remains high. Hence, the evidence argues against the use of LDL cholesterol to identify patients requiring treatment, but rather suggests consideration of absolute risk for coronary events (such as history of known coronary disease, diabetes mellitus, prior ischemic stroke, or estimated 10-year incidence of coronary death or nonfatal MI >10%). Because CKD itself is a risk factor for CV events, a reduced intervention threshold may be appropriate. The KDIGO guidelines take this analysis into account in recommending the routine use of lipid lowering with a statin alone or in combination of ezetimibe in all people older than 50 years with CKD.

ARE STATINS SAFE?

There is ongoing debate in the general community about the safety of statins, and controversies have raised doubts in the mind of patients about whether the risks of statin therapy are outweighed by the benefits. The SHARP study found the risk of myopathy was only 2 additional cases per 10,000 patients per years of treatment with the combination of simvastatin and ezetimibe compared to the placebo (9 [0.2%] vs. 5 [0.1%]), without any evidence of excess risks of hepatitis, gallstones, or cancer. However, the active run-in period employed in this trial could potentially lead to underestimation of this risk. In the high-risk groups (dialysis and renal transplant patients), there was no increase in the incidence of rhabdomyolysis or liver disease in the statin groups as compared to the placebo group in the AURORA, 4D, and ALERT studies. Hence, the Food and Drug Administration has recommended against routine monitoring of liver function, which was once considered standard procedure for statin users for it has not been effective in predicting or preventing the rare occurrences of serious liver injury associated with statin use.

Reports from administrative data have suggested the possibility that high-intensity statins may be associated with an increased risk of admission for acute kidney injury. These findings were not confirmed in analyses of RCT data. A recent pooled analysis of 24 statin placebo-controlled trial specifically looked at renal-associated serious adverse event (SAE). This study showed no difference in the incidence of renal-associated adverse event at 120 days after drug initiation (0.04% vs. 0.10%, $p = 0.162$) between atorvastatin (10,345 patients on atorvastatin [10 to 80 mg per day]) and placebo (8,945 patients on placebo), or in the high-dose versus low-dose statin trials. Results were similar for renal-related SAEs after 120 days. In a review article by Maji et al. on the safety of statins, agents modulating CYP-450 isoenzymes, isoprenoid deficiency, Co-enzymes Q inhibition, selenoproteins, and dolichol deficiency that are more common in patients with CKD, have been proposed as potential pathways behind statins toxicity. Although it occurs infrequently, this may explain why statin toxicity was more common in patients with CKD. Hence, a clinical assessment of risk factors and awareness of drug-to-drug interaction seems like a more sensible approach in predicting risk of adverse effects.

A more recently reported trial raises questions about the equivalence of different agents in people with kidney disease. In this combined data analysis from two concurrent studies (Prospective Evaluation of Proteinuria and Renal Function in Diabetic Patients With Progressive Renal Disease (PLANET) I and II) conducted in proteinuric patients with type 1 and type 2 diabetes mellitus and proteinuric nondiabetic CKD, respectively, individuals were randomized to either atorvastatin 80 mg or rosuvastatin 10 mg or rosuvastatin 40 mg daily with the primary aim of assessing effects on albuminuria. Not only did the participants treated with atorvastatin have lower levels of proteinuria by the end of the 12-month study, they had significantly less decline in kidney function. It is not possible to be certain whether this might reflect a protective effect of atorvastatin or a harmful effect of rosuvastatin, but it does suggest that agents shown at least to be safe from a renal perspective (such as simvastatin–ezetimibe and perhaps atorvastatin) might be preferred in people with CKD. Based on all these reports, the KDIGO work group recommended to prescribe doses of statins that were studied in outcome studies. These doses are equivalent to moderate-intensity statin treatment, and high doses should be avoided in patients with CKD.

ARE PCSK9 OR CHOLESTERYL ESTER TRANSFER PROTEIN INHIBITORS PROMISING CHOLESTEROL LOWERING AGENTS IN CHRONIC KIDNEY DISEASE PATIENTS?

The proprotein convertase subtilisin/kexin type 9 (PCSK9) inhibitors alirocumab and evolocumab reduce LDL cholesterol levels by about 60% when compared to the placebo. In the FOURIER CV outcome study, evolocumab reduced the primary composite endpoint consisting of CV death, MI, stroke, hospitalization for unstable angina, or coronary revascularization by 15% (HR, 0.85; 95% CI, 0.79 to 0.92; $p < 0.001$) in 27,564 patients. So far, no data on subgroup analyses of impaired kidney function have been published. A recent experimental study suggested that podocyte damage triggers marked inductions in plasma PCSK9, and knockout of PCSK9 ameliorates dyslipidemia in a mouse model of nephrotic syndrome. Thus, PCSK9 inhibitors may be beneficial in patients with nephrotic syndrome-associated hypercholesterolemia.

The cholesteryl ester transfer protein inhibitors, such as anacetrapib, reduce LDL cholesterol by around 25% to 40% and more than doubles HDL cholesterol. The vascular effects of HDL differ under certain clinical conditions. The composition of HDL is modified in patients with CKD. As a consequence, uremic HDL induces endothelial dysfunction. Recent data identify symmetric dimethylarginine as a marker of HDL dysfunction and highlight a potential role in mediating premature CV disease in patients with CKD. The clinical outcomes remain to be seen in the Randomized EValuation of the Effects of Anacetrapib Through Lipid-modification (REVEAL) study, which will be published during the second half of 2017.

CONCLUSION

Current evidence suggests that statin therapy reduces the risk of major CV events in patients with CKD across a broad range of kidney function with uncertainty for patients receiving maintenance dialysis. The value of cholesterol lowering in preventing CV disease has been established in patients with CKD, who are intrinsically at high CV risk. Although data from completed studies has clearly demonstrated substantive benefit of statins in early CKD, the effects in ESKD are controversial. Recent studies have also suggested the safety of high-dose statins in this population remains uncertain. The evaluation of risks and benefits for this class of agents is critically dependent on baseline risk.

Suggested Readings

Baigent C, Landray MJ, Reith C, et al. The effects of lowering LDL cholesterol with simvastatin plus ezetimibe in patients with chronic kidney disease (Study of Heart and Renal Protection): a randomised placebo-controlled trial. *Lancet.* 2011;377(9784):2181–2192.

Cholesterol Treatment Trialist (CTT) Collaboration, Herrington WG, Emberson J, et al. Impact of renal function on the effects of LDL cholesterol lowering with statin-base regimens: a meta-analysis of individual participant data from 28 randomised trials. *Lancet Diabetes Endocrinol.* 2016;4:829–839.

Dormuth CR, Hemmelgarn BR, Paterson JM, et al. Use of high potency statins and rates of admission for acute kidney injury: multicenter, retrospective observational analysis of administrative databases. *BMJ.* 2013;346:f880.

Haas ME, Levenson AE, Sun X, et al. The role of proprotein convertase subtilisin/ kexin type 9 in nephrotic syndrome-associated hypercholesterolemia. *Circulation.* 2016;134:61–72.

de Jager DJ, Grootendorst DC, Jager KJ, et al. Cardiovascular and noncardiovascular mortality among patients starting dialysis. *JAMA.* 2009;302(16):1782–1789.

Maji D, Shaikh S, Solanki D, Gaurav K. Safety of statins. *Indian J. Endocrinol. Metab.* 2013;17(4):636–646.

Palmer SC, Craig JC, Navaneethan SD et al. Benefits and harms of statin therapy for persons with chronic kidney disease: a systematic review and meta-analysis. *Ann Intern Med.* 2012;157:263–275.

Robinson JG, Farnier M, Krempf M, et al. Efficacy and safety of alirocumab in reducing lipids and cardiovascular events. *N Engl J Med.* 2015;372(16):1489–1499.

Sabatine MS, Giugliano RP, Keech AC, et al; FOURIER Steering Committee and Investigators. Evolocumab and clinical outcomes in patients with cardiovascular disease. *N Engl J Med.* 2017;376:1713–1722.

Sabatine MS, Giugliano RP, Wiviott SD, et al. Efficacy and safety of evolocumab in reducing lipids and cardiovascular events. *N Engl J Med.* 2015;372(16):1500–1509.

Wanner C, Tonelli M, Kidney Disease: Improving Global Oucomes (KDIGO) Lipid Work Group. KDIGO clinical pracice guideline for lipid management in chronic kidney disease. *Kidney Int.* 2013;3:1–46.

de Zeeuw D, Anzalone DA, Cain VA, et al. Renal effects of atorvastatin and rosuvastatin in patients with diabetes who have progressive renal disease (PLANET I): a randomised clinical trial. *Lancet Diabetes Endocrinol.* 2015;3:687–696.

Zewinger S, Kleber ME, Rohrer L, et al. Symmetric dimethylarginine, high-density lipoproteins and cardiovascular disease. *Eur Heart J.* 2017;38(20):1597–1607.

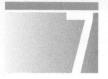

Role of Nutrition in Cardiovascular and Kidney Diseases

Jaimon Kelly, Katrina Campbell, and Juan Jesús Carrero

Dietary habits are known to influence cardiovascular disease (CVD) risk, either through an effect on CVD risk factors such as serum cholesterol, blood pressure, body weight, and diabetes or through effects independent of these. The potential role of a healthy diet is far more complex than delivering a combination of nutrients, and public health recommendations for prevention of CVD have gradually moved from a single-nutrient focus to whole foods and dietary patterns, which are more easily translated into dietary recommendations. The dietary pattern approach can be seen as the equivalent of the shift from evaluating single risk factors to evaluating total risk profiles.

Patients with chronic kidney disease (CKD) are at high risk of CVD complications, which in turn constitute their most common cause of death. Traditional dietary management of CKD focuses predominantly on the quantity within the diet of energy, protein, and the restriction of single micronutrients, with little mention of dietary quality. There is also a tendency to restrict the intake of fruits and vegetables to prevent diet-induced hyperkalemia. Notwithstanding the clinical importance of these practices, the adherence to such restrictive recommendations is difficult and challenging for most patients. This may be explained by financial and social barriers often linked to CKD, an emphasis on restriction of sodium, potassium, and phosphorous at the expense of compromising overall diet quality and simply global dietary changes toward Western diets, with convenience, fast, and ultra-processed foods. Available reports evidence that the overall diet of dialysis patients is of poor quality, at odds with recommendations for CVD prevention.

In this chapter, we will review current recommendations for prevention of CVD. We will elaborate on the suitability of commonly studied dietary patterns for patients with CKD to meet these recommendations and argument on renal-specific adaptations. Next, we will provide a brief overview on the potential positive impact on kidney health of nutrients and foods not currently dealt with by CKD guidelines, namely fruits, vegetables, carbohydrates, and polyunsaturated fat. Finally, we will provide some practical examples of dietary plans that adapt cardioprotective dietary plans to CKD-specific requirements.

DIETARY RECOMMENDATIONS FOR PREVENTION OF CARDIOVASCULAR DISEASE

Healthy dietary practices, at all stages of life, are integral to the prevention and treatment of CVD. American and European Cardiology Societies issued guideline recommendations as to the necessary proportions of specific nutrients in the context of a healthy heart diet (Table 7.1). Both guidelines acknowledge, however, that with few exceptions, evidence is mostly based on observational studies.

The most recent revisions to those recommendations have evolved from nutrient-based to food-based dietary patterns that are more easily translated for

TABLE 7.1	Summary of Single Nutrient Recommendations for Secondary CVD Prevention from the AHA and the ESC

AHA Recommendations *Circulation (2000) 102:2284–2299*	ESC Recommendations *European Heart Journal (2012) 33:1635–1701*
Total fat < 30% of dietary energy	SFA < 10% of total energy intake, through replacement by PUFA
SFA < 10% of dietary energy	Trans-unsaturated fatty acids: as little as possible
MUFA < 30% of dietary energy	Salt < 5 g/d
Cholesterol < 300 mg/d	Fish at least twice a week, one of which to be oily fish
Protein ≥ 15% of dietary energy	Fiber, 30–45 g/d, from whole grains, fruits, and vegetables
Carbohydrate < 60% of dietary energy	Fruit 200 g/d (2–3 servings)
Salt < 2,400 mg/d	Vegetables 200 g/d (2–3 servings)
Fiber > 25 g/d	Alcohol, 2 glasses/d (20 g/d of alcohol) for men and 1 glass/d (10 g/d of alcohol) for women.

AHA, American Heart Association; CVD, cardiovascular disease; ESC, European Society of Cardiology; MUFA, monounsaturated fatty acids; PUFA, polyunsaturated fatty acids; SFA, saturated fatty acids.

counseling patients. This does not diminish the importance of meeting nutrient needs. Rather, for translational purposes, the results from food-based scientific evidence make possible and preferable the opportunity to offer practical recommendations that can readily be applied in the purchasing, preparing, or providing of foods and beverages. To achieve the nutrient goals, the 2013 American Heart Association/American College of Cardiology (AHA/ACC) guidelines on lifestyle management to reduce CVD risk recommend to consume a dietary pattern that emphasizes intake of vegetables, fruits, and whole grains; includes low-fat dairy products, poultry, fish, legumes, nontropical vegetable oils, and nuts; and limits intake of sweets, sugar-sweetened beverages, and red meats.

Dietary patterns aligned with these recommendations include the Dietary Approaches to Stop Hypertension (DASH) diet, the Mediterranean diet, or vegetarian diets. These patterns represent the full preventive potential of diet, because they yield the combined impact of several favorable dietary nutrients and habits. As an example, intake low in sodium also has collateral benefits of reducing intake of ultra-processed food that is high in sodium, increasing fruit and vegetables, and so on. Furthermore, diets rich in omega-3 fatty acids represent increased fish intake, while displace food alternatives with higher content in saturated fat.

Dietary Patterns: Evidence and Practical Applications in Kidney Disease
Cardioprotective dietary patterns when supported by a health care professional represent a practical nutrition prescription in CVD and kidney disease, to improve both short- and long-term outcomes for patients. Evidence for effectiveness of the abovementioned dietary patterns have a large body of evidence in the general population, primarily for mediating cardiovascular risk factors. Therefore, these dietary patterns may offer a novel opportunity for the nutritional management of CVD risk in the CKD population.

Is the Dietary Approaches to Stop Hypertension Diet Relevant in Chronic Kidney Disease?

The DASH diet emphasizes fruits and vegetables, low-fat dairy products, and complex (whole grain) carbohydrates. Furthermore, the DASH diet limits large quantities of meats and discretionary choices. It has a nutrient profile high in fiber, protein, magnesium, calcium, and potassium, yet low in total and saturated fats. As a result, the cardioprotective DASH diet has been previously argued to be inappropriate for patients with CKD, because of the high content of potassium, phosphorus, and protein. However, practical modifications still make achieving a cardioprotective "DASH-type" diet realistic in CKD and are proposed in Table 7.2.

Is the Mediterranean-Style Diet Relevant in Chronic Kidney Disease?

In contrast to the clearly defined DASH dietary pattern, there is no one, standardized Mediterranean diet. Rather, the widely used term Mediterranean diet reflects a variety of eating habits traditionally practiced by populations in countries bordering the Mediterranean Sea, with considerable variability by location. The Mediterranean pattern of eating is in general rich in unsaturated fats, fruits, vegetables, legumes, fiber, and moderate in red wine consumption. This dietary pattern has established evidence for effectiveness in the general population, for reducing the risk of cardiovascular events, and in observational analysis delaying progression to end-stage kidney disease

 TABLE 7.2 Characteristics of the DASH Diet and Key Considerations in CKD

Food Group	Serving Target*	Considerations in CKD
Grains and cereals	6–8/d	At least 50% from wholegrain sources, aim for >6 g fiber per 100 g
Fruits and fruit juice	4–5/d	Low-potassium options encouraged (if required). Fruit juice is not appropriate
Vegetables	4–5/d	Low-potassium alternatives only if required
Meat, poultry, and fish	<2/d	Predialysis: Limit animal protein serves to 2 times 65 g (palm size) servings per day. Dialysis: 2 times 125 g (hand size) servings per day
Dairy products	2–3/d	Low-fat options: 250 mL milk, 40 g cheese, and 200 g yoghurt. Nondairy substitutes are lower in phosphorous if appropriate
Nuts, seeds, and legumes	4–5/wk	Unsalted; 30 g (small handful) is the equivalent for 1 meat serve
Fats and oils	2–3/d	Emphasize healthy oils: target intake of 30–40 g (1 tablespoon) unsaturated fats per day
Sweets, added sugars, and other processed foods	<5/wk	Limit where possible. Be aware: potassium and phosphate additives are abundant in the food supply and highly bioavailable

CKD, chronic kidney disease; DASH, Dietary Approaches to Stop Hypertension.
*Refer to relevant dietary guidelines to determine the quantity of common serving sizes. Shaded sections indicate protein sources that should be monitored for overconsumption.

TABLE 7.3	Characteristics of the Mediterranean Diet and Key Considerations in CKD	
Food Group	**Serving Target**[*]	**Considerations for CKD**
Fruit	1–2/main meal	Low-potassium alternatives only if required
Vegetables	2/main meal	Low-potassium alternatives only if required
Cereals	1–2/main meal	At least 50% from wholegrain sources, aim for >6 g fiber per 100 g
Potatoes	3/wk	1 small potato; boil and discard water prior to further cooking; restriction not necessary unless clinically indicated
Olive oil	1/main meal	Aim for 2–3 times 15 mL (1 tablespoon) serving per day; replace other cooking oils for olive oil
Nuts	1–2/d	Unsalted; 30 g (small handful) is the equivalent for 1 meat serve
Legumes	2/wk	
Dairy products	2/d	Low-fat options: 250 mL milk, 40 g cheese, and 200 g yoghurt
		Nondairy substitutes are lower in phosphorous if appropriate
Eggs	2–4/wk	Aim for <2 in 1 meal
Fish	2/wk	Mediterranean servings practically reflect best-practice guidelines for modified for protein (<1 g/kg/d); monitor for adequacy in dialysis
White meat	2/wk	
Red meat	<2/wk	
Sweets and other processed foods	2/wk	Limit where possible. Be aware potassium and phosphate additives are abundant in the food supply and highly bioavailable
Fermented beverages	1–2 glasses/d	

CKD, chronic kidney disease.

[*]Refer to relevant dietary guidelines to determine the quantity of common serving sizes. Shaded sections indicate protein sources that should be monitored for overconsumption.

Adopted from Bach-Faig A, Berry EM, Lairon D, et al. Mediterranean diet pyramid today. Science and cultural updates. *Public Health Nutr* 2011;14:2274–2284.

(ESKD) in individuals with CKD. However, the benefits of certain foods and nutrients emphasized in the Mediterranean diet do not feature in current best-practice renal nutrition guidelines. Therefore, practical modifications to make achieving a 'Mediterranean-style' diet realistic in CKD are required, and are proposed in Table 7.3.

Modifications of Cardiovascular Disease-Specific Dietary Recommendations in Progressive Chronic Kidney Disease and Dialysis

Maintaining a healthy eating pattern for reducing overall CVD risk is complicated in the advanced stages of CKD and ESKD because of the elevated potassium and calcium content of the DASH, AHA, and Mediterranean diets, as well as the potential risk for hyperkalemia, hyperphosphatasemia, and vascular calcification. In addition, these dietary patterns characteristically are higher in protein than what is recommended for a predialysis CKD diet. As detailed in Table 7.4, the recommended nutrient intakes advised for people

TABLE 74

Typical Nutrient Composition of Dietary Patterns Compared to Evidence-based CKD Guidelines

Nutrient	Mediterranean*	DASH†	AHA*	American Dietary Guidelines‡	CKD Diet§	Dialysis§
Protein (%EEI)	19.7	18	15	10–35	10	15–18
Fat (%EEI)	35.2	27	<30	20–35	<30	<30
Saturated (%EEI)	11.1	7	<10	<10	<7	<7
Monounsaturated fat (%EEI)	15.4	10	>30 Combined	11	>20	>20
Polyunsaturated fat (%EEI)	5	7		NR	>10	>10
Carbohydrates (%EEI)	43.6	58	<60	45–65	50–60	50–55
Fiber (g/d)	36.9	30	>25	20–30	20–30	20–30
Sodium (mg/d)	3,616	2,886	<2,400	<2,300	<2,400	<2,400
Potassium (mg/d)	6,132	4,589	NR	4,700	2,000–4,000	2,000–4,000
Phosphorous (mg/d)	2,226	1,481		700	800–1,000	
Calcium (mg/d)	1,409	1,220		1,000–1,200	700	

AHA, American Heart Association; CKD, chronic kidney disease; DASH, Dietary Approaches to Stop Hypertension; EEI, estimated energy intake; NR, no recommendation.
*Lichtenstein AH, Appel LJ, Brands M, et al. Diet and lifestyle recommendations revision 2006: a scientific statement from the American Heart Association Nutrition Committee. *Circulation* 2006;114:82–96.
†Serra-Majem L, Bes-Rastrollo M, Román-Viñas B, et al. Dietary patterns and nutritional adequacy in a Mediterranean country. *Br J Nutr* 2009;101(Suppl 2):S21–S28.
‡U.S. Department of Health and Human Services and U.S. Department of Agriculture. Available at http://health.gov/dietaryguidelines/2015/guidelines/.
§As recommended by the K/DOQI guidelines.

with CKD are mostly in line with American Dietary guideline recommendations, with minor modifications for nondairy alternatives lower in calcium and low-potassium fruit/vegetables if required. Although DASH and Mediterranean diets are higher in protein (as a percent of total calories consumed), they contain higher plant-based protein ratios that may be kidney sparing and cardiorenal protective. The bioavailability of phosphorous and calcium from plant-based sources is typically poor which strengthens the kidney-sparing potential these diets may possess. Western diets, in comparison, are higher in animal proteins which contain highly bioavailable sources of calcium and phosphorous, and promote gut dysbiosis and the production of uremic toxins, which are known to be associated with CVD.

RATIONALE FOR SELECTED FOOD COMPONENTS OF A CARDIOVASCULAR DISEASE-PROTECTIVE PATTERN IN PATIENTS WITH CHRONIC KIDNEY DISEASE

Fish and Omega-3 Intake

The quality of dietary fat has important implications on CVD prevention. Monounsaturated fat has a positive effect on increasing high-density lipoprotein (HDL) cholesterol when it replaces saturated fat or carbohydrates in the diet. Polyunsaturated fat lowers low-density lipoprotein and HDL cholesterol when it replaces saturated fat. The polyunsaturated can be divided into two main subfamilies: omega-6 fatty acids, mainly from plant foods, and omega-3 fatty acids, mainly from fatty fish. Eicosapentaenoic and docosahexaenoic acids are the most important representatives of this family. The evidence that omega-3 fatty acids can reduce CHD mortality and to a lesser extent stroke mortality in the general population is consistent; and guidelines for secondary CVD prevention recommend frequent fish consumption, at least twice weekly. Mechanisms behind this effect may involve the capacity of omega-3 fatty acids of inhibiting platelet aggregation, as well as anti-inflammatory, antiproliferative, and vasodilatory properties by reducing the availability of arachidonic acid, leukotriene and cytokine production, as well as increasing prostaglandin-I_3 production. These salutary effects may offer additional benefits in patients with advanced kidney disease.

Studies examining the quality of dietary intake show that patients with CKD have very low consumption of fish and omega-3 fat, with a subsequent lower proportion of omega-3 fatty acids in plasma, red blood cells, and tissue. Studies addressing the potential of omega-3 supplementation in patients with CKD suggest capacity to reduce triglyceride levels, reduce CKD progression, improve dialysis access patency, and possibly improve systemic inflammation, oxidative stress, and uremic pruritus. Studies in patients with end-stage renal disease have shown that fish consumption and omega-3 PUFA supplementation is associated with improved vascular access patency and rates of thrombosis and potentially cardiovascular morbidity and mortality risk. Small sample sizes, short intervention periods, and observational nature in most cases render overall evidence, however, inconclusive.

Increased intake of omega-3 supplements or oily fish in patients with CKD should be advocated for cardioprotection. Natural sources of omega-3 (e.g., fatty fish) are preferred to supplements, but considerations are required on the amount of protein ingested for patients with nondialysis CKD or the protein/phosphate ratio of different species (Table 7.5). Wild fatty fish is preferred to farmed fish, because they are often fed with flour and preparations rich in bioavailable phosphorus to promote rapid growth, resulting in unquantifiable phosphorus content. This, together with the alleged elevated costs of fatty fish, may render omega-3 supplements as an attractive alternative. Reported adverse effects associated to these have been minimal in CKD studies and generally limited to gastrointestinal complaints.

Phosphorus to Protein Ratio per 100 g of Selected Species of Wild Fatty Fish

Fatty Fish	Protein (g)	Phosphorus (mg)	Phosphorus/ Protein Ratio
Anchovy	17.6	182	10.34
Mackerel	15.4	157	10.19
Tuna	22.0	230	10.45
Trout	15.7	208	13.24
Salmon	18.4	250	13.58
Sardine	18.1	475	26.24

Modified from Barril-Cuadrado G, Puchulu MB, Sánchez-Tomero JA. Table showing dietary phosphorus/protein ratio for the Spanish population. Usefulness in chronic kidney disease. *Nefrologia* 2013;33(3):362–371.

Optimal Fruit and Vegetable Intake: Balancing Risks and Benefits

Increasing consumption of fruit and vegetables to meet a healthy dietary pattern, particularly those known to be high potassium containing, is typically cautioned owing to the potential to contribute to hyperkalemia. On the other hand, the cardioprotective effects of the associated fiber, base-producing properties, benefits to gut health, and also provision of antioxidants are well established and are important in CVD and kidney disease as detailed in Table 7.6. This needs to be balanced with the potential electrolyte toxicity and thereby monitored regularly.

 Summary of Mechanisms by Which Fruit and Vegetable May Reduce CVD-related Outcomes in CKD

Mechanism	Rationale and Considerations
Base Producing	
Managing metabolic acidosis	Sulfur-containing animal proteins are naturally acid-producing, including alliums and cruciferous vegetables. Potassium salt-containing FV are base producing, and have been established as a safe alternative compared to a standard sodium bicarbonate prescription in Stage 4 CKD, without adverse hyperkalemia.
Increased Fiber, Antioxidants, and Phytochemicals	
Inflammation and oxidative stress	FV are naturally higher in fiber than diets lower in plant-based food. Additionally, FV follows a higher intake of phytochemicals, which have protective effects CRP and ICAM-1 that mediates inflammation and oxidative stress.
Reducing albuminuria	Higher FV diets result in less albumin leakage compared to higher animal protein diets.
Controlling constipation	A higher fiber diet from FV consumption can reduce incidence of constipation which might alleviate risks to increasing serum potassium given the higher fecal excretions as GFR declines.

(*continued*)

	Summary of Mechanisms by Which Fruit and Vegetable May Reduce CVD-related Outcomes in CKD (*continued*)
Mechanism	**Rationale and Considerations**
Production of short-chain fatty acids	Promoting saccharolytic fermentation in the gut produces short-chain fatty acids that can improve lipid profiles and insulin sensitivity.
Uremic toxins	Vegetarian diets are known to manipulate the dysbiotic nature of the kidney gut-axis, and reduce key nephrovascular toxins that contribute to the cardiorenal syndrome.
Bioavailability Nonequivalence	
Preventing malnutrition	Shifting animal–plant protein ratios likely results in consumption of vegetables protein sources that are less bioavailable and may be "kidney sparing," which ensure adequate protein can be consumed in the CKD diet to prevent protein-energy wasting.
Reduced Sodium	
Blood pressure	FV are naturally low in sodium, which can help in the
Endothelial function	control of blood pressure through control of the extracellular volume and elastically of the arteries.
Lower Calorie and Saturated Fat	
Weight management	FV as substituted for high saturated fat food sources
Lipid profiles	manipulates the fatty acid profiles within the diet, having evidence for controlling cholesterol and reducing weight.
Long-term Outcomes	
Delaying dialysis	Large-scale observational evidence supports a
Reduced risk of mortality	healthy eating index (reflective of achieving adherence to dietary guidelines), the DASH diet, and the Mediterranean diet to be protective against renal-related mortality and initiating dialysis.

CKD, chronic kidney disease; CRP, C-reactive protein; CVD, cardiovascular disease; DASH, Dietary Approaches to Stop Hypertension; FV, fruit and vegetables; GFR, glomerular filtration rate; ICAM-1, intercellular adhesion molecule 1.

Carbohydrate Quality: Considerations of Whole Grains, Glycemic Index, and Added Sugars

Intake of energy-dense, nutrient-poor sources of carbohydrates, including refined and highly processed foods with high glycemic index and added sugars may contribute to CVD exacerbation in CKD through a range of mechanisms. Fructose has been investigated in preclinical studies to cause glomerular hypertrophy and accelerate progression of CKD. In clinical trials, a low-fructose diet has in turn demonstrated reduction in inflammation and improved blood pressure control. Added sugars may also contribute to increased hyperglycemia, known to impair nitric oxide-mediated vascular reactivity. Further, phosphorus and other additives presented in ultra-processed, nutrient-poor sources of carbohydrates (such as cola beverages, cookies, and cakes) may also have direct effects on vascular health through exacerbation of hypophosphatemia and vascular calcification risk. However, how this translates to clinical outcome in established CKD is yet to be established.

In turn, the therapeutic benefit of carbohydrate quality, notably dietary fiber content on cardiovascular risk is well recognized. Traditional mechanisms underpinning the benefits of quality carbohydrates, rich in dietary fiber, including delayed gastric emptying, sequestering of bile acids, improved insulin resistance, and weight control are well established. There are numerous meta-analyses summarizing the effect of carbohydrate quality on blood pressure, hyperlipidemia, glycemic control, and diabetes management and inflammation indicating benefit. Importantly, several of the meta-analyses have suggested an enhanced benefit based on dose, duration, and in participants with the highest cardiovascular risk. Studies specific to CKD are limited, however indicate carbohydrate quality may have a role in the development of CKD and influence outcomes (all-cause mortality) in established CKD. Table 7.7 details the potential mechanisms, both traditional (well established in the general population) and novel (associated with the influence of uremia and/or gut microbiota), for the role of carbohydrates in cardiorenal syndrome.

IMPLEMENTATION STRATEGIES: NUTRITION MANAGEMENT PLAN AND ASSESSMENT OF ADHERENCE

Table 7.8 provides example meal plans matched in calories and protein, modified for key features of the DASH diet (increased fruit and vegetables, whole grains, reduced sodium) and Mediterranean-style diet (increased mono- and polyunsaturated fats, increased vegetables, whole grains, olive oil, and nuts). Both adapted meal plans resulted in increased serves of fruit and vegetables and substantially increased fiber and low in sodium. As a result, the traditionally cardioprotective patterns both have increased potassium and phosphorous. Therefore, these options would require further modifications to meet the needs of individuals prescribed a restriction. However, this contrast displays how achievable shifting a few dietary components are to achieving each dietary pattern.

Dietary behavior change is complex. Despite the best intentions, inadequate or incomplete instructions could have adverse effects on patients dietary management. Understanding and addressing barriers which may exist, providing support in a timely manner, and building self-efficacy as a moderator for behavior change are critical and to limit patient frustration that could sabotage adherence. Commonly cited barriers include lack of practical knowledge—the "how to" implement change day to day—including shopping, eating out, and the impact on social life, of being a "burden" on family and friends. Contact with a registered renal dietitian trained in motivational interviewing is strongly recommended to support patient empowerment for making food choices toward a desired healthy dietary pattern.

Patients with CKD prefer nutrition interventions to be individualized, provide peer support, and combine repeated coaching with regular monitoring and feedback. We know from successful studies such as PREDIMED, that a combination of individual and group intervention, at least once every 3 months is necessary to support dietary change. Self-monitoring and feedback strategies are integral to achieving and supporting adherence to the recommended dietary pattern. Although not formally tested in patients with CKD, simplified assessment tools can promote self-monitoring based on dietary pattern recommendations. These include the "Rate Your Plate" (http://www.dashdietoregon.org/Rate-Your-Plate) and the "Your Med Diet Score" (https://oldwayspt.org/system/files/atoms/files/RateYourMedDietScore.pdf), two one-time assessment tools for patients to self-evaluate their adherence to DASH and Mediterranean diets, respectively. General feedback, motivational messages, and tips to increase intake to reach the amount recommended are provided.

	Traditional	**Novel**
Cholesterol	• Bind bile acids and cholesterol (formation of micelles, upregulate LDL receptors, increase clearance) • Reduced glycemic response (lower insulin stimulation of hepatic cholesterol synthesis)	• Inhibition of hepatic cholesterol synthesis by SCFA production • Microbial metabolism of cholesterol and bile
Body weight	• Increased satiety secondary to gastric distension (triggers afferent vagal signals of fullness) • Lower energy density of fiber containing foods	• Appetite regulation (release of gut hormones, and neurotransmitters modulated via SCFA) • Changes in the efficiency of calorie harvest from dietary fiber (via microbiota)
Diabetic control	• Lower glycemic index of food will reduce the glycemic response; hyperglycemia may impact on vascular function. • Delayed gastric emptying • Decreases bioavailability of starch in the lumen	• Improved insulin sensitivity (expression of glucose transporters modulated by SCFAs) • Activation of intestinal gluconeogenesis (via brain–gut axis)
Blood pressure	• Improved insulin resistance • Weight control	• Bacterial production of angiotensin-converting enzyme inhibitory peptides
Uremic toxin management	• Replace other food components, for example,, protein, favoring saccharolytic bacterial fermentation	• Inhibition of bacterial production of uremic toxins • Alteration of the urea enterohepatic cycling (via microbial metabolism of diffused serum urea and creatinine)
Inflammation	• Improved cardiometabolic risk factors	• Increased gut wall integrity via selective growth of beneficial bacteria • Reduction in bacterial-derived nephrovascular toxins

LDL, low-density lipoprotein; SCFA, short-chain fatty acids.

TABLE 7.8   Sample Menus of a Traditional Dialysis Diet and the Cardioprotective Diet Pattern of DASH or Mediterranean Style

Meal	Sample Menu*	DASH-Style Diet Modification	Mediterranean-Style Diet Modification
Breakfast	Cranberry juice, 4 ounces Eggs (2) or ½ cup egg substitute Toasted white bread, 2 slices, with butter or tub margarine or fruit spread	¾ cup cooked oatmeal with ½ cup berries (blueberry, raspberry, or strawberry)	Greek yoghurt ¼ cup with ½ cup berries, ½ toasted oats, and 10 almonds
Lunch	Tuna salad sandwich (3 ounces tuna on a hard roll with lettuce and mayonnaise) Coleslaw, ½ cup Pretzels (low salt) Peaches, ½ cup Ginger ale, 8 oz	Tuna salad sandwich (3 ounces tuna in spring water wholegrain bread [2 regular slices] with mayonnaise and lettuce) Salad 1 cup (snow peas, carrot, peppers) with 1 tab olive oil Creamed rice 1/2	Tuna salad sandwich (3 ounces tuna in olive oil wholegrain bread [2 regular slices] with mayonnaise and lettuce) Salad 1 cup (snow peas, carrot, peppers) with 1 tab olive oil ½ cup peaches and 1 tab yoghurt
Dinner	Hamburger patty, 4 ounces on a bun with 1–2 teaspoons ketchup Salad (1 cup): lettuce, cucumber, radishes, peppers, with olive oil and vinegar dressing Lemonade, 8 ounces	Turkey meatloaf (1 slice) with buttered green beans, peas and broccoli (½ cup of each). Sorbet (2 scoops) or ½ cup peaches and 1 tab cream	Mediterranean pizza with wholewheat base, olive oil and garlic base, sliced chicken breast (3 oz), with roasted peppers, mushroom, and reduced sodium cheese (1 oz)
Snack options	Milk, 4 ounces Slice of apple pie	Handful of mixed nuts (unsalted) 1 Apple or canned and drained fruit, handful of berries or grapes.	Handful of mixed nuts (unsalted) 1 Apple or canned and drained fruit, handful of berries or grapes.
Calories	2,150 cal	2,150 cal	2,150 cal
Protein	91 g	91 g	95 g
Sodium	2,300 mg	920 mg	1,350 mg
Potassium	1,800 mg (46 mEq)	3,300 mg (85 mEq)	3,000 mg (77 mEq)
Phosphorus	950 mg	1,400 mg	1,400 mg
Fiber	16 g	40 g	37 g

DASH, Dietary Approaches to Stop Hypertension.
*Sourced from https://www.kidney.org/atoz/content/dietary_hemodialysis (accessed August 11, 2016).

As a summary, recommendations for supporting dietary change to a healthy eating pattern in kidney disease include:

- Providing individualized, tailored support aligned with patient preferences.
- Select components of the dietary pattern that work best for the individual patient on the balance of dietary restrictions (i.e., increasing olive oil yet maintaining stable calories).
- Supporting frequent contact, at least once every 3 months initially, face-to-face and/or using telehealth (phone call, text messages, e-mail, etc.) methods.
- Managing key barriers such as eating out, including viewing the menu beforehand, and empowering patients with strategies for meal selection.
- Engaging self-monitoring and feedback mechanisms suitable to the individual patient to support long-term self-management.

Suggested Readings

Bach-Faig A, Berry EM, Lairon D, et al. Mediterranean diet pyramid today. Science and cultural updates. *Public Health Nutr* 2011;14(12A):2274–2284.

Eckel RH, Jakicic JM, Ard JD, et al. 2013 AHA/ACC guideline on lifestyle management to reduce cardiovascular risk: a report of the American College of Cardiology/ American Heart Association Task Force on Practice Guidelines. *J Am Coll Cardiol* 2014;63(25 Pt B):2960–2984.

Estruch R, Ros E, Salas-Salvado J, et al. Primary prevention of cardiovascular disease with a Mediterranean diet. *N Engl J Med* 2013;368(14):1279–1290.

Kelly JT, Palmer SC, Wai SN, et al. Healthy dietary patterns and risk of mortality and ESRD in CKD: a meta-analysis of cohort studies. *Clin J Am Soc Nephrol* 2017;12(2):272–279.

Kwasnicka D, Dombrowski SU, White M, et al. Theoretical explanations for maintenance of behaviour change: a systematic review of behaviour theories. *Health Psychol Rev* 2016;10(3):277–296.

Luis D, Zlatkis K, Comenge B, et al. Dietary quality and adherence to dietary recommendations in patients undergoing hemodialysis. *J Ren Nutr* 2016;26(3):190–195.

Palmer SC, Hanson CS, Craig JC, et al. Dietary and fluid restrictions in CKD: a thematic synthesis of patient views from qualitative studies. *Am J Kidney Dis* 2014;65(4): 559–573.

Requirements for Protein, Calories, and Fat in the Predialysis Patient

Jose Perez and William E. Mitch

GOALS OF NUTRITIONAL THERAPY

For patients with chronic kidney disease (CKD), the goals of dietary therapy are: (i) to diminish the accumulation of nitrogenous wastes and limit the metabolic disturbances created by uremia; (ii) to prevent the loss of protein stores; and (iii) to slow the progression of CKD. Fortunately, achieving these goals is possible because protein-restricted, low-protein diets (LPD) can overcome the complications of CKD in patients for two reasons: they reduce the levels of uremic toxins and the accumulation of sulfates, phosphates, potassium, and sodium that are responsible for producing uremic symptoms. Specifically, the source of most uremic toxins arises from the catabolism of dietary protein, whereas a high-protein diet is invariably associated with the accumulation of salt, phosphates, and other minerals in patients with CKD (Fig. 8.1). It follows that a LPD ameliorates specific complications of CKD, including metabolic acidosis, renal osteodystrophy, hyperkalemia, and hypertension. For these reasons, dietary protein restriction has been used for decades to treat chronically uremic patients.

ASSESSING PROTEIN REQUIREMENTS

Nitrogen Balance and Protein Requirements

Nitrogen balance (Bn) is the classic method for assessing dietary protein requirements: a negative Bn means that protein stores are being lost, whereas a neutral or positive Bn indicates that protein stores are stable or increasing. Based on Bn measurements, the World Health Organization (WHO) concluded that the average protein requirement for healthy adults who perform a moderate amount of physical activity and consume sufficient (but not excessive) calories is approximately 0.6 g protein/kg body weight/day (b.w./d). Bn measurements in patients with CKD indicate that the same level of dietary protein will achieve neutral Bn as long as the CKD patient does not have another catabolic condition. Furthermore, the WHO concluded that 0.6 g protein/kg b.w./d diet plus 2 standard deviations of this average value leads to a dietary requirement of 0.75 g protein/kg b.w./d. This amount of dietary protein has been designated as the "safe level of intake" because it meets the dietary requirements of 97.5% or more of healthy adults. Again, patients with CKD have the same requirements. There are two caveats to these recommendations: firstly, for obese or edematous patients, the ideal body weight (IBW) should be based on the patient's height when prescribing a LPD or monitoring compliance with the LPD (see Table 8.1). Secondly, providing levels of dietary protein greater than these amounts simply increases the production and accumulation of toxins and minerals that cause uremic symptoms.

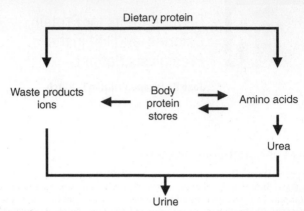

FIGURE 8.1 A flow diagram illustrating the use of foods rich in protein by healthy adults and by patients with chronic kidney disease (CKD). The scheme indicates that dietary protein is converted to amino acids, which can be used to build new stores of body protein. Any excess is converted to urea, which must be excreted by the kidney, and hence, will accumulate with renal insufficiency.

TABLE 8.1	Estimating Compliance with the Dietary Protein Prescription from the 24-Hour Urinary Urea Nitrogen Excretion

Formulas

1. $B_N = I_N - U - NUN$, where $NUN = 0.031$ g N/kg b.w.
2. if $B_N = 0$, then $I_N = U + 0.031$ g N/kg b.w.
3. When BUN is unchanging, then $U = UUN$, and
4. $I_N = UUN + 0.031$ g N/kg b.w.

Example

A 40-year-old woman is seen 1 month after instruction in a diet providing 0.6 protein/kg b.w./d (i.e., 60 kg $\times$ 0.6 protein/kg = 36 g protein)

Weight: 60 kg; UUN = 4.1 g/d; NUN = 0.031 g N $\times$ 60 kg = 1.86 g N/d

if $B_N = 0$, then $I_N = UUN + NUN$
  = 4.1 + 1.86 = 5.96 g N
  = 5.96 g N $\times$ 6.25 g protein/g N
  = 37.3 g protein/d

B_N, nitrogen balance (g N/d); BUN, blood urea nitrogen; I_N, nitrogen intake (g N/d); N, nitrogen; NUN, nonurea nitrogen (g N/d); U, urea nitrogen appearance (g N/d); UUN, 24-hour urinary urea nitrogen (g N/d).

MECHANISMS RESPONSIBLE FOR NEUTRAL NITROGEN BALANCE

Healthy Subjects

In Western societies, the intake of protein by otherwise healthy individuals generally exceeds the minimum or safe level required to achieve neutral Bn. In the absence of anabolic hormones, an excess in dietary protein does not result in muscle growth; instead, the response is to increase urea production plus an increase in adipose tissue resulting from the increase in calories that is associated with a high-protein intake. In contrast, a decrease in protein intake by either normal subjects or patients with CKD stimulates metabolic responses that improve the metabolism of protein. These responses include a reduction in the oxidative destruction of amino acids, which results in more efficient use of essential amino acids (EAAs) that are necessary for building body protein stores (see Chapter 1).

A reduction in the rate of amino acid oxidation is not the only response. A reduction in protein intake below the recommended amounts also leads to changes in the rates of protein synthesis and degradation. In short, there are metabolic changes in protein metabolism that act to improve nitrogen balance (i.e., Bn). Notably, daily rates of protein synthesis and degradation are much larger than rates of amino acid oxidation (Fig. 8.2): approximately 280 g of body protein is synthesized and degraded in a 70-kg adult each day! With such a large amount of protein being degraded and synthesized each day, the rates of protein synthesis and degradation must be precisely regulated to achieve neutral Bn. Specifically, when normal adults or patients with CKD are not eating, protein stores are being degraded. But when dietary protein increases, there is a rapid suppression of protein degradation and a stimulation of protein synthesis that acts to replete body protein stores lost during fasting. In terms of Bn, a diet that is nutritionally adequate will cause Bn to be neutral or positive with preservation of protein stores. A principal modulator of these changes in rates of protein turnover stimulated by eating proteins is insulin because it: (i) suppresses catabolism of EAAs; and (ii) inhibits protein degradation while increasing protein synthesis.

Patients with Chronic Kidney Disease

Patients with advanced but uncomplicated CKD (patients with an estimated glomerular filtration rate [eGFR] of approximately 5 to 15 mL/min) are remarkably efficient in adapting to dietary protein restriction. Specifically, patients with CKD fed a restricted amount of dietary protein rapidly reduce their oxidation of amino acids and the rate of protein degradation just as occurs in normal adults who are fed a restricted amount of dietary protein. These responses are relevant because patients will be in neutral Bn even when the intake of protein or amino acids is barely sufficient. In contrast, when patients with CKD are fed an excess of dietary protein, the excess will be used to produce more urea. If the amount of dietary protein

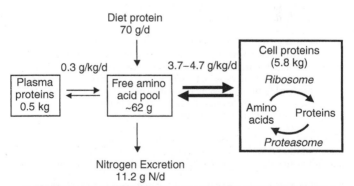

FIGURE 8.2 Results illustrated in this figure are the amounts of protein in the cellular pool and in plasma as well as the amount of free amino acids in the body of an adult weighing approximately 70 kg. A very large turnover of cellular proteins (3.7 to 4.7 g protein/kg b.w./d) occurs, amounting to the protein contained in 1 to 1.5 kg of muscle. This rate is 10-fold higher than the turnover of protein in the plasma pool.

or amino acids is insufficient, patients with CKD (or amino acids) will have incomplete compensatory response(s), leading to negative Bn with loss of lean body mass.

Dietary Protein Restriction and Nephrotic Syndrome

Patients with nephrotic syndrome and >5 g proteinuria per day who are fed a well-designed LPD will experience a decrease in proteinuria plus an increase in serum albumin compared to results in nephrotic patients fed an excessive amount of protein. This occurs because a restricted amount of dietary protein not only suppresses proteinuria but also activates adaptive responses, resulting in positive Bn and improved components of protein turnover. In summary, patients with uncomplicated CKD, including those with proteinuria in the nephrotic range, activate critical compensatory responses to dietary protein restriction by suppressing EAA oxidation and reducing protein degradation. This causes Bn to be neutral, resulting in maintenance of lean body mass during long-term therapy with LPD.

Complications of Chronic Kidney Disease That Impair Adaptive Responses in Protein Turnover

Metabolic acidosis and insufficient insulin develop as complications of CKD, and both limit the ability of patients to adapt their nutritional responses to LPD. For example, in muscles, both metabolic acidosis and a decline in insulin stimulate the oxidation of EAA and accelerate the degradation of protein. Fortunately, the risks of developing metabolic acidosis or insulin resistance are substantially reduced in CKD patients treated with a LPD.

The mechanisms by which metabolic acidosis interferes with achieving Bn involve two catabolic responses. Firstly, the essential, branched-chain amino acids, valine, leucine, and isoleucine, are catabolized by branched-chain keto acid dehydrogenase (BCKAD), and acidosis increases BCKAD activity in skeletal muscle. Acidosis also accelerates protein degradation by increasing the activity of the major proteolytic system in muscle, the adenosine triphosphate–dependent, ubiquitin–proteasome proteolytic pathway. These catabolic cellular responses explain why metabolic acidosis causes negative Bn. Fortunately, the catabolic responses can be overcome because acid is generated by metabolism of animal-derived proteins, resulting in a strong inverse relationship between higher protein intakes and a reduced concentration of serum bicarbonate.

Amelioration of Insulin Resistance

Subjects with CKD frequently develop glucose intolerance, characterized by hyperglycemia and hyperinsulinemia while fasting. One of the major initiators of glucose intolerance is metabolic acidosis that frequently complicates CKD. The development of insulin resistance proceeds by decreasing glucose uptake in skeletal muscle and adipose tissues, whereas glucose production by the liver is normal and suppresses appropriately when insulin is present. The presence of insulin resistance is emphasized because impaired insulin responses will interfere with the adaptive responses that suppress amino acid oxidation and protein degradation that are needed to maintain Bn by patients with CKD who are fed the minimum daily requirement of protein.

Reversing Acidosis-Induced Responses Can Suppress Complications of Chronic Kidney Disease

Recently, the scope of topics associated with correcting metabolic acidosis has grown substantially, in large part because correction of metabolic acidosis by dietary manipulation can effectively suppress the accelerated loss of kidney function that occurs in patients with progressive CKD. Initially, the finding consisted of an inverse correlation between serum levels of bicarbonate and increases in serum creatinine. Subsequently, De Brito-Ashurst and colleagues devised controlled clinical trials to determine if correction of metabolic acidosis in patients with CKD would slow the loss of kidney function (i.e., creatinine clearances or eGFR). Over a 2-year period, the outcomes were positive, documented as a slowing of creatinine clearance ($p < 0.0001$) and the number of patients who required initiation of chronic dialysis therapy ($p < 0.001$). Considering the foregoing discussion, it is not surprising that patients who were treated to correct metabolic acidosis also experienced an improvement in indices of protein nutrition. In another trial, patients were treated with angiotensin-converting enzyme inhibitors (ACEI) and then randomly assigned to receive sodium bicarbonate, an equimolar amount of sodium as sodium chloride, or a placebo. The outcome was positive as the rate of decline of eGFR (estimated from plasma cystatin C levels) was less in patients treated with supplements of sodium bicarbonate compared to results from patients treated with sodium chloride or placebo. These reports might differ if a larger number of patients were studied, but for the present, it is mandatory to correct metabolic acidosis.

How does metabolic acidosis develop? It is established that the catabolism of proteins in the diet is the principal source of acid generation. Consequently, limiting proteins in the diet should reduce the generation of acid and aid in correcting metabolic acidosis. For example, in 2012, Goraya and colleagues reduced the daily amount of acid generated by simply increasing fruits and vegetables in the diet. The strategy was based on adding fruit and vegetables to reduce the daily generation of acid by 50%. Generally, the change amounted to adding two to four cups of fruits and vegetables to the daily diet of hypertensive patients with Stage 1 or 2 CKD being treated with ACEI. The outcome measures included an evaluation of reduced urinary markers of kidney damage, namely N-acetyl beta-D-glucosaminidase and transforming growth factor $\beta 1$. In this trial, patients with CKD who were either treated with sodium bicarbonate or fed an LPD had similarly positive responses. Similar positive responses were achieved during 1 year when patients were given sodium bicarbonate or an LPD: there was an increase in total CO_2. Importantly, markers of kidney injury were lower in patients treated with diets enriched in fruits and vegetables.

Based on these reports and the established benefits of improving nutritional status simply by correcting metabolic acidosis, we recommend treating patients with metabolic acidosis. As a general rule, we maintain that the serum HCO_3 should be ≥ 24 mmol/L. Usually, two or three 650-mg sodium bicarbonate tablets (approximately 8 mEq of sodium and bicarbonate per tablet), given 2 to 3 times daily, are well tolerated and effective.

OTHER ADVANTAGES OF DIETARY RESTRICTION OF PROTEIN

Amelioration of Hyperfiltration, Proteinuria, and Abnormalities in Lipid Profile

In experimental models of CKD and in patients with CKD, excessive dietary protein acutely increases GFR. This response is blocked by reducing protein intake, and it is proposed that a decrease in GFR would be a beneficial response to a LPD. Likewise, there is evidence that restriction of dietary protein will decrease the degree of proteinuria.

In patients with CKD, LPDs will commonly limit animal sources of protein (e.g., meat and dairy products). In this case, the intake of saturated lipids would decrease, and this would result in an improvement in the serum lipid profile. For example, reducing protein intake from 1.1 to 0.7 g/kg b.w./d over 3 months was found to increase the levels of serum lipoprotein A-1 and the apolipoprotein A-1:apoprotein B ratio.

Effect on Mineral and Bone Disorder

Phosphates are an integral constituent of animal-derived proteins (1 g of protein contains about 13 mg of phosphorus), so limiting protein intake automatically reduces phosphate intake (Chapter 5). This response in turn will reduce serum levels of parathyroid hormone and an improvement in renal osteodystrophy. These benefits were extended to include an improvement in renal osteomalacia and osteofibrosis during a 12-month trial in which CKD patients were fed a LPD that included a supplement of ketoanalogs of EAAs.

Improvement in Blood Pressure and Erythropoietin Responsiveness

Another unexpected advantage of LPD is an improvement in blood pressure (BP). For example, it was found that BP decreased on the order of 15 mm Hg in systolic BP and 6 mm Hg in diastolic BP in patients with CKD who were treated with a very low-protein diet supplemented with ketoanalogs of EAAs. These responses were attributed at least in part to a 28% decrease in sodium intake that was associated with a 30% decrease in protein intake (Chapter 17).

As with improvements in mineral metabolism and hypertension, dietary protein restriction in patients with advanced CKD (creatinine clearance ≤ 25 mL/min/1.73 m^2) was associated with an improvement in the response to erythropoietin. Specifically, the erythropoietin dose required to maintain a constant level of hemoglobin progressively decreased in patients who were treated with a LPD plus ketoanalogs.

CONCERNS ABOUT DIETARY PROTIEN RESTRICTION IN PATIENTS WITH PROGRESSIVE CHRONIC KIDNEY DISEASE

Two observations have raised concerns about prescribing LPDs in the treatment of patients with CKD. Firstly, there was an association between hypoalbuminemia and increased mortality in patients being treated with maintenance hemodialysis. It was suggested that the restricted diets were the cause of hypoalbuminemia via a mechanism that led to malnutrition. Secondly, there was concern that patients with advanced CKD were starting chronic dialysis therapy and this led to worse outcomes, and it was suggested that LPDs should be used cautiously or avoided in patients with CKD. The first concern was principally linked to the finding that dialysis patients often do have low levels of serum proteins. The second concern arose because patients with CKD can undergo a spontaneous decrease in protein intake in association with deterioration of certain nutritional indices. It was suggested that patients with CKD should begin dialysis therapy at an "early" stage. In contrast, evaluation of the development of hypoalbuminemia in patients with advanced CKD was found to be linked more closely to inflammation or excessive accumulation of fluid than changes induced by treatment with a LPD. In fact, results from patients with advanced CKD being treated with LPDs or with more restricted diets that are supplemented with ketoanalogs of EAAs were found to have stable or increased serum concentrations of different proteins, including serum albumin when compared to levels of serum albumin that were found in patients initiating chronic maintenance dialysis therapy. Moreover, there have been no reports that indicate survival is improved in patients who were treated with an "early" initiation of dialysis (Chapter 11).

The greatest challenge for physicians and dieticians is achieving compliance with LPD. For this reason, we believe it is essential for a skilled dietician to be involved in the treatment of patients with CKD. The dietician/nutritionist is needed because he/she will be familiar with problems that are specific to patients with CKD. In addition, the dietician will have knowledge about the use of seasonings and supplements that can make meals appetizing and pleasant.

In summary, there is substantial evidence indicating that when properly applied, LPDs do not lead to protein-energy wasting, even in patients with advanced CKD. Such diets must, however, emphasize dietary education for patients with CKD. When patients do not understand the goals and implementation of LPDs, it will not be possible to ensure that the diet is adequate and that foods that increase the accumulation of nitrogenous wastes are avoided in order to avoid aggravating uremic symptoms.

ENERGY METABOLISM IN PATIENTS WITH CHRONIC KIDNEY DISEASE

Energy Metabolism and Protein Turnover

In clinical studies of patients with CKD and a protein intake that was constant at 0.60 g protein/kg b.w./d, variation in the patient's energy intake from 15 to 45 kcal/kg b.w./d led to more positive Bn in patients with higher levels of energy intake. Moreover, patients fed higher levels of energy experienced a decrease in urea appearance (i.e., net urea production calculated as the sum of urea nitrogen excreted plus accumulated). These results indicate that dietary protein was being used efficiently, resulting in building of body protein stores.

The rate of energy expenditure (and hence, the energy requirement) at rest and with exercise is similar in patients with uncomplicated CKD and healthy subjects. Thus, an energy intake of approximately 35 kcal/kg b.w./d maintains normal levels of serum proteins, anthropometric values, and Bn in patients with CKD who are consuming protein-restricted diets. Importantly, the recommended level of energy intake is commonly calculated using the patient's IBW, because *actual* body weight may over- or underestimate energy requirements if the subject is edematous or obese, or malnourished. For patients with CKD who are exercising vigorously, the energy content of the diet must be raised to maintain a stable weight. Given the relationship between obesity and the presence of CKD-related metabolic abnormalities such as inflammation and oxidative stress, the energy intake for patients with Stage 1–5 CKD could be kept at 30 kcal/kg b.w./d. This level of calories is suggested in order to avoid having patients develop obesity that would complicate treatment of CKD. As with manipulation of protein intake, the first step in achieving sufficient dietary energy is to interact with a renal dietician (Chapters 2, 20, and 21).

GLUCOSE AND LIPID METABOLISM IN CHRONIC KIDNEY DISEASE

Patients with CKD and almost normal levels of eGFR can develop insulin resistance leading to glucose intolerance and fasting hyperglycemia and hyperinsulinemia, especially in patients with CKD and metabolic acidosis. The major metabolic abnormality in glucose intolerance resides in peripheral tissues; there is decreased glucose uptake by skeletal muscle and adipose tissue, whereas hepatic glucose production is normal and appropriately suppressed by insulin. Thus, the abnormality in insulin resistance develops following interaction between insulin and its receptor; this postreceptor defect consists of suppression of phosphatidylinositol-3 kinase activity. This is relevant because insulin resistance is common in patients with CKD, and it can interfere with the metabolism of skeletal muscle as well as other organs.

Lipid Metabolism

The predominant lipid abnormality in non-nephrotic patients with CKD who are not being treated by chronic dialysis therapy is hypertriglyceridemia. There is also an increase in very low-density lipoprotein (VLDL) levels, a decrease in high-density lipoprotein (HDL) cholesterol levels, and normal to below-normal levels of LDLs. This lipoprotein pattern is consistent with a type IV hyperlipoproteinemia; this pattern can be aggravated by genetic predisposition, male gender, steroid therapy, and proteinuria (see Chapter 6).

The mechanism causing hypertriglyceridemia in patients with CKD is mainly defective catabolism of triglyceride-rich lipoproteins, and this in turn is related to decreased activity of lipoprotein lipase and hepatic triglyceride lipase. Complications of CKD, including metabolic acidosis or hyperinsulinemia, can depress lipoprotein lipase activity, and even secondary hyperparathyroidism can contribute to the development of hypertriglyceridemia in patients with CKD. Another mechanism is an increase in triglyceride production that reflects insulin resistance. Thus, conversion of triglyceride-rich VLDL to LDL is defective, leading to accumulation of potentially atherogenic, intermediate-density lipoproteins.

Patients with the nephrotic syndrome generally have high plasma levels of total cholesterol consisting of LDL and VLDL cholesterol, normal or low levels of HDL cholesterol, and normal or elevated triglycerides, that is, type IIa, IIb, or V patterns of hyperlipoproteinemia. The major factors that increase the risk of atherosclerosis in patients with nephrotic syndrome include hypoalbuminemia and hyperlipidemia, which lead to dysregulation of 3-hydroxy-3-methyl-glutaryl-coenzyme A reductase and 7α-hydroxylase expression (Chapters 6 and 10).

ASSESSING DIETARY ADEQUACY AND COMPLIANCE

A key component in designing a successful plan of dietary therapy for a patient with CKD is regular assessment of dietary adequacy and compliance. Although changes in serum visceral protein concentrations such as albumin, prealbumin, or transferrin can be included, they should not be the sole indicators of the adequacy of a diet because other factors, including the presence of inflammation, also lead to low values of serum proteins. Our approach is to monitor serum albumin and serum transferrin plus anthropometric indices of muscle mass with serial evaluations, coordinated with measures of dietary compliance (Chapters 2, 20, and 21).

Monitoring Compliance with the Diet Prescription
Protein Intake
For inpatients and outpatients, the protein–calorie content of meals should be evaluated by the dietician and the nephrologist. In both cases, compliance with a dietary protein prescription can be estimated because the waste nitrogen released following degradation of dietary proteins is excreted either as urea or as nonurea nitrogen (NUN). The concentration of urea rises because it is the principal end product of amino acid degradation and because the urea appearance rate (or net urea production rate) parallels protein intake. The urea nitrogen appearance rate is equal to the amount of urea excreted in urine plus the urea that is accumulated in body water. In contrast, NUN excretion (i.e., nitrogen contained in feces and urinary creatinine, uric acid, amino acids, peptides, and ammonia) does not require measurement, because it varies minimally with dietary protein. Instead, NUN averages 0.031 g N/kg b.w./d and is calculated from the patient's weight (Fig. 8.3). To estimate dietary compliance, it is assumed that Bn is neutral (i.e., nitrogen intake equals output and there is no loss or gain of protein). In this case, nitrogen intake (I_N) equals urea nitrogen appearance (U) plus the estimated NUN losses (Table 8.1, equation 2). Notably, the intake of nitrogen can be converted to the intake of dietary protein by multiplying I_N by 0.16 (i.e., protein is 16% nitrogen). To calculate nitrogen intake (and hence, protein intake), the patient should be in the steady state with constant values of blood urea nitrogen (BUN) and weight. This allows an initial calculation of the urea nitrogen appearance

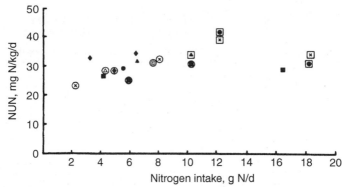

FIGURE 8.3 Nonurea nitrogen (NUN) losses measured in healthy subjects (*solid triangles, circles,* and *squares*) and patients with chronic kidney disease (CKD) being treated with low-protein diets (LPD) (*solid diamonds, open circles with cross,* and *open triangle*), by hemodialysis (*open circle with solid square* and *open square with solid triangle*) or continuous ambulatory peritoneal dialysis (CAPD) (*open square with cross* and *open square with solid circle*). These results indicate that NUN losses (i.e., nonurea urinary nitrogen plus fecal nitrogen) are relatively constant despite large variations in nitrogen intake and renal function. (From Maroni BJ, Steinman TI, Mitch WE. A method for estimating nitrogen intake in patients with chronic renal failure. *Kidney Int* 1985;27:58–65, with permission.)

(U) rate from the urea nitrogen contained in a 24-hour urine collection. If the BUN and weight are constant, then the 24 hour urine urea nitrogen measurement equals the urea nitrogen appearance rate. In this case, I_N will equal the 24 hour urea nitrogen excretion plus 0.031 g N/kg b.w. (Table 8.1, equation 4). On the other hand, if weight or BUN is changing, there should be an additional calculation of changes in the accumulation of urea nitrogen in body water as shown in Table 8.1.

The importance of calculating protein intake is that the dietician can assist a patient with CKD in his/her understanding of the goals of nutritional therapy and guide the patient in making changes in the diet. For example, if the calculated protein intake is found to be less than prescribed, patients should meet with the dietician to determine how the patient can increase his/her protein intake. Conversely, if the estimated protein intake exceeds that prescribed by more than 20%, there should be recognition that the patient is not compliant with the diet or there could be a superimposed, catabolic illness or condition (e.g., gastrointestinal bleeding or metabolic acidosis).

The formula for estimating protein intake can also be used for other clinical tasks: for example, the steady-state BUN for any prescribed protein intake can be calculated when the value of the urea clearance is known (Table 8.2). This calculation can be useful because it provides an index of the severity of renal insufficiency; a BUN > 70 mg/dL can identify patients with CKD who are likely to develop complications of CKD.

Energy Intake
Unlike calculating dietary protein, there is no simple method for the estimation of the calorie intake. Instead, dietary diaries are used to assess energy intake of outpatients with CKD. Unfortunately, the accuracy of diary estimates depends on knowing all foods consumed, the portion size, their energy contact, and the number of days each food was eaten. In short, the energy intake derived

| | Relationship between Nitrogen Balance, Urea Nitrogen Appearance Rate, and Steady-State Blood Urea Nitrogen |

Dietary Protein (g/d)	IN–NUN (g N/d)	Steady-State BUN (mg/dL)
80	10.6	123
60	7.4	86
40	3.9	49

where

$$BUN = \frac{I_N - g\ N/kg\ body\ weight}{C_{UREA}} \times 100$$

Calculated for a 70-kg person with a urea clearance of 6 mL/min (8.6 L/d). BUN, blood urea nitrogen; C_{UREA}, urea clearance (L/d); I_N, nitrogen intake (16% of protein intake); N, nitrogen; NUN, nonurea nitrogen, which averages 0.031 g N/kg b.w./d.

from dietary records must be interpreted with considerable caution. We use a 3-day food diary that is completed every 3 to 4 months in order to monitor the energy intake of patients with CKD. This information can be integrated with the calculated protein intake. For example, if protein intake is calculated from urea and nonurea excretion, the dietician/nutritionist can use records of foods eaten to estimate the percentage of calories from protein. With this information, the total dietary calories can be estimated.

The role of the dietician/nutritionist is discussed in Chapters 2 and 21. Besides planning the diet and monitoring compliance, a dietician can provide sample menus to assist in education of the patient and monitoring his/her protein intake, nutritional status, and dietary compliance. We suggest these tasks are undertaken every 3 months. At each visit, we estimate protein intake (see Table 8.1) and calorie intake from food recall or diaries, and we monitor serum albumin, prealbumin, and transferrin concentrations and anthropometrics.

PROTEIN REQUIREMENTS OF PREDIALYSIS PATIENTS

As noted earlier, two dietary regimens have been used most commonly to treat patients with progressive CKD: (i) a diet based on common foods and restricted to provide approximately 0.6 g protein/kg b.w./d; or (ii) a very low-protein diet that contains approximately 0.3 g protein/kg b.w./d, supplemented with a mixture of EAA or their nitrogen-free ketoanalogs (i.e., keto acids or KAs). The latter diet is often described as a vegetarian diet. It is not widely used because KAs (the nitrogen-free analogs of EAAs) are not available in the United States; they are available and used in Europe, Asia, and Latin America. Because energy expenditure (and hence, energy requirements) of patients with CKD is comparable to those of healthy subjects, 30 to 35 kcal/kg b.w./d is recommended to achieve maximal use of the dietary protein.

DIETARY PROTEIN PRESCRIPTION

There are several reasons to limit the dietary protein of patients with CKD: (i) providing more than the required amount simply increases the accumulation of unexcreted waste products, aggravating uremic symptoms; (ii) the severity of acidosis, secondary hyperparathyroidism, and insulin resistance is reduced; and (iii) proteinuria is reduced. The effect of reducing dietary protein on the progression of CKD is discussed in Chapter 11.

Recommended Nutrient Intake in Patients with Chronic Kidney Disease

Chronic Kidney Disease	Daily Recommendations
Protein*	
GFR (mL/min/1.73 m^2)	Amount of protein (g/kg of ideal body weight)
>50	No restriction recommended
25–50	0.6 to 0.75 controlled
<25	0.6 or 0.3 plus supplementation†
Renal transplant recipient	
Early phase or acute rejection	1.3
Stable phase	As CKD
For nephrotic patient	0.8 plus 1 g of protein/g of proteinuria
Energy	(kcal/kg of ideal body weight)
<60 yr	≥35
>60 yr	30–35
Carbohydrates	35% of nonprotein calories
Fat	Polyunsaturated to saturated ratio of 2:1
Phosphorus	800–1000 mg
	No restriction in transplant recipient if serum phosphorus is normal
Calcium	Should not exceed 2.5 g (dietary plus calcium-based binders)
Potassium	Individualized
Sodium and water	As tolerated, to maintain body weight and blood pressure

*At least 50% of proteins should be of high biologic value.
†Mixture of essential amino acids and ketoacids.[51]
CKD, chronic kidney disease; GFR, glomerular filtration rate.

Generally, we begin dietary protein restriction when patients develop symptoms or complications of uremia such as edema or poorly controlled hypertension that is related to salt intake (Chapter 17). In addition, we institute LPD for patients who continue to exhibit progressive renal insufficiency despite control of BP and the use of ACEI or angiotensin II receptor blocker. After discussing the goals and the participation required by the patient, we use the guidelines outlined below and in Table 8.3.

Moderate Chronic Renal Failure (Estimated Glomerular Filtration Rate, 25 to 60 mL/min)

Dietary therapy for patients with moderate CKD begins with a LPD that provides approximately 0.6 g protein/kg b.w./d, of which approximately two-thirds is provided as high-biologic-value protein (meat, fish, eggs, etc.; Table 8.3). The advantage of this strategy is that the goals of dietary restriction can be achieved using traditional foods. For patients that develop additional symptoms or have problems with compliance, we prescribe an essentially vegetarian diet that contains approximately 0.3 g protein/kg b.w./d (approximately 15 to 25 g protein per day) supplemented with a mixture of EAA; in other areas of the world, investigators use ketoacids. The purpose of either regimen is to provide the daily requirements of EAA while reducing dietary protein. The latter is possible because there is a variety of low-protein, high-calorie food products that can be used to achieve calorie requirements. Examples of calorie-rich products include glucose polymers (Polycose) that can be added to beverages, high-density oral supplements (Suplena), and low-protein breads, pastas, and cookies (see Chapter 21).

Fortunately, the LPD invariably limits the intake of phosphates, as long as milk-based products and high-phosphate foods are avoided. The rationale for dietary phosphorus restriction is discussed in more detail in Chapters 5 and 16.

Advanced Chronic Renal Failure (Estimated Glomerular Filtration Rate, 5 to 25 mL/min)

The dietary regimens outlined in Table 8.3 can also be beneficial for patients with advanced CKD because the patients will develop fewer uremic symptoms and metabolic complications of CKD. Albeit controversial, these diets may also slow the rate at which kidney function is lost (Chapter 11). Because the very low-protein dietary regimens supplemented with EAAs or their keto-analogs will have a lower nitrogen content, waste nitrogen will accumulate and phosphates and acids will accumulate to a lesser degree. At least in the latter case, the requirement for phosphate binders will be reduced.

Nephrotic Syndrome (Glomerular Filtration Rate <60 mL/min)

A LPD can reduce proteinuria and ameliorate hypercholesterolemia in patients with nephrotic syndrome (Chapter 10). Emphasis is placed on reducing proteinuria because it is an important risk factor for progressive kidney disease and cardio-vascular complications. For nephrotic patients, a safe regimen that produces neutral Bn responses is 0.8 g protein (plus 1 g protein per g proteinuria) and 35 kcal/kg b.w./d because this diet produces neutral Bn in patients with nephrotic syndrome, regardless of the level of renal function (i.e., GFR: 19 to 120 mL/min). With such diets, serum albumin levels remain stable or increase. We do not recommend LPD for patients with extremely high levels of pro-teinuria (more than 15 g per day) or in patients with catabolic illnesses (e.g., vasculitis and systemic lupus erythematosus), or those receiving catabolic medications (e.g., glucocorticoids). These catabolic illnesses are emphasized because there are no measurements of the safety of LPDs in patients with these problems. Until appropriate measurements are available, we recommend that patients with CKD who are infected or who are receiving prednisone should not be restricted below the "safe" level of protein intake (0.75 g protein/kg b.w./d). It is also necessary to measure the urea appearance rate regularly as part of the monitoring progress. Specifically, if the urea appearance rate is declining, there is evidence that protein stores are being built. But if urea appearance rises, it means that a patient is catabolic. Consequently, rising dietary protein is unlikely to reverse the problem, and efforts should be directed at correcting catabolic illnesses.

Why is careful monitoring of dietary protein/energy intakes so critical for success in using LPD to treat patients with CKD? First, there are inter-relationships among different nutrients and a reduction in dietary protein must be accompanied by a concomitant increase in the intake of other nu-trients to provide calorie requirements. The difficulty in meeting this goal is compounded by the development of insulin resistance that interferes with the utilization of carbohydrates and lipids. Moreover, it is difficult to provide the proper amounts of ions and minerals because a high-protein diet is accompanied by an increase in the amounts of phosphates, salt, and other minerals. This difficulty was highlighted when the interrelationships among the intakes of ions and minerals and the ability of ACEI to slow progression of CKD were examined. The evaluation concluded that unregulated amounts of either dietary phosphates or sodium chloride will interfere with the ability of

ACEI to suppress the progression of CKD. The initial investigation revealed that changes in the levels of serum phosphorus were positively correlated with values of serum creatinine in patients who were participating in the prospectively designed Ramipril Efficacy in Nephropathy (REIN) trial. Specifically, patients with serum phosphorus levels in the two highest quartiles (3.45 to 4.00 mg/dL and >4.00 mg/dL) experienced significantly faster progression of CKD, compared to results from patients with serum phosphorus levels <3.45 mg/dL. Importantly, renoprotective responses to ACEI decreased as serum phosphorus levels increased ($p \leq 0.008$). The authors concluded that reducing serum phosphorus by changing the diet should be the principal goal in planning the diets of patients with CKD. Unfortunately, this can be very difficult because phosphates are added to processed grocery products. It is well described that diets rich in animal proteins are also rich in phosphates, which can impair the benefits of ACEI therapy on progression of CKD as well as the prevention of renal bone disease. Besides phosphates, sodium chloride is often added to processed foods to improve their "shelf life" and tastiness. Just as with the high phosphate content of protein-rich foods, responses to a high-salt diet include suppression of the ability of ACEI to suppress progression of CKD. Evaluation of results of the REIN trial revealed that a high intake of sodium (>14 g of salt per day) led to a three-fold higher risk of progression to end-stage renal disease (ESRD) compared to subjects in the same trial who were using <7 g of salt daily. The increased risk of developing ESRD was independent of BP control. Instead, the risk was largely because of blunting of the ability of ACEI to suppress proteinuria. In short, diets containing an excess of sodium chloride or phosphates can blunt the antiproteinuric effectiveness of ACEI and increase the risk for developing ESRD.

Role of Phytoestrogens and Vegetable-based Proteins
Evidence from animal experiments and small groups of patients indicates that consumption of soy proteins, which are rich in isoflavones, or flaxseed, including lignans, may prevent progressive CKD. As noted, there are reports that outcomes achieved with a diet based on vegetables compared to results with animal proteins. The vegetarian-like diet not only improved indices of bone disease but also significantly lowered the BUN and 24-hour excretions of creatinine and phosphate. These benefits in patients with CKD have been linked to responses that prevent metabolic acidosis.

FAT REQUIREMENTS IN CHRONIC KIDNEY DISEASE

Even in healthy individuals, there is insufficient evidence defining the optimal intake of dietary fat. The Food and Nutrition Board of the Institute of Medicine suggests that an acceptable range of total fat intake should be 20% to 35% of energy. This is controversial, however, and should be tested thoroughly by clinical trials.

CONCLUSION

In summary, manipulation of the diet remains a critical aspect of the armamentarium for treating patients with progressive CKD. A properly designed diet for these patients is both safe and effective in ameliorating uremic symptoms and metabolic complications. The dietary prescription should include plans for serial assessments of each patient's calculated protein and energy intake. Dietary adherence and nutritional adequacy of the LPD must be monitored regularly, and therapeutic success requires motivation by the patient and nephrologist. Tangible rewards of nutritional therapy include reduced uremic symptoms and metabolic complications, plus at least the potential for slowing the progression of CKD. Fortunately, many patients welcome the opportunity to have "control" over their illness.

Suggested Readings

Banerjee T, Crews DC, Wesson DE, et al. High dietary acid load predicts ESRD among adults with CKD. *J Am Soc Nephrol* 2015;26:1693–1700.

Chauveau P, Couzi L, Vendrely B, et al. Long-term outcome on renal replacement therapy in patients who previously received a keto acid-supplemented very-low-protein diet. *Am J Clin Nutr* 2009;90:969–974.

de Brito-Ashurst I, Varagunam M, Raftery MJ, et al. Bicarbonate supplementation slows progression of CKD and improves nutritional status. *J Am Soc Nephrol* 2009;20:2075–2084.

Garneata L, Stancu A, Dragomir D, et al. Ketoanalogue-supplemented vegetarian very low-protein diet and CKD progression. *J Am Soc Nephrol* 2016;27:2164–2176.

Goraya N, Simoni J, Jo CH, et al. A comparison of treating metabolic acidosis in CKD stage 4 hypertensive kidney disease with fruits and vegetables or sodium bicarbonate. *Clin J Am Soc Nephrol* 2013;8:371–381.

Mahajan A, Simoni J, Sheather SJ, et al. Daily oral sodium bicarbonate preserves glomerular filtration rate by slowing its decline in early hypertensive nephropathy. *Kidney Int* 2010;78:303–309.

Mitch WE. Malnutrition: a frequent misdiagnosis for hemodialysis patients. *J Clin Invest* 2002;110:437–439.

Moe SM, Zidehsarai MP, Chambers MA, et al. Vegetarian compared with meat dietary protein source and phosphorus homeostasis in chronic kidney disease. *Clin J Am Soc Nephrol* 2011;6:257–264.

Thomas SS, Zhang L, Mitch WE. Molecular mechanisms of insulin resistance in chronic kidney disease. *Kidney Int* 2015;88:1233–1239.

Vegter S, Perna A, Postma MJ, et al. Sodium intake, ACE inhibition, and progression to ESRD. *J Am Soc Nephrol* 2012;23:165–173.

Zoccali C, Ruggenenti P, Perna A, et al. Phosphate may promote CKD progression and attenuate renoprotective effect of ACE inhibition. *J Am Soc Nephrol* 2011;22:1923–1930.

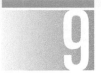

Nutritional Considerations in Patients with Diabetes and Kidney Disease

Biruh Workeneh and Mandeep Bajaj

There are few conditions in medicine that are more influenced by nutrition than diabetes and chronic kidney disease (CKD), both of which result in changes in macronutrient balance and processing. Abnormalities in glucose metabolism develop during the course of kidney disease in many patients, even at an early stage of CKD. This is manifested by insulin resistance, which occurs as a part of the uremic syndrome and was first suggested by Neubauerer over a century ago. This was later shown to result from peripheral insensitivity to insulin in the uremic milieu. The nexus between overt diabetes and CKD is even clearer; diabetes accounts for 44% of incident CKD cases and is implicated as an etiology of end-stage renal disease (ESRD) in almost half of prevalent dialysis patients in the United States. Internationally, diabetic renal disease is rising sharply, with more than 382 million people living with diabetes because of the rapid rise in obesity worldwide and changes in living standards. It is estimated that by 2,035 there will be a 55% increase in the prevalence of diabetes, and global health expenditures for treating diabetes will be over 600 billion dollars. The development of nephropathy in diabetic patients results in higher rates of cardiovascular events and mortality, and even the most advanced health care systems will be strained economically. Developing a better understanding about nutritional approaches in patients with diabetic CKD is essential and timely.

DIABETIC NEPHROPATHY

Diabetes is a multisystem disease; among other consequences, it affects vision, causes muscle atrophy, neuropathy, nephropathy, raises risk for cardiovascular events (myocardial infarction and stroke), and ultimately increases mortality. Historically, the risk of diabetic kidney disease among type 1 diabetic patients was ~50%, but with medical innovation and better access to treatment, the cumulative risk of nephropathy has declined to 20% to 30%. The rate of nephropathy in type 2 diabetic patients is more difficult to ascertain, but the prevalence increases with age, reaching roughly 20% by the eight decade of life. The difficulty accurately characterizing type 2 diabetes arises from a long-standing illness because patients could have been diabetic for years prior to being diagnosed in majority of the patients. Both type 1 and type 2 diabetes contribute to the profound changes in metabolism and body composition that are observed in CKD, and amplify prevalent cardiovascular morbidity and mortality among these patients. Clues to the diagnosis of diabetic kidney disease in lieu of a kidney biopsy are the presence of albuminuria or retinopathy and complications with substantial concordance with diabetic nephropathy.

Diabetes, particularly type 2 diabetes, is associated with several metabolic abnormalities besides hyperglycemia, but hyperglycemia is a necessary precondition for diabetic nephropathy. The development of hallmark renal lesions, such as Kimmelsteil-Wilson nodules, however does not fully

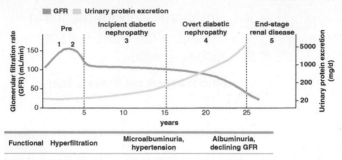

FIGURE 9.1 The typical course of diabetic nephropathy: initial hyperfiltration followed by progressive decline in GFR. GFR, glomerular filtration rate.

correlate with glycemic control. Evidently, there is a strong genetic component that predisposes to these lesions; glomerular volume and podocyte numbers are important determinants. Hyperfiltration is a hallmark of diabetic nephropathy that disrupts the elegant three-layered filtration system that comprises the glomerular ultrafiltration barrier, and is key to understanding how diabetic nephropathy progresses. Early in the course of diabetic nephropathy, glomerular hyperfiltration develops, often resulting in a decline in serum creatinine and an increase in glomerular filtration rate (GFR), a phenomenon that may persist for years. In the latter phase of diabetic nephropathy, proteinuria develops with a progressive decline in renal function (Fig. 9.1). Untreated, the average GFR declines ~5 mL/min/1.73 m^2 every year once overt diabetic nephropathy is present and this is accompanied by mesangial matrix expansion and hyperfiltration damage ultimately leading to glomerulosclerosis, fibrosis, and ESRD. All of these glomerular abnormalities observed in diabetic nephropathy can be affected by diet, serving as a basis for using nutritional interventions to modify the course of diabetic nephropathy. The major progression factor in diabetic kidney disease is blood pressure, which has a number of physiologic and nutritional determinants: the Kidney Disease Improving Global Outcomes (KDIGO) workgroup provides recommendations regarding blood pressure control in patients with diabetic CKD (Table 9.1). A formal evaluation for blood pressure control should be performed in all diabetic patients along with dietary counseling. The evaluation should be comprehensive, addressing behavioral, dietary, lifestyle, and pharmaceutic interventions to manage these chronic conditions.

Protein Intake

Thomas Addis, in the first half of the 20th century, introduced and developed the concept of "osmotic work" in laboratory animals-fed diets with varying amounts of protein. He demonstrated that in animals fed with a higher dietary content of protein, there was increasing hypertrophy, suggesting that there was increased osmotic work. His research led to the conclusion that high-protein diets resulted in faster progression and death of animal CKD models, and suggested a mechanism by which protein *restriction* preserved renal function.

The possibility that loss of kidney mass stimulated progression of kidney damage was subsequently extended leading to the conclusion that an increase in glomerular hypertension causes vascular intimal tension and injury, which induces progressive glomerulosclerosis. This maladaptation

TABLE 9.1 KDIGO Blood Pressure Recommendations in Diabetic CKD Patients

Recommendation

- We recommended that adults with diabetes and CKD with urine albumin excretion < 30 mg per 24 h whose office BP is consistently > 140 mm Hg systolic or > 90 mm Hg diastolic be treated with BP lowering drugs to maintain a BP that is consistently < 140 mm Hg systolic or <90 mm Hg diastolic

- We suggest that adults with diabetes and CKD with urine albumin excretion >30 mg per 24 h whose office BP is consistently >130 mm Hg systolic and >80 mm Hg diastolic be treated with BP-lowering drugs to maintain a BP that is consistently <130 mm Hg systolic and <80 mm Hg diastolic

- We suggest that an ARB or ACE-I be used in adults with diabetes and CKD with urine excretion of 30–300 mg per 24 h

- We recommend that an ARB or ACE-I be used in adults with diabetes and CKD with urine excretion >300 mg per 24 h

- Encourage lifestyle modification in patients with CKD to lower BP and imrove long-term cardiovascular and other coutcomes; maintain a healthy weight (BMI 20–25)

From Kidney Disease: Improving Glnbal Outcomes (KDIGO) CKD Work Group. KDIGO 2012 clinical practice guideline for the evaluation and management of chronic kidney disease. *Kidney Int Suppl* 2013;3:1–150. ACE-I, angiotensin-converting enzyme inhibitor; ARB, angiotensin receptor blocker; BMI, body mass index; BP, blood pressure; CKD, chronic kidney disease.

has led to effective therapies targeting glomerular hypertension, such as angiotensin-converting enzyme inhibitors (ACE inhibitors) for patients with diabetic nephropathy. Data from the National Health and Nutrition Examination Survey (NHANES) showed that individuals with an eGFR 55 to 80 mL/min/1.73 m^2 at baseline, protein intake was significantly correlated with a reduction in eGFR of almost 2 mL/min/1.73 m^2 for every 10 g increase in protein consumption. The effect of protein on GFR was greatest in adults with the highest intake of nondairy animal protein.

Consuming a high-protein diet is also associated with a high-salt intake, which could raise the blood pressure in patients with CKD. In experimental kidney disease, there is an association between an increase in dietary protein and a higher blood pressure although reducing dietary protein has been effective in reducing systemic arterial pressure. Moreover, dietary protein restriction slows renal progression, even in the event blood pressure does not decrease, which indicates that the beneficial effects of protein restriction do not exclusively depend directly on reducing blood pressure. The effect of dietary protein on blood pressure appears to increase as GFR falls, suggesting that either alterations in the diseased nephrons create sensitivity to dietary protein or that other constituents of the diet that are accumulated in CKD (e.g., phosphorous, acid, uric acid, or other uremic toxins) cause hypertensive effects.

Retained uremic toxins in CKD affect the function of the kidney vasculature and interfere with the functioning of the kidney and nearly every organ. Protein and its various metabolites are responsible for most of the known uremic toxins, a comprehensive list of uremic toxins can be found in a database maintained by the European Uremic Toxin (EuTox) workgroup at http://uremic-toxins.org. Many of the identified uremic solutes are generated from protein metabolism by colonic microbiota and absorbed systemically. A diet high in protein, especially in a patient with a low GFR, will contribute to uremic signs and symptoms. Therefore, patients with advanced CKD, especially in predialysis patients, should be advised to limit protein in their diet.

It is apparent that protein restriction limits the negative responses to a high-protein diet in adults with diabetic nephropathy. However, it must be emphasized that in children low-protein diet strategy should be used with caution because there is a concern for impairing growth. The American Diabetes Association (ADA) recommendations regarding protein restriction in diabetic nephropathy are as follows:

> 1) We suggest lowering protein intake to 0.8 g/kg/day in adults with diabetes or without diabetes and GFR <30 ml/min/1.73 m^2, with appropriate education. 2) We suggest avoiding high protein intake (>1.3 g/kg/day) in adults with CKD at risk of progression.

The World Health Organization (WHO) also has commissioned studies that reach the conclusion that a protein intake <0.4 g/kg/d may result in protein malnutrition, unless the patients also ingest a supplement of essential amino acids or ketoacids. Otherwise, recommendations for dietary therapy that are aimed at slowing progression is to maintain protein intake in the range of 0.6 g/kg/d.

Protein–Energy Wasting

Muscle wasting in patients with CKD is a prevalent and often underappreciated problem that results in significant weakness, reduced mobility, and decreased quality of life. There are publications based on measurements of protein turnover and imaging techniques that dialysis patients can lose up to 3 kg of lean mass per year and the loss can be even greater in patients who are diabetic. The presence of diabetes accentuates the process of muscle wasting. Although uremic myopathy and neuropathy contribute to muscle weakness, it is clear from histologic evaluation of muscle architecture that the predominant mechanism underlying muscle weakness in CKD is loss of muscle protein and infiltration with fat tissue. As a consequence of the negative effect of CKD on skeletal muscle, patients endure a sedentary and inactive lifestyle, and the inactivity jeopardizes cardiovascular health. In addition, impaired physical functioning in patients with CKD with muscle wasting is correlated with a low quality of life, loss of independence, and an increased mortality. There is concern that a vicious cycle develops in patients with CKD in which inactivity as a result of muscle weakness worsens the muscle wasting that is present in patients with ESRD.

The influence of diabetes and the effects of insulin action on skeletal muscle have been studied extensively, and it is clear that insulin withdrawal results in muscle wasting. Therefore, it is doubly important for patients with type 1 diabetes to maintain strict control of their insulin regimen. In patients with type 2 diabetes, the link between impaired insulin signaling and muscle degradation is less direct, but is present.

Hyperglycemia

A deficiency of insulin or impaired insulin action results in hyperglycemia and chronically, this leads to hemodynamic, structural, and ultrastructural changes in the kidney. Chronic hyperglycemia affects all the components of the glomerular tuft. Hyperglycemia induces nonenzymatic glycosylation of proteins, injury to mesangial cells, and leads to mesangial proliferation and matrix expansion. Increased matrix production in the mesangium and basement membrane thickening decreases filtration surface area and results in progressive decline in GFR. Frequently, because of the nature of diabetic nephropathy, the kidneys by imaging appear to have enlarged or are large relative to the magnitude of renal dysfunction in advanced disease. These changes are attributed to an increase in activity of growth factors, activation of inflammatory cytokines, formation of reactive oxygen species, accumulation of advanced glycosylation end products, and collagen in glomerular tuft and surrounding structures. Hyperglycemia also injures arterioles and the vascular bed, causing hyalinosis and further decline in renal function. The net effect of these changes are glomerular hypertrophy and later in the course, glomerulosclerosis and renal fibrosis.

Glycemic control has been evaluated as strategy to limit the complications of diabetes. A pair of seminal trials, the Diabetes Control and Complications Trial (DCCT) and United Kingdom Prospective Diabetes Study (UKPDS) studied type 1 and type 2 diabetes, respectively by randomly assigning them to intensive therapy versus conventional therapy. Both studies demonstrated that intensive therapy reduced microalbuminuria, albuminuria, and progression of diabetic nephropathy. Moreover, early recognition of incipient nephropathy is crucial because intensive control was unlikely to alter course of advanced diabetic nephropathy. There is also increasing evidence that diets with a high-fructose content worsens insulin resistance and promotes fat storage. Based on the ADA recommendations, patients should be encouraged to undertake exercise, follow a disciplined diet as well as oral/injectable diabetes medications and/or insulin to control hyperglycemia.

Salt

Arterial hypertension arises in the course of most cases of CKD, and generally becomes more prevalent as renal damage progresses. It is known that blood pressure control can reduce the rate of loss of residual kidney function as well as reductions in cardiovascular morbidity and mortality. It is important to recognize the primary role that sodium retention plays in the hypertension seen in CKD (see Chapter 17). The role of sodium intake on blood pressure and mechanisms of hypertension-related renal damage an increase in salt intake not only raises blood pressure in humans with mild CKD but also increases glomerular hydrostatic pressure leading to vascular injury. KDIGO recommends salt restriction in patients with CKD:

> We recommend lowering salt intake to <90 mmol (<2 g) per day of sodium (corresponding to 5 g of sodium chloride), unless contraindicated.

Because limiting dietary salt can decrease total body sodium, which is associated with improved control of blood pressure, patients with diabetic nephropathy and especially those with hypertension must control their intake of salt. Indeed, the association between salt and blood pressure can be attributed in part to the blood pressure reduction that was observed in the Dietary Approaches in Systolic Hypertension (DASH) diet. This diet limits salt and substitutes fruits, vegetables, and low-fat dairy foods to reduce blood pressure. This is a strategy that should be considered in patients with diabetic kidney disease.

Potassium

Patients with progressive CKD are often encouraged to eat a low-potassium diet, but such diets can be associated with faster progression of CKD. Thus, if hyperkalemia can be avoided, a diet rich in fruits and vegetables can have measurable benefits. For example, potassium-rich fruits and vegetables also have a high content of citrate and other weak acids. These compounds can be converted to bicarbonate, which benefits muscle metabolism while slowing progression of CKD. Fortunately, potassium hemostasis can be maintained until GFR is very low, especially if metabolic acidosis is controlled. However, patients who have developed hyperkalemia or are on dialysis should restrict potassium to 2 g per day.

Acid Load

Two factors account for the development of acidosis in CKD: excess dietary protein because it generates more fixed acid and second, a reduced GFR, which limits acid excretion. Excess in dietary protein increases the intake of sulfa-containing amino acids plus phosphorylated proteins and lipids, and these substrates are metabolized to sulfuric and phosphoric acids. There is also emerging evidence that high acid load diets can contribute to CKD injury despite having normal serum bicarbonate levels. Unfortunately, as renal function declines, the acids accumulate unless bicarbonate, intracellular proteins, and bone buffer them. Diabetics are at additional risk for developing acidosis because they frequently develop aldosterone resistance and renal tubular acidosis (type 4 RTA), although this can be difficult to diagnose separately when GFR falls significantly.

For years, it has been known that correcting metabolic acidosis allows for normal growth in in CKD affected children because growth hormone is not effective in an acidic milieu. In adult patients with CKD and ESRD, the correction of acidosis improves or slows the devastating effects of muscle wasting. Some of these results are outlined in Table 9.2. Fortunately, patients with CKD experienced an increase in muscle mass and fewer hospitalizations, but did not develop hypertension even though sodium in their diets was increased. Moreover, recent reports conclude that correcting acidosis in patients with CKD can slow the loss of their kidney function. Results of several retrospective analyses and prospective clinical trials suggest that alkali therapy benefits patients with progressive diabetic kidney disease (Table 9.2).

Fat Intake

Fat in the diet of patients with diabetes and CKD should be limited because the patients are already at the highest risk for developing cardiovascular complications. Energy is stored primarily as triglycerides and when fat depots are exhausted, fat is deposited ectopically in muscle, liver, myocardium, and other organs. This complication results in inflammation, insulin resistance, and specific abnormalities, including nonalcoholic fatty liver disease and obstructive sleep apnea.

The quality of fat in foods is an aspect of dietary counseling that should be given careful consideration. There are several types of dietary fats: saturated fat, trans fat, monounsaturated fat, and polyunsaturated fat. Saturated fat and trans fat can worsen cholesterol and exacerbate cardiovascular risk profiles. Monounsaturated fats and chiefly polyunsaturated fats, the latter including essential ω-3-fatty acids, should be encouraged. Sources of different types of fat are shown in Table 9.3.

TABLE 9.2   Benefits of Acidosis Correction

Citation	Subjects Investigated
Kalhoff H et al. Paediatr 1997;86:96-101	Infants
Boirie Y et al. Kidney Int 2000;58:236-41	Children with CKD
Reaich D et al. Am J Physiol 1993; 265:E230-5	Adults with CKD
Williams B et al. kidney Int 1991;40:779-86	Adults with CKD
Graham KA et al. J Am Soc Nephrol 1997;8:632-7	Hemodialysis
Graham KA et al kidney Int 1996;49:1396-400	Peritoneal dialysis
de Brito-Ashust I et al. J Am Soc Nephrol 2009;20(9):2075-84	Adults with stage 4 CKD
Mahajan at el. kidney Int 2010; 78:303-9	Adults with stage 2 CKD

CKD, chronic kidney disease.

TABLE 9.3 Types of Fat

Saturated Fats	Trans Fats	Monounsaturated Fats	Polyunsaturated Fats
Beef; Chicken skin; butter; chocolate; lard(pork fat); ice cream; whole milk	Margarine; Shortening; Imitation Cheese; pastries; other processed foods	Olive oil; canola oil; olives; cashews; oatmeal; avocados	Flax seed oil; soybean; salmon; mackerel; beans; eggs; poultry; strawberries; broccoli

Diabetes and CKD are considered coronary equivalents; they share the similar risk for fatal stroke and myocardial infarction as patients with existing heart disease. Therefore, targets for cholesterol should be aggressive; low-density lipoprotein (LDL) less than 70 mg per dL. Statins are recommended for patients with diabetes, and the presence of CKD is not a contraindication for including them. Beyond the cardiovascular benefit, there may be an additional renal benefit in terms of progression because of the pleotropic effects of statins. Statins are associated with reduced inflammatory biomarkers, inhibition of platelet adhesion, increased synthesis of nitric oxide, and inhibition of transforming growth factor β1 (TGF-β1) expression in the glomerular cells. The Greek Atorvastatin and Coronary Heart Disease Evaluation (GREACE) study enrolled over 1,500 patients with coronary artery disease (CAD) in a randomized controlled design targeting LDL < 100 using atorvastatin versus usual care; patients were followed for 3 years. The results demonstrated benefits of aggressive lipid lowering versus usual care on renal function in diabetic and nondiabetic patients. Therefore, the risks and benefits of statin therapy should be weighed in patients with diabetic kidney disease.

Energy Balance

Energy is required for growth, development, and the normal functioning of all of our body processes. Energy balance is the difference between the energy derived from macronutrients consumed and energy expenditure over a given period of time. Daily energy expenditure consists of three components: basal metabolic rate, energy cost of physical activity, and diet-induced thermogenesis. The basal metabolic rate is the energy consumed during the normal functioning of cells and organs. Interestingly, diabetic patients consistently have higher basal energy expenditure than demographically matched nondiabetics, and this may be caused by increased hepatic glucose production, which requires a significant investment of energy. Despite the increased basal energy expenditure, weight loss is more difficult to achieve in diabetics, suggesting other mechanisms such as orexigens and hormones that interfere with the process of weight loss. It is notoriously difficult to alter eating behavior once it has been established in adults, but equipping patients with information and knowledge about nutrition and energy balance can change mental firing patterns, alter habitual eating, and allow patients to be more receptive to effective dietary intervention.

Current recommendations in overweight and obese diabetic patients are to tip energy balance in the direction that promotes weight loss and improves insulin sensitivity, either by decreasing caloric intake or increasing expenditure. Diet-induced thermogenesis is roughly 10% of the energy consumed and is dependent of the source macronutrients. The relative energy required for digesting, absorbing, and storing energy from protein is higher than carbohydrates, and fat requires the least energy required to process. In the modern era with fad diets, many individuals try to lose weight by promoting a high-protein intake. However, such diets may be raising their cardiovascular risk and acceleration of renal disease. Increasing physical exercise can also help improve energy balance and achieve healthy weight, and a clear relationship has been demonstrated between blood pressure and improved blood pressure control. KDIGO recommends the following:

> We recommend undertaking an exercise program compatible with cardiovascular health and tolerance, aiming for at least 30 minutes 5 times per week.

A balanced approach of limiting caloric intake and encouraging exercise can be tremendously beneficial in patients with diabetic kidney disease.

Formulas that approximate caloric requirements can aid in achieving energy balance. The Harris-Benedict equation is a frequently used equation that estimates energy requirements in men and women. This and other equations for estimating energy requirements are limited because of differences in demographics, body habitus, and comorbidities, including diabetes. Physical activity monitors are limited because they do not provide information about basal metabolic weights. The gold standard measure for measuring total energy expenditure is the doubly labeled water technique, but this technique is limited to only a few centers.

Bariatric Surgery

Maintaining a healthy weight (body mass index [BMI] 20 to 25) can reduce blood pressure and blood glucose while conferring other health benefits in patients with diabetic CKD. For this reason, bariatric surgery can result in significant improvements in obese patients with diabetes and the metabolic syndrome. It must be mentioned that bariatric surgery is generally reserved for obese individuals with BMI >35 kg per m^2 with type 2 diabetes, but the STAMPEDE (Surgical Treatment and Medications Potentially Eradicate Diabetes Efficiently) trial showed metabolic benefits in patients with type 2 diabetes and BMI ≥27 kg per m^2. The complications of bariatric surgery must be considered before recommending this intervention. Nevertheless, there is evidence now that bariatric surgery can mitigate and even reverse end-organ damage, including CKD. In several studies, it has been shown that Roux-en-Y gastric bypass in obese diabetic patients can improve blood pressure, albuminuria as well as an improvement in insulin sensitivity. A meta-analysis has even shown that there is suppression of albuminuria and a decline in the progression of CKD. Some reports of events in morbidly obese ESRD patients receiving maintenance dialysis also show that bariatric surgery can improve outcomes and help patients develop weight loss required for eligibility for kidney transplantation.

Diabetes and End-Stage Renal Disease

The medical and nutritional management of diabetic patients on hemodialysis is complicated by several factors. First, the most common glycemic control measurements in diabetic patients, such as hemoglobin A1c, systematically underestimate blood glucose levels in the majority of hemodialysis patients. This occurs because there is chronic blood loss with each dialysis treatment plus there is decreased red blood cell survival. Alternatives to the use of hemoglobin A1c as a monitor of blood glucose have not been widely tested. In patients treated by peritoneal dialysis, there is also a daily loss of protein, including albumin, making measurements of glycosylated albumin unreliable as a measure of long-term glucose control.

Diabetes management is also complicated in patients with ESRD because oral agents or even insulin can develop an increase in the risk of hypoglycemia because of altered pharmacokinetics in the uremic milieu. Furthermore, patients with ESRD are often ill or hospitalized and have fluctuations in their diets related to uremia.

Regarding the use of peritoneal dialysis, diabetes control can be complicated because the dialysate infused into the abdomen uses dextrose as the osmotic agent to remove fluid and toxins. The use of dextrose can cause increases in blood sugars and can damage the peritoneum or failure to remove fluid adequately (i.e., ultrafiltration failure). Despite these challenges, a multidisciplinary approach by the dietician, nephrologist, and endocrinologist can successfully manage diabetic patients and achieving results similar to outcomes recommended national guidelines. In our experience, the principle reasons for decreased technique survival and withdrawal from peritoneal dialysis are because of repeated bouts of peritonitis, catheter dysfunction, ultrafiltration failure, patient choice or lack of support and hernia, and leak or other surgical complications. Obviously, poor control of diabetes can increase the risk of peritonitis, ultrafiltration failure while contributing to central adiposity, and problems related to catheters and hernias. Some have advocated using intraperitoneal insulin in diabetic peritoneal dialysis patients, but this may result in increased rate of peritonitis.

CONCLUSION

Patients with type 1 and type 2 diabetes are living longer and hence, their lifetime risk of developing kidney disease is significant. Nutritionists, physicians, and other care providers must focus on what can be done to ameliorate this growing condition that is enormously expensive for patients and the economy. Dietary interventions can be very effective and carry few "downside risks." Sadly, many patients with CKD exacerbate their disease because they are ill informed about the consequences of their diets on the course of their disease. A prime example is that protein loading should be used because it avoids the sugar spiking of carbohydrates. Changes in diet outlined in this chapter, such as limiting salt, liberalizing fruits and vegetables, and striking the right energy balance, can result in significant improvement in the progression of diabetic kidney disease as well as the risks of cardiovascular morbidity and mortality. Multifactorial risk reduction including dietary intervention is imperative and has paramount importance in diabetic kidney disease.

Suggested Readings

Addis T. The osmotic work of the kidney and the treatment of glomerular nephritis. *Trans Assoc Am Phys* 1940;55:223–229.

American Diabetes Association. Classification and diagnosis of diabetes. Sec. 2. In Standards of Medical Care in Diabetes–2016. *Diabetes Care* 2016;39(Suppl 1): S1–S112.

Athyros VG, Mikhailidis DP, Papageorgiou AA, et al. The effect of statins versus untreated dyslipidaemia on renal function in patients with coronary heart disease. A subgroup analysis of the Greek atorvastatin and coronary heart disease evaluation (GREACE) study. *J Clin Pathol* 2004;57:728–734.

Brenner BM, Lawler EV, Mackenzie HS. The hyperfiltration theory: a paradigm shift in nephrology. *Kidney Int* 1996;49(6):1774–1777.

de Brito-Ashurst I, Varagunam M, Raftery MJ, et al. Bicarbonate supplementation slows progression of CKD and improves nutritional status. *J Am Soc Nephrol* 2009;20:2075–2084.

Kidney Disease: Improving Global Outcomes (KDIGO) CKD Work Group. KDIGO 2012 clinical practice guideline for the evaluation and management of chronic kidney disease. *Kidney Int Suppl* 2013;3:1–150.

Meyer TW, Hostetter TH. Uremia. *N Engl J Med* 2007;357(13):1316–1325.

Pupim LB, Flakoll PJ, Majchrzak KM, et al. Increased muscle protein breakdown in chronic hemodialysis patients with type 2 diabetes mellitus. *Kidney Int* 2005;68:1857–1865.

UK Prospective Diabetes Study Group. Tight blood pressure control and risk of macro-vasclar and microvasclar complications in type 2 diabetes. *BMJ* 1998313:703–713.

U.S. Renal Data System. USRDS 2013 Annual Data Report: Atlas of Chronic Kidney Disease and End Stage Renal Disease in the United States. Bethesda, MD: National Institutes of Health, National Institute of Diabetes and Digestive and Kidney Diseases; 2013.

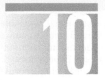

Nephrotic Syndrome:
Nutritional Consequences
and Dietary Management

**Monica Cortinovis, Norberto Perico,
and Giuseppe Remuzzi**

Nephrotic syndrome is the collective name given to a group of diseases characterized by heavy proteinuria, hypoalbuminemia, hyperlipidemia, and edema. Quantifying the loss of tissue protein is much more difficult than measuring the urinary loss of albumin and other plasma proteins. However, muscle protein wasting has been documented in patients with persistent proteinuria. Moreover, micronutrients such as vitamin D, iron, and zinc, which are bound to plasma proteins, may be lost in the urine leading to depletion syndromes in patients with long-lasting and massive proteinuria. Nephrotic syndrome can also result in hyperlipidemia, thereby potentially accelerating atherosclerosis and renal damage. Thus, the major rationales for changing a patient's diet are to blunt manifestations of the syndrome (e.g., edema and hyperlipidemia), replace nutrients lost in the urine, and reduce risks for renal disease progression and atherosclerosis. It should be mentioned that specific food allergens (e.g., milk protein and gliadin) have been involved in the development of nephrotic syndrome in some adult and pediatric patients, and in these cases, dietary manipulation may have a beneficial effect on the disease course.

PROTEINS

Metabolic abnormalities in nephrotic syndrome include depletion of plasma and tissue protein pools. At first glance, nephrotic syndrome resembles protein–calorie malnutrition, also known as kwashiorkor, because they both involve reduction in plasma albumin concentration. However, in the case of kwashiorkor, it is possible to correct all the manifestations of malnutrition by providing the needed proteins and calories. On the contrary, clinical studies documented that in patients with nephrotic syndrome a high dietary-protein intake (i.e., 1.6 to 2.0 g/kg/d) failed to restore the plasma albumin pool and further increased proteinuria. The latter, apparently paradoxic finding, can be explained by glomerular hyperfiltration and hypertrophy induced by dietary proteins. By contrast, a lower protein regimen (i.e., 0.8 g/kg/d) in nephrotic patients induced a significant reduction of urinary protein excretion eventually improving circulating albumin concentrations. The increase in plasma albumin levels was also favored by a complex adaptive response to reduced protein intake involving postprandial stimulation of protein synthesis, inhibition of whole body proteolysis, and suppression of amino acid oxidation. Thus, nephrotic patients can reduce dietary protein intake while maintaining a neutral nitrogen balance and an adequate nutritional status. It is noteworthy that the concept of low-protein diet is undergoing a substantial change, mainly as a consequence of the revision in the definition of normal-adequate protein intake in the overall population, which has shifted from 1.0 to 0.8 g/kg/d, according to the most recent guidelines. Hence, low-protein regimens are currently featured by dietary protein intake of 0.6 to 0.8 g/kg/d. Besides the absolute amount of protein in the diet, its source and composition have important implications in renal disease. Indeed, vegetable proteins have a lower impact on glomerular permeability and hemodynamics compared to those of animal origin. Along the same line, the implementation of a vegetarian diet using soy as a main protein source in patients with nephrotic syndrome led to a significant decline in proteinuria while improving the lipid pattern. Nevertheless, because this diet was low in fat (28% of calories) and protein (0.71 g/kg/d), it was not possible to establish whether the favorable effects were because of the special amino acid composition or the reduced fat and protein content. The addition of 5 g per day of fish oil to this soy-based diet did not provide additional benefits on either proteinuria or blood lipid levels and, in fact, tended to raise low-density lipoprotein (LDL) cholesterol and apolipoprotein B (apo B) concentrations. Another vegetarian low-protein (0.7 g/kg/d) diet has been proposed for nephrotic patients, even with preserved renal function. This low-protein diet was supplemented with essential amino acids and ketoanalogues to partially cover the protein losses, thereby protecting against nutritional impairment. Urinary protein excretion decreased as well as LDL cholesterol levels, without detrimental effects on plasma albumin levels.

Blockade of the renin–angiotensin system (RAS) by means of angiotensin-converting enzyme (ACE) inhibitors and/or angiotensin II type 1 receptor blockers (ARBs) is the first-line treatment in proteinuric chronic kidney disease (CKD), even in the absence of hypertension. Intriguingly, in patients with nondiabetic renal disease and heavy proteinuria, the combination of an ACE inhibitor and a low-protein diet (target, 50% reduction in protein intake) reduced urinary protein excretion more effectively than either intervention alone. Such an additive antiproteinuric effect was ascribed to the different renal hemodynamic actions induced by ACE inhibitors and dietary protein restriction, resulting in glomerular afterload and preload reduction, respectively, both improving glomerular barrier selectivity function. Another nutritional intervention that should be implemented in nephrotic patients is dietary sodium restriction because it has a beneficial effect on proteinuria, either by itself or additive to that of RAS blockers.

Recommendations

A diet providing 0.7 to 0.8 g/kg/d of proteins seems to be the most feasible and safest strategy for nephrotic patients. At least 50% of the protein should come from high-biologic value sources, such as meat, dairy products, and soybean, to ensure provision of essential amino acids. Adequate calorie intake (i.e., 30 to 35 kcal/kg/d) is needed to spare proteins from being used as energy substrates and prevent vitamin and mineral deficiencies. It is noteworthy that if urinary protein excretion exceeds 3 g per day, 1 g per day of high-biologic value protein should be added to the diet for each gram of proteinuria. In this context, it is important to assess 24-hour urinary protein excretion during the follow-up to guarantee adequate adjustment. Adherence to the proposed diet should be monitored every 2 to 3 months by means of 24-hour urinary urea nitrogen excretion, which enables to estimate dietary protein intake. When the actual protein intake exceeds the target threshold, patient referral to a dietician may be considered.

LIPIDS

Nephrotic syndrome results in hyperlipidemia and profound alterations in lipid and lipoprotein metabolism. The magnitude of these changes is proportional to the degree of proteinuria. Plasma concentrations of cholesterol, triglycerides, apo B-containing lipoproteins (i.e., very low-density lipoprotein

[VLDL], intermediate-density lipoprotein [IDL] and LDL), and lipoprotein(a) are increased in nephrotic syndrome. High-density lipoprotein (HDL) cholesterol levels are usually unchanged or reduced, leading to an increase in LDL/HDL ratio. In addition to these quantitative changes, the lipoprotein composition is markedly altered in the setting of nephrotic syndrome. Both increased synthesis and impaired catabolism/clearance of serum lipids and lipoproteins contribute to nephrotic dyslipidemia. Hyperlipidemia in nephrotic syndrome is of considerable clinical significance because it contributes to the increased cardiovascular morbidity and mortality in these patients. Moreover, evidence is accumulating, at least in experimental models, that dyslipidemia plays a role in the progression of renal damage. Therefore, correcting lipid abnormalities, or their prevention when possible, has become a prominent goal in the management of the abovementioned pathologic conditions. A number of dietary and pharmacologic strategies have been proposed to reduce blood lipid levels in nephrotic syndrome. For instance, in patients with idiopathic membranous nephropathy, the introduction of a diet low in fat (<30% of calories) and cholesterol (<200 mg per day), but rich in polyunsaturated fatty acids (PUFA) and linoleic acid (10% of energy) for 6 months reduced total and LDL cholesterol levels by 24% and 27%, respectively. However, there is no long-term experience with the use of low-fat diets in the management of nephrotic hyperlipidemia. As with protein intake, the lipid composition in the diet may turn out to be as important as the total fat content. Eicosapentaenoic acid (EPA) and docosahexaenoic acid (DHA), the essential omega-3 (ω-3) PUFA purified from fish oils, serve as substrates for cyclooxygenase and lipoxygenase pathways leading to less potent inflammatory mediators than those produced through the ω-6 PUFA substrate, arachidonic acid. Dietary supplementation with ω-3 PUFA, especially as fish oils, has been shown to provide a number of beneficial cardiovascular effects, including systolic blood pressure and triglyceride lowering as well as reduction in the risk of sudden cardiac death in patients with established coronary heart disease. Based on this evidence, a handful of small studies explored the efficacy of dietary supplementation with ω-3 PUFA in nephrotic syndrome. In patients with hyperlipidemia associated with nephrotic syndrome, 6-week treatment with 15 g per day of fish oil (2.7 g of EPA and 1.8 g of DHA) added on to an unrestricted diet resulted in a significant decline in plasma levels of total triglycerides and VLDL-triglycerides, even though LDL cholesterol increased. Similarly, a more recent study reported that in nephrotic patients 8-week treatment with 4 g per day of ω-3 PUFA led to a significant reduction in plasma triglyceride and VLDL cholesterol levels along with an increase in LDL cholesterol. The latter effect was accompanied by LDL cholesterol redistribution to larger, lighter, and therefore potentially less atherogenic particles. However, it remains unclear whether the LDL raising effect induced by ω-3 PUFA coupled with redistribution of LDL profile would eventually increase the risk of cardiovascular disease. Perhaps, the most prominent clinical studies on ω-3 PUFA in nephrotic syndrome involved their use in immunoglobin A (IgA) nephropathy, under the rationale that these fatty acids inhibit cytokine and eicosanoid production, thereby reducing intrarenal inflammation. A pivotal randomized, placebo-controlled trial including 106 patients with IgA nephropathy showed that fish oil (daily dose of 1.87 g of EPA and 1.36 g of DHA) supplementation for 2 years reduced renal disease progression, even though proteinuria remained unchanged. A follow-up of this study extending beyond 6 years confirmed the beneficial influence of fish oil on renal function preservation, but the results did not improve with the administration of higher dosages of ω-3 PUFA. In a more recent trial encompassing 30 patients with biopsy-proven IgA nephropathy, the addition of ω-3 PUFA (3 g per day) on top of dual RAS blockade for 6 months was more effective in reducing proteinuria and erythrocyturia than dual RAS blockade alone. Unfortunately, other randomized clinical trials found no benefits of fish oil supplementation on renal outcomes in patients with IgA nephropathy. As pointed out by a meta-analysis on this topic, possible explanations for the inconsistent findings include differences in patient populations, composition of the fish oils used, and duration of treatment.

Statins (hydroxymethylglutaryl-coenzyme A reductase inhibitors) are well tolerated and effective in correcting the lipid profile in nephrotic patients. However, clinical trial evidence supporting the use of these agents to slow down CKD progression or reduce cardiovascular events in nephrotic syndrome is limited. Given the central role of proteinuria in the pathogenesis of lipid disorders in nephrotic syndrome, therapeutic interventions targeting proteinuria can also improve hyperlipidemia. Indeed, the reduction in urinary protein excretion induced by ACE inhibitors in nephrotic patients has been associated with a 10% to 20% decline in the plasma levels of total and LDL cholesterol levels and lipoprotein(a), even though plasma albumin concentrations did not increase.

Recommendations

Restriction of fat (<30% of total calories) and cholesterol (<200 mg per day) intake along with an increase in the proportion of PUFA should be encouraged in patients with nephrotic syndrome. However, nutritional measures alone are usually inadequate to control nephrotic hyperlipidemia. If dietary fat restriction and proteinuria reduction do not effectively reduce blood lipid levels, statin therapy should be instituted. There is not yet compelling evidence to prescribe fish oil supplementation for the management of hyperlipidemia due to nephrotic syndrome. Nevertheless, the Kidney Disease: Improving Global Outcomes guidelines suggested optional use of fish oil (3.3 g of ω-3 PUFA per day) in the treatment of patients with IgA nephropathy and persistent proteinuria greater than 1 g per day despite 3 to 6 months of optimized RAS blockade. Although these supplements appear to be safe, fishy aftertaste is a common complaint limiting adherence. Thus, it seems reasonable to let patients decide for themselves whether the tolerability issues and cost of fish oil therapy overweigh uncertain renal benefits.

SODIUM AND WATER

Edema is a major clinical feature of nephrotic syndrome. Although it is widely accepted that nephrotic edema is caused by extravascular fluid accumulation secondary to sodium and water retention, the status of intravascular volume is somewhat controversial. Two hypotheses have been posited in this field (Fig. 10.1). The classic, or underfill hypothesis, postulates that the effective circulating blood volume is decreased in the setting of nephrotic edema. In particular, the reduced plasma oncotic pressure induced by hypoalbuminemia promotes fluid shift from the intravascular to the interstitial compartment. The decrease in plasma volume stimulates activation of the RAS and vasopressin release, which result in water and sodium retention by the kidney. In contrast, according to the overfill hypothesis the intravascular volume is expanded in nephrotic edema. Proponents of this hypothesis postulate that in nephrotic patients sodium retention reflects an intrinsic renal defect in sodium excretion, which in turn induces an expansion in plasma volume. It should be noted, however, that the underfill and overfill hypotheses are not mutually exclusive, because the volume status may depend on the stage of disease. Management of nephrotic edema may be different in the context of intravascular volume expansion compared to volume contraction. Indeed,

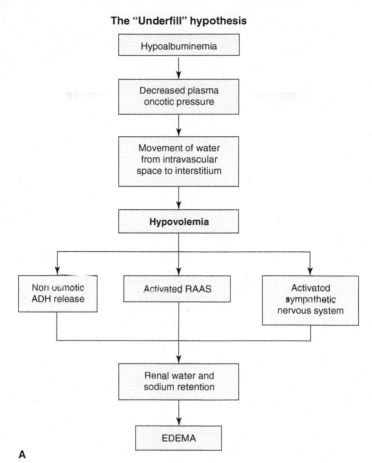

FIGURE 10.1 The "underfill" and "overfill" mechanisms of edema formation. According to the underfill hypothesis **(A)**, hypovolemia induced by reduced oncotic pressure is the key event that signals the kidney to retain the filtered sodium and water. By contrast, the overfill hypothesis **(B)** postulates that the abnormal renal sodium retention in nephrotic syndrome is the consequence of the blunted natriuretic response to ANP and increase in activity of ENaC and Na^+/K^+ ATPase. The resulting hypovolemia alters Starling's forces across the capillary wall at local tissue level, leading to overflow edema. ADH, vasopressin; ANP, atrial natriuretic peptide; cGMP, cyclic guanosine monophosphate; ENaC, epithelial sodium channel; RAAS, renin–angiotensin–aldosterone system.

albumin infusion should be tried to expand plasma volume only if symptomatic hypovolemia is present. Nevertheless, dietary sodium restriction is effective in treating edema associated to either hypovolemia or defects in renal sodium excretion.

Recommendations
Edema in nephrotic syndrome is primarily because of sodium and water retention. Thus, the aim of treatment is to create a negative sodium and water

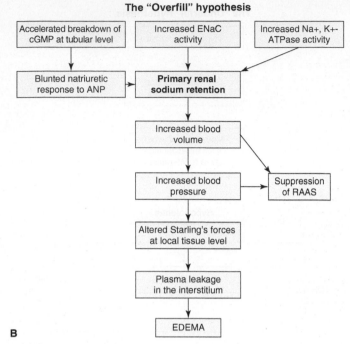

The "Overfill" hypothesis

FIGURE 10.1 *(continued)*

balance. Patients often need to limit dietary intake of sodium (target, 1.5 to 2 g per day) and fluids (<1.5 L per day) and use diuretics. It is recommended to reverse edema slowly, with a target weight loss of 0.5 to 1.0 kg per day, because aggressive diuresis can lead to electrolyte disturbances, acute kidney injury, and thromboembolic complications as a result of hemoconcentration.

MINERALS AND VITAMINS

Abnormalities in circulating levels of iron, copper, zinc, and calcium observed in nephrotic syndrome can be directly related to the urinary loss of plasma proteins that either carry divalent cations or to some way regulate their metabolism. For example, urinary excretion of the iron-binding protein transferrin accounts for reduced plasma iron concentrations in patients with proteinuria. This provides a potential mechanism for iron-deficiency anemia that can develop in nephrotic syndrome. Notably, iron released from filtered transferrin can catalyze the generation of oxygen-free radicals, eventually promoting tubulointerstitial injury. Thus, care should be exercised when iron supplementation is undertaken to manage iron-deficient anemia in nephrotic patients. Urinary losses of erythropoietin can also contribute to anemia in nephrotic syndrome.

Approximately 95% of circulating copper is bound to ceruloplasmin, and urinary loss of this protein can induce a decrease in serum copper levels. However, this does not result in clinical manifestation of nephrotic syndrome. Therefore, copper supplementation is not necessary.

Albumin is the main zinc-carrying protein, and its urinary loss can lead to substantial zinc depletion. Nevertheless, zinc deficiency in nephrotic syndrome probably stems from both reduced intestinal absorption and excessive urinary loss of this mineral. The involvement of zinc depletion in the clinical manifestations of nephrotic syndrome is as yet unclear. It is noteworthy that in children with steroid-sensitive nephrotic syndrome, zinc supplementation (at the recommended dietary allowance, 10 mg per day) for 12 months reduced the frequency of relapse. This finding could be ascribed to the documented role of zinc in preventing respiratory infections, which are the most predominant infectious triggers of relapse.

Patients with nephrotic syndrome often exhibit disturbances in vitamin D metabolism. Serum concentrations of 1,25-dihydroxyvitamin D [$1,25(OH)_2D$], the active metabolite of vitamin D, are decreased or in the normal range. More importantly, serum levels of 25-hydroxyvitamin D [25(OH)D], the best marker of vitamin D nutritional status, are reduced in patients with nephrotic syndrome. Urinary loss of vitamin D-binding protein secondary to proteinuria accounts for reduced 25(OH)D concentrations. Deficiency in 25(OH)D may lead to hypocalcemia, hyperparathyroidism, and reduced bone mineral density. This picture can be complicated by repeated exposure to glucocorticoids, which are known to adversely impact bone health, especially in pediatric patients. In this regard, a recent randomized controlled trial showed that in children with idiopathic nephrotic syndrome treated with prednisone for 12 weeks, supplementation with vitamin D_3 (1,000 IU per day) and calcium (500 mg per day) significantly improved bone mineral density.

Recommendations

Oral iron supplementation should be prescribed with caution in nephrotic patients with severe transferrinuria and iron-deficiency anemia because of the possible tubular injury induced by free iron. Subcutaneous administration of recombinant erythropoietin can be used for the treatment of erythropoietin-deficiency anemia in nephrotic syndrome. However, correction or amelioration of the underlying proteinuria would be the ideal approach to reverse these complications. In case of zinc deficiency, oral replacement is indicated. Nephrotic patients likely to be treated for at least 3 months with corticosteroids should receive daily supplements of oral calcium and vitamin D to ameliorate bone mineral density.

CONCLUSION

In patients with nephrotic syndrome, a comprehensive nutritional approach should embrace control of the amount and quality of protein and fat intake, dietary sodium restriction along with an adequate provision of energy and other nutrients, such as vitamins and minerals. However, practical fulfillment of these recommendations in the long run proved to be far from theory. Thus, a major goal is to improve patient's adherence to dietary prescriptions while averting the risk of nutritional impairment. Various strategies can be employed to pursue this aim, including counseling by skilled dietitians, individualization of dietary programs and intensive educational programs. Regular monitoring of nutritional status is also needed to assess compliance with the proposed diet and to detect signs of malnutrition as soon as possible.

Suggested Readings

Arun S, Bhatnagar S, Menon S, et al. Efficacy of zinc supplements in reducing relapses in steroid-sensitive nephrotic syndrome. *Pediatr Nephrol* 2009;24:1583–1586.

Bell S, Cooney J, Packard CJ, et al. The effect of omega-3 fatty acids on the atherogenic lipoprotein phenotype in patients with nephrotic range proteinuria. *Clin Nephrol* 2012;77:445–453.

Bellizzi V, Cupisti A, Locatelli F, et al. Low-protein diets for chronic kidney disease patients: the Italian experience. *BMC Nephrol* 2016;17(1):77. doi:10.1186/s12882-016-0280-0.

Cravedi P, Ruggenenti P, Remuzzi G. Proteinuria should be used as a surrogate in CKD. *Nat Rev Nephrol* 2012;8:301–306.

Denburg MR. Skeletal manifestations of renal disease in childhood. *Curr Opin Nephrol Hypertens* 2016;25:292–300.

Ferraro PM, Ferraccioli GF, Gambaro G, et al. Combined treatment with renin–angiotensin system blockers and polyunsaturated fatty acids in proteinuric IgA nephropathy: a randomized controlled trial. *Nephrol Dial Transplant* 2009;24: 156–160.

Kidney Disease Improving Global Outcomes (KDIGO) Glomerulonephritis Work Group. KDIGO clinical practice guideline for glomerulonephritis. *Kidney Int* 2012;2 (Suppl 2):139–274.

Perico N, Remuzzi A, Remuzzi G. Chapter 53: Mechanisms and consequences of proteinuria. Skorecki K, Chertow GM, Marsden PM, Taal MW, Yu ASL. In: *Brenner and Rector's The Kidney*. 10th ed. Philadelphia, PA: Elsevier Saunders; 2015:1780–1806.e8.

Vaziri ND. Erythropoietin and transferrin metabolism in nephrotic syndrome. *Am J Kidney Dis* 2001;38:1–8.

World Health Organization. *Protein and Amino Acid Requirements in Human Nutrition: Report of a Joint WHO/FAO/UNU Expert Consultation*. Geneva, Switzerland: WHO Press; 2007. Report 935.

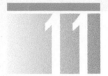

Nutritional Intervention in Progressive Chronic Kidney Disease

Fitsum Guebre-Egziabher
and Denis Fouque

Lipids and carbohydrates are completely processed or stored in the body, so protein and its nitrogen derivatives are the most important food-derived compounds handled by the kidney. At equilibrium, every gram of nitrogen from the diet is absorbed and rapidly eliminated into the urine. This property allows easy monitoring of protein intake by measuring excreted nitrogen (or urea) in urine. In healthy adults, increasing protein intake is associated with a concomitant increase in nitrogen output, whereas a diet with inadequate protein is associated with a markedly reduced urinary urea nitrogen output. This adaptive ability is limited because the body has obligatory daily nitrogen losses that are not influenced by protein intake, for example, nitrogen losses in feces, perspiration, hair, and nails. In patients with kidney disease, this loss has been estimated to be approximately 0.031 mg nitrogen per kg body weight (b.w.).

Protein requirements are estimated by standard methods, such as nitrogen balance or labeled *amino acid turnover*. These methods can characterize body nitrogen metabolism and the optimal level of protein intake for healthy adults and patients with chronic kidney disease (CKD). From these data, safe diets are devised for patients with varying levels of kidney disease.

Protein intake influences the degree of proteinuria (Fig. 11.1). Because proteinuria has been identified as one of the most important and independent risk factors for CKD progression, every attempt to lower proteinuria to minimal levels seems worthwhile. We address the potential influence of protein intake on kidney function, the optimal dietary protein for patients with CKD who have various levels of kidney function, the ways to monitor such diets, the potential side effects, and the results of large clinical trials and meta-analyses of low-protein dietary interventions on the course of CKD.

PROTEIN METABOLISM AND KIDNEY DISEASE

The typical Western diet contains about twice the protein intake recommended by the dietary guidelines. Overnutrition is associated with altered renal hemodynamics, particularly when there is a high level of protein or amino acid intake. Whether lipids or carbohydrates directly affect kidney function or disease is unclear, but there is ample evidence that a high animal protein intake will increase both renal blood flow and glomerular filtration rate (GFR) as well as urinary albumin excretion. In the long term, protein intake also influences the degree of glomerulosclerosis. By contrast, reducing the protein load may stop or even induce remission in the progression of experimental renal scarring. The impact of excessive animal protein intake on kidney function decline is multifactorial. Multiple humoral and local mediators triggered by amino acids or derived from their metabolism have been proposed to explain these alterations, including glucagon, insulin, insulin-like growth factor-1, angiotension II, prostaglandins, kinins and the potential increase in uremic toxins derived from the digestion of certain amino acids in the gastrointestinal tract. Furthermore, dietary protein is

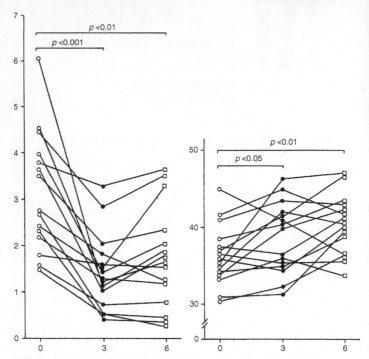

FIGURE 11.1 The decrease in proteinuria **(left panel)** and the concomitant increase in serum albumin **(right panel)** during 3 and 6 months' treatment with a very–low-protein diet (0.3 g/kg b.w./d) in 15 patients with Stage 4 CKD. CKD, chronic kidney disease. (From Aparicio M, Bouchet JL, Gin H, et al. Effect of a low-protein diet on urinary albumin excretion in uremic patients. *Nephron* 1988;50:288–291, with permission.)

the source of phosphate and acid load and sodium intake parallels protein ingestion. Sodium retention may also be associated with protein-induced hyperfiltration via activity of the proximal, sodium–amino acid cotransporter. Protein restriction ablates hemodynamic changes related to 5/6 nephrectomy because it reduces glomerular pressure and flow.

Glomerular protein trafficking induces hypermetabolism and oxidant stress, while a low-protein diet (LPD) reduces oxygen consumption and malondialdehyde production. The nature of protein absorbed may also influence the renal response because the GFR of vegetarians is reportedly lower than that of omnivores. One hypothesis is that animal source proteins produce greater amount of acids than plant source proteins. When rats with CKD were fed casein or soy proteins, proteinuria and histologic renal damage were always more severe compared with results in rats fed protein of vegetable origin. In humans, studies have shown that addition of plant source proteins in patients with CKD preserves GFR.

Levels of growth factors and profibrotic agents, such as transforming growth factor-β, fibronectin, and plasminogen activator inhibitor-1, are modulated by an LPD, resulting in reduced proteinuria and kidney injury. Finally, albuminuria per se possesses pathogenic effects promoting tubulointerstitial scar and apoptosis, and LPD can independently decrease glomerular capillary pressure and albuminuria, adding a protective antifibrotic and antiapoptotic effect.

OPTIMAL LEVEL OF DIETARY PROTEIN AND ENERGY INTAKE

A Western diet contains approximately 1.4 g protein/kg/d; women have a daily protein intake that is 35% to 50% lower than men because of their lower b.w., and aging also affects protein intake; it is spontaneously reduced 15% by the age of 70 years. The median optimal protein intake according to the World Health Organization and Food and Agriculture Organization in 2007 is 0.66 g protein/kg/d. The safe level was identified as the 97.5th percentile of the population distribution of requirement, that is, 0.83 g/kg/d. These values for average and safe intakes are about 10% higher than the values proposed in 1985 (0.6 g). There is a Gaussian distribution of protein requirements, however, explaining why some patients do well with protein intakes below the average recommended values. Finally, the protein requirements have been estimated in healthy adults or in patients with kidney disease who were receiving a controlled energy intake of at least 35 kcal/kg/d, and the diet may not be applicable to healthy adults or patients with CKD with a reduced energy intake. Interestingly, the basal metabolic rate and energy requirements in patients with CKD who are not on maintenance dialysis do not differ from those in healthy adults, and nitrogen balance is obtained when a protein intake is 0.6 g/kg/d. In 2012, the Kidney Disease Improving Global Outcomes of the National Kidney Foundation recommended that protein and energy intake should be 0.8 g protein/kg/d in adults with diabetes or without diabetes and GFR <30 mL/min/1.73 m^2 with appropriate education and to avoid protein intake >1.3 g/kg/d in adults with CKD at risk of progression. These recommendations change when maintenance dialysis treatment is initiated. However, there are spontaneous reductions in energy and protein intake when kidney function decreases, leading to intake values as low as 21 kcal and 0.85 g protein/kg b.w./d in patients with Stage 3 CKD (estimated GFR <30 mL per minute). Notably, for an equal amount of protein, a diet with 70% of protein from vegetable sources enables a greater amount of calories to be consumed than a diet consisting of 70% of its protein from animal sources. Because energy intake may decrease when kidney function falls, a defect in protein metabolism may occur with an inadequate dietary energy intake. Obviously, patients with CKD will need instruction in methods for achieving an optimal, moderately low-protein intake and adequate energy intake.

METABOLIC CONSEQUENCES OF REDUCED PROTEIN INTAKE IN CHRONIC KIDNEY DISEASE

Nature of Protein-Restricted Diets

Healthy adults or patients with CKD have been shown to adapt to a dietary protein intake as low as 0.3 g protein/kg/d (very–low-protein diet, VLPD), if energy and essential amino acid (EAA) requirements are met. To avoid nutritional deficits, supplements of EAA or keto acids (KA) of amino acids have been suggested; the KAs are synthesized into the corresponding EAAs. Without these supplements, intakes as low as 0.6 g protein/kg/d can be safely used if at least 50% of the protein is of high biologic value (e.g., principally from animal sources) and energy intake meets the recommended goal (i.e., 35 kcal/kg/d for patients younger than 65 years and 30 to 35 kcal/kg/d for those >65 years). If lower levels of protein intake are prescribed, supplements (EAA or KA) should be considered to avoid inducing an EAA deficit. The potential benefits are that low dietary protein intake can slow the progression of CKD and alleviate uremic symptoms and postpone the start of maintenance dialysis or prolong survival when dialysis opportunities are limited.

Adaptation to Protein Metabolism

An adaptive response (i.e., a decrease in whole body leucine flux and oxidation) occurs in patients with Stages 3 and 4 CKD who had a 40% reduction in their dietary protein intake (i.e., from 1.1 to 0.7 g/kg/d) during a period of 3 months; body composition is maintained. This adaptive response was also observed with a more restricted protein intake (0.35 g/kg/d supplemented with KA) treated over an extended period of 16 months. The adaptation has also been observed in patients with CKD with nephrotic syndrome when their protein intake was reduced from 1.85 to 1.0 g protein/kg/d. The LPD was even more beneficial in nephrotic patients with CKD who were tested while their intake was reduced from 1.20 to 0.66 g protein/kg/d; amino acid metabolism improved, and there was a strong reduction in proteinuria, leading to increased serum albumin concentrations. Thus, with adequate energy supply, patients with CKD correctly adapt their protein metabolism.

Glucose Metabolism

Insulin resistance is common during the course of CKD, and glycemic control can improve with attention to nutrition. After 3 months of an LPD, insulin sensitivity improved and there was reduced fasting serum insulin or daily insulin needs and blood glucose values and endogenous glucose production. The mechanisms for these benefits are unclear, but the results are encouraging.

Control of Chronic Kidney Disease—Mineral and Bone Disorders

Because proteins of animal origin are strongly associated with phosphate (1 g protein approximately contains 13 mg of phosphorus), limiting dietary protein intake reduces the phosphate intake and hence the amount that must be excreted. With calcium salts of KA as a supplement, there also is extra calcium. Both low phosphate intake and calcium supplements reduce serum parathormone levels and improve renal osteodystrophy, and this has been shown during 12 months of an LPD supplemented with KA. Given the adverse effects of excessive calcium intake in patients with advanced CKD, calcium containing KA supplements must be used with caution.

Improvement in Lipid Profile

The reduced protein intake of animal origin (e.g., meat and dairy products) generally entails a decrease in saturated lipids, leading to an improvement in the overall serum lipid profile. For example, reducing protein intake for 3 months from 1.1 to 0.7 g/kg/d resulted in an increase in serum lipoprotein AI and in the Apo-AI–Apo-B ratio, changes considered to reduce the cardiovascular risk in general population. Likewise, a 6-month LPD regimen decreased red cell malondialdehyde and increased polyunsaturated fatty acids, particularly C22:4 and C22:5, thereby limiting oxidative stress.

Correction of Metabolic Acidosis

Correction of acidosis and a decreased need of bicarbonate supplementation have been documented for patients on VLPD supplemented with KA, an effect that may also be related to the nature of the ingested protein.

Reduction in Proteinuria and Improvement of Kidney Injury

Lowering dietary protein intake induces a decrease in proteinuria (see Fig. 11.1). Because proteinuria is now identified as an independent risk factor for progression of CKD, every attempt to reverse proteinuria is worthwhile. Whether reducing protein intake will protect the kidney from progressive injury in humans is less clear. First, experimental studies used diets with extreme differences in protein intake. Obviously, the clinical use of these diets does not allow this much variation. Second, protein in food is associated with other factors such as phosphorus, sodium, energy, and water that could affect kidney function. Third, a single intervention can be studied experimentally, but in clinical practice, patients generally receive several nephroprotective interventions that may mask the true effect of the diet as a single intervention. Besides angiotensin-converting enzyme (ACE) inhibitors, AT1 receptor blockers, or both, and LPD might confer additional protection against progression of kidney disease and may potentially postpone end-stage renal disease (ESRD).

Hypocaloric Risk

Without adequate counseling, too few calories may be contained in the protein-restricted diet. With adequate supervision, however, energy intakes are usually greater than 30 kcal/kg/d, and body composition is unchanged during long-term LPD therapy. However, clinical trials have led to the conclusion that even at fairly low energy intake, long-term nutritional status, as measured by dual-energy x-ray absorptiometry or anthropometry, does not reveal significant changes. Furthermore, patients treated with LPD for years had a survival rate during maintenance dialysis similar to that achieved by other therapies.

MONITORING NUTRITIONAL INTAKE

Protein intake can be estimated from two sources: (i) intake from dietary reports and (ii) output from urinary urea excretion in patients without ESRD, or protein nitrogen appearance (PNA), formerly called protein catabolic rate. Two formulas are routinely used to assess nitrogen (N) and thus protein intake in CKD:

$$\text{N intake (g/d)} = \text{UNA (g/d)} + 0.031 \times \text{b.w. (kg)} \ (1)$$

$$\text{N intake (g/d)} = 1.20 \times \text{UNA (g/d)} + 1.74 \ (2)$$

where b.w. is the patient's edema-free body weight (Table 11.1).

Adherence to an LPD is defined by an intake equal to ±20% of prescribed intake. In well-controlled studies, protein intake tends to be greater than the prescribed amount by 10% to 20%, with 40% to 70% of patients meeting the required intakes. Thus, repeated efforts are needed to support the nutritional care of patients with CKD.

TABLE 11.1	Estimation of Dietary Protein Intake Based on a Daily Urinary Nitrogen Appearance in a Stable, 80-kg Adult Patient Prescribed with a 0.6 g protein/kg/d Diet

Patient's UNA = 5.2 g/d and protein is 16% nitrogen (nitrogen intake × 6.25 protein intake)

UNA + 0.031 × 80 kg = 5.2 + 2.48 = 7.68 g N DPI = 7.68 g × 6.25 = 48 g; thus, DPI/kg = 48 g / 80 kg = 0.60 g/kg b.w./d (1)

Or

1.2 × UNA + 1.74 = 6.24 + 1.74 = 7.98 N DPI = 7.98 × 6.25 = 49.9 g; thus, DPI/kg = 49.9/80 = 0.62 g/kg b.w./d (2)

Protein intake <20% more than prescribed intake, is considered acceptable (i.e., a UNA = 6.3 g/d for this patient).

DPI, dietary protein index; UNA, urinary nitrogen appearance.

From Masud T, Manatunga A, Cotsonis G, et al. The precision of estimating protein intake of patients with chronic renal failure. *Kidney Int* 2002;62:1750–1756, with permission.

	Nutritional Follow-up and Dietary Counseling in Patients with Chronic Kidney Disease Stages 3B-4 and 5 before End-stage Renal Disease	
Time Span	**To Do**	**Result**
Every 6 mo; then every 12 mo	Dietary interview	Develop a care plan; tailor diet to patient taste and economic situation
	Home 3-d food record	Record energy intake; verify adequate understanding of diet and adherence from urinary urea
	24-hr urinary urea	Estimate protein intake
Every 12 mo	Body mass index, anthropometry (optional), subjective global assessment (optional)	
Every 6–12 mo	Serum albumin, serum, prealbumin, serum cholesterol	
	C-reactive protein	

If glomerular filtration rate is <15 mL/min, the nutritional survey should be more frequent, particularly if a superimposed disease occurs; consider starting dialysis treatment if follow-up does not show improvement in nutritional status or laboratory markers.

Energy expenditure can be reliably assessed through indirect calorimetry, the Harris–Benedict formula, or physical activity questionnaires. The optimal energy intake is 35 kcal/kg/d and 30 to 35 kcal/kg/d in patients older than 60 years, but energy intake can only be deduced from dietary interviews or records. We estimate that at least four interviews are necessary to ensure an understanding by the patient of the goals and requirements of an LPD and an optimal energy intake as well as how an adequate home food record should be kept. A general system for patient follow-up is proposed in Table 11.2.

EVIDENCE FOR AN OPTIMAL PROTEIN INTAKE FOR PATIENTS WITH PROGRESSIVE CHRONIC KIDNEY DISEASE

Numerous trials have tried to assess the relationship between the level of protein intake and the potential deleterious or protective effects on the kidney. Some concessions have to be made when interpreting the findings of these trials.

Assessing Kidney Tissue Damage and Estimating Kidney Function

A major caveat for quantifying renal damage in humans is that repeated histologic analyses are not available. In addition, serial measures of kidney function over time are difficult because of the interaction between kidney function markers (e.g., serum creatinine, 1/serum creatinine, urinary creatinine clearance, or creatinine-based formula to estimate GFR) and protein intake. Indeed, variations in dietary protein intake with changes in creatine and creatinine intake can interfere with estimates of kidney function. Serum creatinine and creatinine clearance can also be affected by several medications, such as cimetidine, interfering with tubular excretion of creatinine. Third, and more importantly, a large change in dietary protein index (DPI) can acutely change GFR. Reducing DPI may initially lower GFR by 10% to 20%

until a new equilibrium is reached. Consequently, a delay of 3 to 4 months is mandatory before an effect of protein intake on GFR can be identified as beneficial on CKD progression.

Methodological Caveats

An important aspect of clinical research relies on the methodological quality, design, and reports of trials. Several criteria now exist for rating trials, generating evidence, and producing clinical guidance: Evidence level A is obtained from the best-quality, large, randomized controlled trials (RCT) and meta-analyses (Grades 1 and 2). Evidence level B is from prospective controlled clinical trials (Grade 3), and Evidence level C, the lowest ranking, is information acquired from retrospective trials, case reports, or expert opinion (Grades 4 and 5). We extensively searched the literature published since 1974 and excluded more than 50 low-quality studies (too small in size or uncontrolled), leaving only 11 RCT and 5 meta-analyses that were suitable for evaluating the influence on dietary protein and changes in kidney function.

Results of Major Randomized Clinical Trials and Meta-analyses
Randomized Clinical Trials

Rosman et al. studied the influence of protein restriction in 247 patients over 4 years. Protein intake was 0.90 to 0.95 g/kg/d in patients whose GFR was between 60 and 30 mL per minute and was reduced to 0.70 to 0.80 g/kg/d in patients whose GFR was between 30 and 10 mL per minute; protein intake for the control groups was not restricted. After 2 years, the loss of GFR was significantly slowed. After 4 years, a marked improvement in survival was observed in patients treated with the more restricted protein intake (survival without requiring dialysis was 60% for the dietary protein-restricted group and 30% for the dietary protein unrestricted patients, $p < 0.025$). Adherence to the LPDs was very good after a short period of training and was sustained over time without evidence of malnutrition.

Ihle et al. studied 72 patients with advanced kidney disease for 18 months. The patients were randomized to a protein-unrestricted control diet or 0.4 g protein/kg/d. Actual protein intake, estimated from urinary urea, was 0.8 or 0.6 g/kg/d. The GFR decreased only in the control group and the number of patients who initiated dialysis during the trial was significantly greater in this group ($p < 0.005$). There was no decrease in GFR in the LPD group. Body composition varied, with a loss of b.w. in the LPD group, but no change in other anthropometric measures or in serum albumin levels occurred in either group. The authors concluded that moderate reduction in protein intake exerts a beneficial effect.

Williams et al. studied the three different interventions in 95 patients with Stage 4 and 5 CKD over 18 months. Patients were randomly assigned to receive a diet of 0.6 g protein/kg/d and 800 mg phosphate (LPD group), a diet of 1,000 mg phosphate per day plus phosphate binders but no specific dietary protein restriction (low-phosphate group), or a diet with no protein or phosphate restriction. Dietary adherence, estimated by urinary urea output and diet recalls, averaged 0.7, 1.02, and 1.14 g protein/kg/d and 815, 1,000, and 1,400 mg phosphorus per day, respectively. Slight weight losses were observed in the protein- and phosphate-restricted groups (-1.3 and -1.65 kg for the LPD and low-phosphate group, respectively). No difference was observed in any of the three groups in the rate of decrease in creatinine clearance over time. Death or the initiation of dialysis therapy did not differ among the three groups. Both the small size of the study and the GFR estimation by creatinine clearance greatly limit the value of this study.

The Northern Italian Cooperative Study Group studied 456 patients with GFRs <60 mL per minute during 2 years. Patients were randomly prescribed 1 g protein/kg/d (control group) or 0.6 g/kg/d (LPD). The main outcome was "renal survival," defined as dialysis initiation or doubling of the serum creatinine. The control group ate 0.90 g protein/kg/d, and the LPD group ate 0.78 g/kg/d with a large overlap between groups. Only a borderline difference existed between control and LPD groups, with slightly fewer patients in the LPD group reaching a renal endpoint ($p = 0.059$).

Malvy et al. examined a diet with more severe protein restriction (0.3 g protein/kg/d) supplemented with a mixture of EAA and KA supplements (Ketosteril, 0.17 g/kg/d) and compared results from patients eating 0.65 g protein/kg/d. Fifty patients with severe kidney disease (GFR $\leq$ 20 mL per minute) were followed until dialysis or until GFR was <5 mL per minute. For patients with advanced disease at inclusion, the "half-life" for renal death was 9 months in those prescribed 0.65 g protein/kg/d; it was 21 months in those treated with the most restricted diet. There was a loss of 2.7 kg over 3 years in the group assigned to the VLPD; no weight loss or body composition change occurred with those assigned to the 0.65 g protein/kg diet.

Mirescu et al. assessed a VLPD (0.3 g/kg/d) diet supplemented with KAs (Ketosteril, 1 pill/5 kg b.w./d) and compared results with those from patients assigned to 0.6 g/kg/d; 53 nondiabetic patients with Stage 4 CKD with moderate proteinuria were studied. The VLPD was associated with an increase in serum bicarbonate and serum calcium and a reduction in blood urea nitrogen and serum phosphate. There were significantly fewer patients entering dialysis in the very–low-protein group (4%) compared with the low-protein group (27%; $p = 0.01$).

Cianciaruso et al. reported on 423 patients with Stages 4 and 5 CKD who received either a 0.8 or a 0.55 g protein/kg/d diet for 18 months. Actual protein intakes estimated from urinary nitrogen were 0.92 versus 0.72 g protein/kg/d, respectively. There were 9 renal deaths in the 212 patients in the protein-restricted group versus 13 in the 211 patients assigned to the 0.8 g/kg/d group ($p =$ NS). Most metabolic parameters and/or medications were improved with the lower protein intake group.

The MDRD study tested the effects of low-protein intake and strict blood pressure control on the progression of kidney disease in more than 800 patients (Study A, GFR: 25 to 55 mL/min/1.73 m^2 and Study B, GFR: 13 to 24 mL/min/1.73 m^2). In Study A, patients received 1 g protein/kg/d or more and were treated to a mean blood pressure of 105 mm Hg. The LPD patients received 0.6 g protein/kg/d and a mean blood pressure of 92 mm Hg. In Study B, patients received 0.6 or 0.3 g protein/kg/d plus a KA supplement and were treated to blood pressure goals comparable to those in Study A. The mean follow-up was 2.2 years, and achieved protein intakes were 1.11 g versus 0.73 g protein/kg/d in Study A (n = 585), and 0.69 versus 0.46 g protein/kg/d in Study B (n = 255). No difference was observed in GFR decline between groups in Study A. There was a trend for a faster GFR decline in the 0.60 g protein/kg/d diet group as compared with the 0.46 g/kg/d plus KA group of Study B ($p = 0.07$).

During the first 4 months in Study A, a sharp decrease in GFR was observed in the group with the more restricted protein intake (0.73 g/kg/d). This difference was attributed to the physiologic reduction in glomerular hemodynamics that follows protein restriction. Subsequently, there was a slower GFR decline compared with results from the group eating the higher protein intake (1.11 g/kg/d). If the initial hemodynamic effect is eliminated (from 4 months after the start until 3 years), the slope of GFR decrease was significantly lower in patients assigned to more restricted protein group; renal survival also improved ($p = 0.009$). These analyses support the conclusion that there is a moderate beneficial effect of reduced protein intakes in patients with CKD. A long-term evaluation of the MDRD study showed that patients assigned to the VLPD didn't have a lower progression of their function but had increased death, but this study was limited by the absence of control during follow-up.

More recently, Garneata et al. reported a single-center study with 207 nondiabetic CKD patients (eGFR < 30 mL/min/1.73 m^2 and urinary protein per creatinine ratio <1 g per g) who were randomly assigned to a conventional low-protein diet (0.6 g/kg/d) or SVLPD (0.3 g/kg/d vegetable protein) supplemented with ketoanalogues (Ketosteril) 1 cp/5 kg b.w. for 15 months. They were able to show a reduction of primary end point (renal replacement therapy or >50% reduction of initial eGFR) with correction of most metabolic abnormalities in the SVLPD group without detrimental effect on nutritional status estimated by subjective global assessment. The compliance for the diet was good (3% of selected subjects left the study) but only 44% of the initial population was selected after a 3 months run in period for their compliance for such a diet. Furthermore, it cannot be excluded that some of the effects might also be related from the nature of the protein that was ingested because they compared a conventional protein-restricted diet to a vegetarian diet.

Meta-analyses

To clarify these issues, a series of meta-analyses have been performed (Fig. 11.2). The criterion analyzed was renal death (i.e., the occurrence of death, the need to start dialysis, or a given GFR decrease during the course of the study). Literature published since 1974 was examined, and only RCT with a follow-up of at least 1 year were included. Among 2,000 patients (1,002 in LPD groups and 998 in control or larger protein intake groups), there were 281 renal deaths (113 in the low-protein diet and 168 in the larger protein intake) and the risk ratio was in favor of low-protein diet (RR 0.68, 95% confidence interval 0.55 to 0.84, $p = 0.0002$). When using a meta-analysis to address the effect of LPDs on GFR, Kasiske et al. reported that in more than 1,900 patients, a beneficial effect for patients with lower protein intake spared 0.53 mL/min/yr of GFR ($p < 0.05$).

The effects of protein restriction in patients with diabetes are somewhat less clear. Indeed, some clinical trials included participants with large varying degrees of CKD stages and proteinuria, different types of protein diets and are of shorter duration, during which renal death cannot be taken into account. Furthermore, they address surrogate criteria such as reductions in microalbuminuria, proteinuria, and creatinine clearance. In addition, in many older trials, ACE inhibitors were not equally distributed, and blood pressure control was not strictly comparable between groups. Zeller et al. compared 1 g protein/kg/d versus 0.6 g protein/kg/d in 36 patients with insulin-dependent diabetes mellitus (IDDM) for at least 1 year (mean follow-up, 35 months). Actual protein intake was 1.08 g protein/kg/d versus 0.72 g protein/kg/d. The investigators observed a substantial reduction in GFR (iothalamate method) decline in the group treated with an LPD ($p < 0.02$) but only in the subgroup of patients with a GFR greater than 45 mL per minute. Hansen et al. reported the longest randomized trial to date in patients with IDDM. Patients were given their usual protein intake or 0.6 g protein/kg/d and were followed for 4 years. Actual protein intake during the entire trial duration was 1.02 g/kg/d versus 0.89 g/kg/d, a slight but significant difference. No difference in proteinuria was observed, but renal death was reduced by 36% in patients treated with moderately restricted dietary protein. Cox analysis was performed after adjusting for cardiovascular disease, and the difference was even more significant ($p = 0.01$). Koya et al. conducted

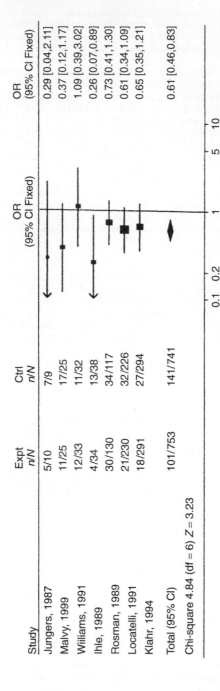

Study	Expt n/N	Ctrl n/N	OR (95% CI Fixed)	OR (95% CI Fixed)
Jungers, 1987	5/10	7/9		0.29 [0.04,2.11]
Malvy, 1999	11/25	17/25		0.37 [0.12,1.17]
Wiiliams, 1991	12/33	11/32		1.09 [0.39,3.02]
Ihle, 1989	4/34	13/38		0.26 [0.07,0.89]
Rosman, 1989	30/130	34/117		0.73 [0.41,1.30]
Locatelli, 1991	21/230	32/226		0.61 [0.34,1.09]
Klahr, 1994	18/291	27/294		0.65 [0.35,1.21]
Total (95% CI)	101/753	141/741		0.61 [0.46,0.83]

Chi-square 4.84 (df = 6) Z = 3.23

FIGURE 11.2 Meta-analysis of the results of low-protein diets in patients with CKD. A *square* denotes the odds ratio (treatment/control) for each trial, and *diamonds* indicate overall results of trials combined. 95% CI are represented by *horizontal lines.* Overall "common" OR = 0.68 (95% CI 0.55 to 0.84), p = 0.00024. CI, confidence interval; CKD, chronic kidney disease; OR, odds ratio. (From Fouque D, Laville M. Low protein diets for chronic kidney disease in non diabetic adults. *Cochrane Database Syst Rev* 2009;(3):CD001892. doi:10.1002/1465 1858.CD001892, with permission.)

a randomized trial in type 2 diabetic subjects with a 5-year follow-up. The achieved protein intake from dietary record in the restricted diet was 0.9 g/kg/d versus 1.1 g/kg/d in the control group ($p < 0.0001$) without difference in protein intake estimated from 24-hour urinary nitrogen excretion. The dietary intervention didn't confer renal protection effect. In a meta-analysis of a subgroup of patients with diabetes, Pedrini et al. showed that a combined criterion of increasing microalbuminuria and reducing kidney function was improved by 44% ($p < 0.001$) in subjects assigned to an LPD. Robertson et al. performed a systematic review of RCT (nine studies) and before and after studies (three studies) of modified or restricted protein diet of at least 4 months in types 1 and 2 diabetic patients' renal function. The results show that reducing protein intake is associated with a lower but not significant decline of GFR in both types 1 and 2 diabetic patients but there was concern on the level of protein intake and compliance to the diet. Pan et al. conducted a meta-analysis on eight RCT trials assessing the effect of LPD on both types 1 and 2 diabetic nephropathy and weren't able to show any beneficial effect of the protein-restricted diet on kidney function, although both HbA1c and proteinuria were decreased. It is difficult to make strong conclusions from these results because Pan et al. included diabetic patients with mostly Grades 1 and 2 CKD with microalbuminuria, proteinuria, and nephrotic syndrome with most studies that were limited to 6 to 12 months of intervention that may not be long enough to observe benefits specially for those with higher degree of proteinuria. Furthermore, the reduction of GFR that may be seen in subjects with higher GFR may be related to a hemodynamic change. Moreover, protein intake for more than 50% of the subjects assigned to LPD was too high and ranged from 0.7 to 1.1 g/kg/d. Another systematic review and meta-analysis of RCT (13 studies enrolling 779 patients) evaluating the effect of low-protein diet on kidney function of patients with diabetic nephropathy has reported a significant improvement in GFR (5.8 mL/min/1.73 m^2) that was consistent across subgroups of type of diabetes and GFR category and intervention period. However, this improvement was demonstrated only for subjects that were compliant for the diet. A recent meta-analysis of 15 RCT with dietary intervention of at least 1 year and including 1,965 subjects has shown a beneficial effect of protein restriction on the progression of CKD only in type 1 diabetic subjects. The achieved protein intake of the restricted group was 0.83 g/kg/d versus 1.07 g/kg/d for the control arm.

CONCLUSION

Patients with impaired kidney function must have dietary adjustments to avoid the complications of CKD. There is convincing evidence that during Stages 3 and 4 CKD (i.e., for a GFR between 60 and 15 mL per minute), protein intake should be reduced from a typical Western diet to 0.6 to 0.8 g/kg/d. The diet must be tailored to meet individual requirements, adherence, and body composition by regular support and education of nutritional principals and dietary advice.

Suggested Readings

Fouque D, Laville M. Low protein diets for chronic kidney disease in non diabetic adults. *Cockrane Database Syst Rev* 2009;(3):CD001892.

Garneata L, Stancu A, Dragomir D, et al. Ketoanalogue-supplemented vegetarian very low-protein diet and CKD progression. *J Am Soc Nephrol* 2016;27:2164–2176.

Goodship TH, Mitch WE, Hoerr RA, et al. Adaptation to low-protein diets in renal failure: leucine turnover and nitrogen balance. *J Am Soc Nephrol* 1990;1:66–75.

Ikizler TA, Greene JH, Wingard RL, et al. Spontaneous dietary protein intake during progression of chronic renal failure. *J Am Soc Nephrol* 1995;6:1386–1391.

Kasiske BL, Lakatua JD, Ma JZ, et al. A meta-analysis of the effects of dietary protein restriction on the rate of decline in renal function. *Am J Kidney Dis* 1998;31:954–961.

Kidney Disease Improving Global Outcomes. 2012 Clinical Practice guideline for the evaluation and management of chronic kidney disease. *Kidney Int Suppl* 2013;3: 19–62.

Klahr S, Levey AS, Beck GJ, et al; Modification of Diet in Renal Disease Study Group. The effects of dietary protein restriction and blood-pressure control on the progression of chronic renal disease. *N Engl J Med* 1994;330:877–884.

Nezu U, Kamiyama H, Kondo Y, et al. Effect of low-protein diet on kidney function in diabetic nephropathy: meta-analysis of randomised controlled trials. *BMC Open* 2013;28:pii:e002934.

Rughooputh MS, Zeng R, Yao Y. Protein diet restriction slows chronic kidney disease progression in non-diabetic and in type 1 diabetic patients, but not in type 2 diabetic patients: a meta-analysis of randomized controlled trials using glomerular filtration rate as a surrogate. *PLoS One* 2015;10:e0145505.

12

Nutritional Requirements in Hemodialysis Patients

T. Alp Ikizler

Patients with end-stage renal disease (ESRD) receiving maintenance hemo-dialysis (MHD) are among the highest risk for protein–energy wasting (PEW) of chronic kidney disease (CKD). Given the strong association between the extent of PEW and major adverse clinical outcomes, the prevention and treatment of PEW is imperative in MHD patients. Multiple factors not only related to advanced kidney disease but also inherent to hemodialysis therapy affect nutritional and metabolic status of MHD patients, necessitating a comprehensive combination of strategies to diminish protein and energy depletion, and to institute therapies that will avoid further losses (Fig. 12.1).

DIAGNOSIS OF PROTEIN–ENERGY WASTING IN MAINTENANCE HEMODIALYSIS PATIENTS

A summary of nutritional parameters for detecting PEW in MHD patients and their applicability for guiding nutritional therapies is provided in Table 12.1. Detailed discussion related to diagnosis of PEW can be found in Chapter 2. Issues only pertinent to MHD patients will be discussed in this chapter.

Assessment of Visceral Protein Stores

Serum albumin has been used most widely as a nutritional marker in MHD patients. This is primarily due to its easy availability and strong association with hospitalization and death risk. Unfortunately, there are many nonnutritional factors that influence serum albumin concentrations such as decreased synthesis from liver diseases, increased transcapillary losses, increased losses from the gastrointestinal tract and kidneys and from tissue injuries such as wounds, burns, and peritonitis. Serum albumin has also been shown to decrease with volume overload, which is a highly prevalent condition in MHD patients. Serum albumin (a "negative acute-phase reactant") is also affected by conditions such as inflammation, infection, and trauma, which decrease albumin synthesis, leading to prompt decreases in serum albumin concentration. Consequently, the decrease in serum albumin can reflect the degree of illness and inflammation, rather than nutritional status. Because a low serum albumin is highly predictive of poor clinical outcomes at all stages of CKD, it is still considered a reliable screening index that there can be abnormalities in a patient's nutritional status.

Serum transferrin is another potential nutritional biomarkers, but its concentration is influenced by changes in iron stores, the presence of inflammation and changes in extracellular volume. Consequently, it is not a good indicator of nutritional status when used alone. Although very responsive to dietary nutrient intake, serum prealbumin may rise because of decreasing kidney function. In addition, prealbumin is a negative acute phase reactant so its utility in monitoring nutritional status is questionable in MHD patients. Since serum albumin is also a negative acute phase reactant like prealbumin, it is reasonable to measure the C-reactive protein (CRP), an acute phase

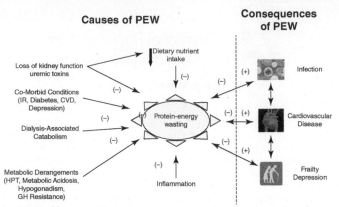

FIGURE 12.1 The conceptual model for etiology and consequences of PEW in chronic kidney disease. CVD, cardiovascular disease; GH, growth hormone; HPT, hyperparathyroidism; IR, insulin resistance; PEW, protein–energy wasting. (Modified with permission from Ikizler TA, Cano NJ, Franch H, et al. Prevention and treatment of protein energy wasting in chronic kidney disease patients: a Consensus Statement by the International Society of Renal Nutrition and Metabolism. *Kidney Int* 2013;84:1096–1107.)

reactant and an index of inflammation when serum concentrations of albumin or prealbumin are low or decline from normal over a period of time.

Assessment of Body Composition

The assessment of body composition and somatic protein stores is based on the measurement of different body compartments (water, fat, bone, muscle, and visceral organs). The fat-free mass (mainly composed of muscle) is the major somatic protein mass. Generally, somatic protein stores are preserved in MHD patients but when there are catabolic illnesses, depletion of fat-free mass will occur. We use body composition techniques to diagnose protein depletion and to monitor efficacy of nutritional therapies. Simple anthropometric measures can provide a guide over long term treatment and bioelectrical impedance analysis and dual-energy x-ray absorptiometry (DEXA) can be used for research purposes as long as it is recognized that both of these techniques are greatly influenced by changes in body water, a complication that is common in MHD patients.

Composite Indices of Nutritional Status

The diagnostic measures based on changes in body composition and dietary intake assessment has been accompanied by a subjective assessment of overall nutritional status, especially when large numbers of patients are being evaluated. The most commonly used composite indices include subjective global assessment (SGA) or its modified or expanded indices such as the composite nutritional index and the malnutrition–inflammation score (MIS). These measures can only provide a general assessment because they evaluate nutritional status from a broader perspective, including medical history, symptoms, and physical parameters.

The Kidney Disease Outcome Quality of the National Kidney Foundation (NKF K/DOQI) guidelines included a recommendation that the modified SGA should be performed every 6 months in MHD patients. However, its subjective nature, the absence of measures of visceral protein stores and

TABLE 12.1 Suggested Table to Monitor Nutritional Status and Guide Therapy in Kidney Failure

Simple (Monthly) Assessment	Findings	Possible Interventions
BW	Continuous decline or <85% IBW	Suspect of PEW and perform more detailed nutritional assessment
Serum albumin	<4.0 g/dL	Consider preventive measures
Serum creatinine	Relatively low predialysis values	No specific intervention needed at this point

Detailed Assessment	Findings	Possible Interventions (Simple)
Serum prealbumin	<30 mg/dL, and/or	Dietary counseling: DPI ≥1.2 g/kg/d, energy intake 30–35 kcal/d
Serum transferrin	<200 mg/dL, and/or	
LBM and/or fat mass	Unexpected decrease	Increase dialysis dose to Kt/V >1.4
SGA	Worsening	Use biocompatible membranes
		Upper GI motility enhancer
		Consider timely initiation of CDT

Repeat Detailed Assessment (2–3 mo from Previous)	Findings	Possible Interventions (Moderate to Complex)
Serum prealbumin	<30 mg/dL, and/or	Nutritional supplements: Oral, enteric tube feeding, IDPN (requires Medicare approval)
Serum transferrin	<200 mg/dL, and/or	
IGF-I	<200 ng/mL, and/or	Anabolic factors:
Serum creatinine	Relatively low predialysis values, and/or	Anabolic steroids
LBM and/or fat mass	Unexpected decrease	rhGH (*experimental*)
C-reactive protein	>10 mg/L	Appetite stimulants: Megase; Ghrelin (experimental)
		Anti-inflammatory (experimental)

Adapted from Pupim LB, Cuppari L, Ikizler TA. Nutrition and metabolism in kidney disease. *Semin Nephrol* 2006;26:134–157, with permission.
BW, body weight; CDT, Chronic Dialysis Treatment; DPI, dietary protein index; GI, gastrointestinal; IBW, ideal body weight; IDPN, intradialytic parenteral nutrition; IGF-1, Insulin like growth factor-1; LBM, lean body mass; PEW, protein–energy wasting; rhGH, recombinant human growth hormone; SGA, subjective global assessment.

its relative insensitivity to small changes in nutritional status greatly limit the usefulness of the SGA. The MIS incorporates components of the SGA and includes components related to nutritional status (body mass index) and inflammation (serum albumin concentration and total iron binding capacity) plus indices that are not directly related to nutritional status, such as comorbidities and functional status. We believe that if used, the SGA or MIS should be accompanied by parameters that include body weight and

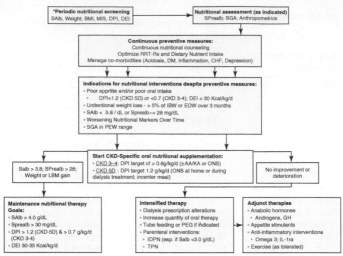

FIGURE 12.2 Algorithm for nutritional management and support in patients with chronic kidney disease. *Minimum every 3 months, monthly screening recommended. ^Only for ESRD patients without residual renal function. SAlb, serum albumin (measured by bromo-cresol green); BMI, body mass index; MIS, malnutrition–inflammation score; DPI, dietary protein index; DEI, dietary energy intake; SPrealb, serum prealbumin; SGA, subjective global assessment; RRT-Rx, renal replacement therapy prescription; DM, diabetes mellitus; CHF, congestive heart failure; CKD, chronic kidney disease; PEW, protein–energy wasting; LBM, lean body mass; ONS, oral nutritional supplement; PEG, percutaneous endoscopic gastrostomy; IDPN, intradialytic parenteral nutrition; TPN, total parenteral nutrition; GH, growth hormone; IL-1ra, interleukin-1 receptor antagonist. (Reprinted with permission from Ikizler TA, Cano NJ, Franch H, et al. Prevention and treatment of protein energy wasting in chronic kidney disease patients: a Consensus Statement by the International Society of Renal Nutrition and Metabolism. *Kidney Int* 2013;8:1096–1107.)

weight-for-height, skinfold measures, and serum albumin concentration (for SGA) plus other estimates of protein stores.

The critical point is that the nutritional status of MHD patients should be monitored regularly to detect nutritional disturbances early. In addition, regular monitoring is needed to evaluate the response of nutritional interventions and to motivate and improve patient's compliance to the dietary therapy. Overall, we recommend routine follow-up measurements that include body weight and nPNA plus values of serum albumin, prealbumin, and cholesterol every 3 months in clinically stable patients. Some investigators include anthropometric measurements, dietary interviews and SGA every 6 months for those patients who are at risk of developing PEW or with established PEW, but the utility of this strategy has not been evaluated carefully. Figure 12.2 depicts a proposed algorithm the assessment and management of nutritional status in MHD patients.

EPIDEMIOLOGY OF PROTEIN–ENERGY WASTING IN MAINTENANCE HEMODIALYSIS PATIENTS

Virtually every study evaluating the nutritional status of MHD patients report some degree of abnormalities in the nutritional status. Unfortunately, many different diagnostic tools were used in the separate studies so the actual prevalence of PEW in MHD patients varies widely, ranging from 20% to 60%. Although there is evidence that nutritional parameters improve within 3 to 6 months following initiation of hemodialysis, there also is evidence that PEW is present in up to 40% or more of the MHD population; the prevalence seems to increase with time of MHD treatment.

The relevance of these findings is that practically every nutritional marker has been associated with hospitalization and death risk in MHD patients. Recent epidemiological data also indicate there is an improvement in survival when these markers are corrected via nutritional interventions.

ETIOLOGY OF PROTEIN–ENERGY WASTING IN MAINTENANCE HEMODIALYSIS PATIENTS

The mechanisms leading to PEW in advanced kidney disease are still being elucidated; they can not be attributed to any single factor in MHD patients (Fig. 12.1). Still, it appears that the common pathway for all the metabolic derangements is related to exaggerated protein degradation relative to protein synthesis. There are no agreed upon mechanisms relating dietary energy intake and the development of nutritional and metabolic abnormalities in MHD but there is a an association between inadequate energy intake and the abnormalities associated with PEW.

Dietary Nutrient Intake in Maintenance Hemodialysis Patients

The observation that patients with CKD decrease their protein and energy intake as they progressively lose kidney function has led some to conclude that uremia per se causes protein catabolism stimulated by decreased nutrient intake. This conclusion has been challenged because even in patients with advanced CKD, nitrogen balance studies show that there is a concomitant decrease in both protein synthesis and degradation in patients with advanced CKD that is uncomplicated by acidosis or another catabolic illness. The dual change in protein synthesis and degradation results in a net nitrogen balance that is not different from matched healthy controls. Accelerated protein degradation stimulated by acute illnesses or stress conditions is not suppressed and there is no adequate compensatory increase in protein synthesis. For example, hospitalized MHD patients can be eating inadequate protein and energy and not be able to adjust rates of protein turnover leading to loss of cellular protein stores.

An additional stimulus for protein losses is the dialytic treatment per se. Recent measurements of protein synthesis and degradation unequivocally demonstrate the catabolic effects of hemodialysis. Both whole-body and skeletal muscle protein homeostasis are disrupted and there is a consistent finding of decreased protein synthesis at the whole-body level and an additional increase in whole-body protein breakdown. There also is evidence for a significant increase in net skeletal muscle protein breakdown. Notably, these undesirable effects persist for at least 2 hours following the completion of hemodialysis.

Systemic Inflammation as a Catabolic Stimulus in Advanced Chronic Kidney Disease

Epidemiologic studies have pointed out that there is a high prevalence of increased levels of inflammatory markers in patients with advanced CKD. The metabolic and nutritional responses to chronic inflammation are many (vide infra) and closely mimic the PEW that appears to be common in patients with advanced CKD, including exaggerated protein catabolism. This raises the question whether there is a "cause and effect" relationship between inflammation and loss of protein stores in patients with ESRD. Inflammation, more correctly termed the systemic inflammatory response syndrome, is a complex combination of physiological, immunological, and metabolic effects occurring in response to a variety of stimulators such as tissue injury or disease processes. Certain cytokines such as interleukin-1 (IL-1), IL-6, and tumor necrosis factor-alpha (TNF-α) are the potential mediators of these effects. Therefore, it is important to limit their biological activities but in conditions where the inflammatory response is ongoing and cannot be controlled effectively, adverse effects are highly likely.

Etiology of Chronic Inflammation in Maintenance Hemodialysis Patients

The etiology of inflammation is multifactorial in patients with advanced CKD (Fig. 12.3). For example, the kidney disease in patients with CKD who are not yet receiving MHD, the progression of kidney disease is associated with inflammatory response. Secondly, moderate to advanced CKD can be associated with increased oxidative stress burden leading to formation of advanced glycosylation end products (AGEs). The interaction of AGE with its RAGE receptor stimulates the production of IL-6 by monocytes and indirectly to excess production of CRP in the liver. Besides the accumulation of proinflammatory compounds in advanced CKD, the hemodialysis procedure is associated with activation of an inflammatory cascade with increases in the synthesis of CRP, IL-6, and fibrinogen. The activation of the inflammatory cascade has been attributed to exposure of blood to dialysis membranes and/or back-leakage of lipopolysaccharide through the dialysis membranes from the use of less-than-sterile dialysate. Indeed, it has been shown that use ultrapure, endotoxin-free dialysate is associated with reduced blood concentrations of proinflammatory cytokines. Infection is another common occurrence in MHD patients which can cause significant inflammation; this is especially common in patients with a hemodialysis catheter.

Effects of Inflammatory Response on Metabolism and Nutrition

Pro-inflammatory cytokines are thought to play an integral role in the muscle catabolism of MHD patients. Injection of animals with TNF-α stimulates skeletal muscle protein breakdown but exposure of the muscle to TNF-α does not cause protein catabolism. This indicates the complexity of these interactions. Anorexia or suppressed nutrient intake is a well-established metabolic response to inflammation; IL-1 and TNF-α can cause anorexia through their

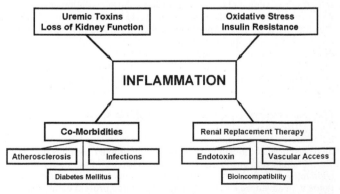

FIGURE 12.3 A number of modifiable and nonmodifiable factors lead to the chronic inflammatory state of advanced kidney disease.

effects on the satiety center in the central nervous system. Again, this is complicated because prostaglandins may be involved since prophylactic use of anti-inflammatory agents blunts the anorectic effects of cytokines. There are hormonal derangements associated with systemic inflammation. These include disruption of the growth hormone and insulin like growth factor 1 (IGF-1) axis leading to decreased anabolism and increased leptin concentrations (a potential contributor to anorexia). It should be noted that the combined presence of decreased nutrient intake plus increased protein breakdown or decreased anabolism worsens overall nitrogen balance, predisposing MHD patients to accelerated loss of skeletal muscle mass and overall poor nutritional state.

Insulin Resistance and Deprivation as Catabolic Stimuli in Advanced Chronic Kidney Disease

Patients with CKD secondary to diabetes mellitus, the leading cause of ESRD in the United States, have a higher incidence of PEW when compared to nondiabetic patients. The degree of insulin resistance and/or insulin deprivation seems to play the most critical role in this process (see Chapter 20 for additional discussion of *Sarcopenia of Obesity*).

As with inflammation, decreased insulin or decreased sensitivity to insulin are the cause of muscle protein losses. Multiple in vitro and in vivo studies have demonstrated the metabolic effects of insulin extend beyond carbohydrate metabolism; specifically, insulin deprivation stimulates protein breakdown and administration of insulin suppresses protein degradation. With adequate amino acid availability, insulin also regulates protein synthesis. These actions are mediated through insulin receptor substrate-1-associated PI3K activity. A deficiency of insulin stimulates the ubiquitin proteasome system (UPS) and caspase-3 activity to breakdown muscle protein. It is believed that regulatory abnormalities in these pathways are responsible for the muscle catabolism observed in MHD patients with diabetes or insulin resistance. Several reports demonstrate that among MHD patients, muscle protein breakdown is enhanced in patients with type II DM when compared to MHD patients without DM. This abnormality translates into a greater loss of lean body mass within the first year of MHD in diabetic MHD patients compared to nondiabetic MHD patients. In the absence of severe obesity, insulin resistance is still detectable in CHD patients and is strongly associated with increased muscle protein breakdown, even after controlling for inflammation.

The Dose of Dialysis and Protein–Energy Wasting Development in Maintenance Hemodialysis Patients

Underdialysis can lead to anorexia and decreased taste acuity and there does appear to be a relationship between underdialysis and decreased dietary protein intake. Not surprisingly, patients with Stage 5 CKD experience a significant improvement in their protein intake within 3 to 6 months of initiation of MHD. Because uremic anorexia usually develops when the dose of dialysis is below acceptable levels (single pool Kt/V < 1.2), it follows that adequate dialysis will raise appetite and improve overall nutritional status.

Metabolic and Hormonal Derangements Leading to Protein–Energy Wasting in Maintenance Hemodialysis Patients

Metabolic acidosis, a common abnormality in patients with progressive CKD promotes PEW, by increasing protein catabolism, especially in muscle. In addition, acidosis stimulates the oxidation of essential amino acids (as shown for leucine oxidation) to raise protein requirements in MHD patients. Even a small correction of a low-serum bicarbonate concentration will improve nutritional status by correcting essential amino acid catabolism and downregulating muscle proteolysis via the ubiquitin–proteasome system.

As with the other abnormalities that stimulate muscle protein catabolism, metabolic acidosis acts in large part by suppressing insulin/IGF-1 signaling in muscle. Currently, we recommend that the predialysis serum bicarbonate level should be greater than 22 mmol per L in MHD patients.

Increased concentrations of parathyroid hormone have been implicated as a protein catabolic factor in ESRD, although evidence for this response in humans is sparse. In addition, there are abnormalities in thyroid hormone-stimulated metabolism in MHD patients, specifically, low circulating thyroxine and triiodothyronine concentrations. Because similar changes resemble those found in patients with prolonged malnutrition, it has been suggested that the thyroid hormone responses to malnutrition (and possibly to advanced CKD), is a maladaptive response to a decrease in energy intake. There are no trials of correcting thyroid hormone levels with documentation of improved nutritional improvements in MHD patients. Finally, abnormalities in the growth hormone and IGF-I axis could be important factors in the development of PEW in MHD patients. For example, growth hormone administration does improve the growth of children with CKD. Growth hormone stimulates beneficial responses such as enhancing protein synthesis, reducing protein degradation, increasing fat mobilization and increasing gluconeogenesis. Administration of recombinant human growth hormone can induce a net anabolic effect in MHD patients.

NUTRITIONAL SUPPORT IN MAINTENANCE HEMODIALYSIS PATIENTS

The prevention and treatment options of PEW in MHD patients are complex. There is no single treatment approach that will alleviate the multiple adverse consequences of PEW. Table 12.2 provides an overview of prevention and treatment options for patients with CKD with PEW plus specific therapeutic options for MHD patients.

General Aspects of Nutritional Management

Management of nutritional aspects of MHD patients includes a comprehensive combination of preventive maneuvers to diminish protein and energy depletion. Unfortunately, for some therapies, there are only empiric data suggesting benefits. Standard therapies for MHD patients with PEW include provision of adequate dialysis, treatment of metabolic acidosis, adjustments of dietary factors and treatment of infections. Factors that are not so closely linked to the nutritional status but could be very useful include correction of fluid overload and treatment of comorbid conditions such as diabetes, cardiovascular diseases, and salient infectious diseases. Likewise, a search for signs of chronic inflammation is required, and all attempts must be made to eliminate inflammatory responses, especially the use of central venous catheters.

Oral Nutritional Supplementation

The susceptibility toward PEW fro decreased protein and energy intake could be ameliorated by increasing nutrient intake through dietary supplements, especially during hemodialysis. Nutritional supplementation of MHD patients should be delivered by the oral route if at all possible but if not, parenteral nutritional supplements can be provided.

Both the short- and long-term benefits of oral nutritional supplements for MHD patients can be accomplished especially when the supplements are provided around the time of hemodialysis, including intradialytic administration. For example, oral feeding can be associated with a robust improvement in whole-body and skeletal muscle protein balance. There are now studies suggesting beneficial responses to prolonged oral nutritional supplementation

TABLE 12.2	Proposed Nutritional and Anti-Inflammatory Interventions in Chronic Disease States

Nutritional interventions:

Chronic kidney disease (Stages 3–5, not on dialysis)

- Close supervision and nutritional counseling (especially for patients on protein restricted diets)
- Initiation of maintenance dialysis or kidney transplant in advanced CKD patients with apparent protein–energy wasting despite vigorous attempts

Maintenance hemodialysis patients

- Continuous dietary counseling
- Appropriate amount of dietary protein and calorie intake (dietary protein and energy intake >1.2 g/kg/d and >30 kcal/kg/d, respectively)
- Optimal dose of dialysis
- *Nutritional support in chronic dialysis patients who are unable to meet their dietary needs
  - Oral supplements
  - Tube feeds (if medically appropriate)
  - Intradialytic parenteral nutritional supplements
  - Resistance exercise combined with nutritional supplementation
- *Anabolic steroids
- *Appetite stimulants (not proven or experimental)
  - Megestrol acetate, dronabinol, melatonin, thalidomide, and ghrelin
- Growth factors (experimental)
  - Recombinant human growth hormone

Anti-inflammatory interventions*:

- Targeted anticytokine therapy
  - IL-1 receptor antagonist
  - TNF-α blocker
- Fish oil
- Pentoxifylline
- Statins
- Thiazolidinediones
- ACE-inhibitors
- Resistance exercise

*Applicable to CKD patients not on maintenance dialysis as well.
CKD, chronic kidney disease; IL-1, interleukin-1; TNF-α, tumor necrosis factor-alpha.

in MHD patients. In brief, the outcome measures examined included clinical (quality of life, complications, and mortality), biochemical (serum albumin and electrolyte levels), and nutritional (dietary intake and anthropometry). The analysis indicated that enteral nutritional support can increase total (energy and protein) intake and raise serum albumin concentrations by an average of 0.23 g per dL, with no adverse effects on electrolyte status (serum phosphate and potassium). The practical implication is that oral nutritional supplementation is effective, especially when administered during hemodialysis and is practical, convenient, and well tolerated.

Intradialytic Parenteral Nutrition

While the gastrointestinal route is always preferred for nutritional supplementation, parenteral provision of nutrients, especially during the dialysis procedure

(IDPN), is safe, effective, and convenient for individuals who can not tolerate oral or enteral administration of nutrients. Several but not all reports provide evidence that nutritional status can improve with IDPN. Unfortunately, the sample size in most reports has been small and did not allow appropriate stratification of MHD patients. They were also carried out over a short period of time. Results from the FINE study have provided insights into effects from long-term use of nutritional supplementations in MHD patients with PEW. In this study, 186 MHD patients with PEW were randomly assigned to receive intradialytic parenteral nutrition (for 1 year) plus standard oral supplements providing 500 kcal per day and 25 g per day protein and were compared to those receiving oral supplements only. The nutritional goal was to bring the intakes up to the recommended amounts of 30 to 35 kcal/kg/d and 1.2 g/kg/d, respectively. The primary outcome, 2-year mortality, was similar in the two groups (39% in the control group and 43% in the IDPN group), suggesting that oral nutritional supplementation is equally effective as IDPN when oral intake is possible. When there was an increase in serum prealbumin, it was associated with a decrease in the 2-year mortality and hospitalization rate.

This large study provides the first prospective evidence of a link between a positive response to nutritional therapy and improved outcomes. The other conclusion is that oral or combined oral–parenteral methods of delivering supplements are the same in terms of mortality of MHD patients with PEW, if equal and adequate amounts of protein and calories are provided. Despite the lack of an appropriate control group, these results imply that nutritional supplementation can improve nutritional markers in CHD patients with PEW; and this conclusion is consistent with the recommendations of the NKF K/DOQI ($>$1.2 g/kg/d and $>$30 kcal/kg/d, respectively). Although these results imply that nutritional interventions can improve the survival of MHD patients, caution is needed in this interpretation because the study lacked a no-intervention arm and the nutritional improvements may just reflect a regression-to-the-mean phenomenon.

Pharmacological Interventions for Treatment of Protein–Energy Wasting in Maintenance Hemodialysis Patients
Growth Hormone
Growth hormone and its major mediator, IGF-1, could have several anabolic properties. Besides the well documented benefits of growth hormone in children with CKD, short-term administration of the hormone to MHD patients can have anabolic responses. Most if not all long-term studies indicate there is a significant increase in lean body mass in the growth hormone-treated MHD patients. For example, growth hormone was associated with statistically significant gains in lean body mass in a trial consisting of 139 patients. There also were statistically significant beneficial changes in other biomarkers of mortality (homocysteine, transferrin, and high-density lipoprotein) as well as quality of life. Finally, there was a trend toward increased levels of serum albumin as compared to placebo administration.

Appetite Stimulants
Examples of pharmacologic agents that may stimulate appetite include megestrol acetate, dronabinol, cyproheptadine, melatonin, thalidomide, and ghrelin. Most of these drugs have not been studied systematically in MHD patients with PEW but have been used in other catabolic illnesses. For example, megestrol acetate, a steroid-like progestagen, led to increased appetite and weight gain in breast cancer patients. In elderly men, the orexigenic and weight-gaining effects of megestrol acetate have been recently attributed to its anticytokine effects via reduced levels of IL-6 and TNF-α. The increase in appetite was associated with an increase in weight, mainly due to increased

fat and not lean body mass. Moreover, megestrol acetate has been associated with side effects including hypogonadism, impotence, and increased risk of thromboembolism. In MHD patients, megestrol acetate can stimulate appetite and induce small increases in serum albumin but large-scale prospective studies are needed to assess whether these drugs provide adjunctive nutritional therapy for MHD or CKD patients. We know of no systematic evaluation of other appetite-stimulating and weight gain responses to dronabinol, cypro-heptadine, melatonin, and thalidomide in MHD patients.

Anabolic Steroids

There are reports of significant improvements in body composition and physical function of MHD patients who are given nandrolone decanoate. In addition, there was an increase in quadriceps muscle cross-sectional area (magnetic resonance imaging measurements) and an increase in lean body mass by DEXA. Curiously, the combination of resistance exercise with nandrole deaconate did not improve the beneficial effects of the drug.

Exercise as an Anabolic Intervention in Maintenance Hemodialysis Patients

Exercise training can maintain and/or improve exercise capacity and endurance in the general population. In addition, resistance exercise can increase muscle mass, strength, and appetite as well as lessen muscle weakness and frailty in elderly patients (see Chapter 21). Resistance exercise can increase oxygen consumption but whether this response only occurs when there is a positive muscle protein balance is unknown. The rates of both muscle synthesis and breakdown increase during a resistance exercise session in normal adults and if resistance exercise is combined with nutrient supplementation, anabolism is maximized while muscle breakdown declines somewhat. Short-term (i.e., a single HD session) metabolic studies indicate that exercise when combined with intradialytic oral or parenteral nutrition will increase net protein balance in MHD patients but longer term evaluations of resistance exercise performed during hemodialysis in MHD patients have not shown significant nutritional benefits. Nonetheless, the beneficial effects of exercise on quality of life and physical functioning must be taken into account when considering an exercise regimen for a MHD patient. We recommend an adequate nutritional supplement during exercise unless the patient is considered for supervised weight loss.

Anti-inflammatory Interventions

Anti-inflammatory interventions aimed at ameliorating the changes in nutritional status in MHD patients (Table 12.2) include interlekin-1 receptor antagonists (IL-1ra), pentoxifylline, fish oil and resistance exercise. Pentoxifylline, a drug that blocks TNF-α release was administered intravenously to patients with Stages 4 and 5 CKD. There was not only an improvement in protein breakdown, but also improvement in the anabolic effects of a balanced amino acid mixture given concurrently. While pentoxifylline did not significantly affect TNF-α levels, it did decrease TNF-α soluble receptors and hence could block the influence of TNF-α. In a study of resistance exercise training over 12 weeks, there was simultaneous improvements in whole-body protein balance and inflammatory markers in patients with Stages 3 and 4 CKD.

Besides pentoxifylline and resistance exercise, thalidomide, IL-1 receptor antagonists, TNF-α receptor blockers, fish oil, statins, ACE inhibitors, PPAR-γ agonists, plus certain antioxidants have been tested. IL-1ra administration over 4 weeks results in statistically significant improvements in hsCRP and IL-6 and trends toward improvement in serum albumin and prealbumin concentrations. Combined administration of γ-tocopherol and docosahexaenoic acid over 3 months was associated with a significant decrease in IL-6 and the white blood cell count in MHD patients. A small study showed significant suppression of skeletal muscle protein breakdown in response to 3-month administration of high-dose fish oil, but there was no effect on net protein balance. These results indicate the need for further, larger-scale studies using various anti-inflammatory interventions in MHD patients with PEW or underlying systemic inflammation.

Suggested Readings

Cano NJ, Fouque D, Roth H, et al. Intradialytic parenteral nutrition does not improve survival in malnourished hemodialysis patients: a 2-year multicenter, prospective, randomized study. *J Am Soc Nephrol* 2007;18:2583–2591.

Deger SM, Hung AM, Ellis CD, et al. High dose omega-3 fatty acid administration and skeletal muscle protein turnover in maintenance hemodialysis patients. *Clin J Am Soc Nephrol* 2016;11:1227–1235.

Fouque D, Kalantar-Zadeh K, Kopple J, et al. A proposed nomenclature and diagnostic criteria for protein–energy wasting in acute and chronic kidney disease. *Kidney Int* 2008;73:391–398.

Hung AM, Ellis CD, Shintani A, et al. IL-1beta receptor antagonist reduces inflammation in hemodialysis patients. *J Am Soc Nephrol* 2011;22:437–442.

Ikizler TA, Cano NJ, Franch H, et al. Prevention and treatment of protein energy wasting in chronic kidney disease patients: a consensus statement by the International Society of Renal Nutrition and Metabolism. *Kidney Int* 2013;84:1096–1107.

Lim VS, Ikizler TA, Raj DS, et al. Does hemodialysis increase protein breakdown? Dissociation between whole-body amino acid turnover and regional muscle kinetics. *J Am Soc Nephrol* 2005;16:862–868.

Pupim LB, Majchrzak KM, Flakoll PJ, et al. Intradialytic oral nutrition improves protein homeostasis in chronic hemodialysis patients with deranged nutritional status. *J Am Soc Nephrol* 2006;17:3149–3157.

Siew ED, Ikizler TA. Determinants of insulin resistance and its effects on protein metabolism in patients with advanced chronic kidney disease. *Contrib Nephrol* 2008;161:138–144.

Stratton RJ, Bircher G, Fouque D, et al. Multinutrient oral supplements and tube feeding in maintenance dialysis: a systematic review and meta-analysis. *Am J Kidney Dis* 2005;46:387–405.

13

Nutritional Considerations for Patients on Peritoneal Dialysis

Jie Dong

Peritoneal dialysis (PD) is the most commonly used home dialysis modality in patients with end-stage renal disease (ESRD). Numerous studies have shown that poor nutritional status independently predicts higher hospitalization rates, lower patient and technique survival, and poor quality of life in patients on PD. The prevalence of protein–energy wasting (PEW) is high for patients undergoing PD similar to ones on hemodialysis (HD), that is, 18% to 56%, because of persistence of mechanisms applicable across the stages of chronic kidney disease (CKD). Comprehensive nutrition management is necessary to prevent PEW along with appropriate interventions in order to improve overall nutrition status. Of note, because the process of PD therapy per se is quite different from HD, the mechanisms leading to PEW, evaluation of nutrition status, and interventions to prevent the PEW in PD patients may differ significantly.

General concepts on PEW have been comprehensively reviewed in Chapters 2 and 3 for patients CKD and in Chapter 12 for patients on HD. In this chapter, we focus on specific nutritional considerations in patients undergoing PD. We also briefly discuss the metabolic syndrome (MS) in PD patients.

ASSESSMENT OF PROTEIN–ENERGY WASTING IN PATIENTS ON PERITONEAL DIALYSIS

The basic concepts related to evaluation of nutrition status in advanced CKD are also applicable in PD patients and are not discussed herein. Given the relevance to PD therapy, we only discuss specific issues related to serum albumin and body composition in the setting PD.

Serum Albumin

Hypoalbuminemia is a powerful predictor of poor survival in CKD, including those on PD, HD, and transplantation. Among PD patients, the extent of volume overload and protein loss is more obvious, especially in high transporters and those with systemic or local inflammation. This could explain the higher prevalence of hypoalbuminemia in PD patients compared to ones on HD. Switching from PD to HD has been reported to increase plasma albumin concentration by 3 to 4 g per L. Incident PD patients with a high peritoneal large pore flux have been reported to display a decrement in serum albumin concentrations, aptly named as iatrogenic "nephrotic" syndrome. Despite lower serum albumin concentrations in general, an observational study reported differing thresholds for death risk in HD patients versus PD patients, that is, serum albumin concentrations less than 4.0 and less than 3.8 g per dL, respectively. For each serum albumin category, the overall death risk for PD patients was lower than for HD patients. This suggests that the level of serum albumin that mandates clinical evaluation and intervention by the nephrologists and the criteria used by regulators to judge the quality of care should vary by dialysis modality.

BODY COMPOSITION

Assessments for Body Composition

Body composition consists of fat mass and nonfat mass. Nonfat mass includes lean body mass (LBM) and bone mineral tissues. LBM is the sum of total body water, skeletal muscle mass, and the fat-free part of organs. Each part of body composition has its significant physiologic effect. LBM reflects muscle protein stores, which is an important nutrition marker and prognostic index for patient outcomes.

The LBM by bioelectrical impedance (BIA) is generally influenced by hydration status. In addition, BIA measurements made in PD patients with dialysate instilled can overestimate LBM. Anthropometry is an easy and noninvasive method, which measures four or more site skinfolds to evaluate fat mass. However, low precision, high inter- and intraobserver variation, and hydration status also influence anthropometry measurements and equations derived from these data. Creatinine kinetics is used to calculate the LBM by measurements for creatinine in serum, 24-hour dialysate, and urine sample. It has been shown that LBM estimated from creatinine kinetics independently predicts all-cause mortality in PD patients. However, LBM estimated from creatinine kinetics has wide variation and may be underestimating actual LBM as shown by several studies. This method is affected by the quality of 24-hour urine and dialysate collection, dietary protein intake, and by creatinine degradation and elimination.

As compared to HD patients, the distribution of LBM and fat mass in PD may be different. A study in 491 PD patients compared body composition to HD patients matched by country, age, gender, and dialysis vintage and showed that PD patients have significantly higher lean tissue index and volume overload as measured by BIA. Another study indicated that PD patients have the greatest increase in total body fat measured by dual-energy x-ray absorptiometry (DEXA) and visceral fat by computed tomography (CT) in the first year of maintenance dialysis, as compared to HD patients. The potential causes for these differences are not clear. One study indicated incident PD patients experience weight gain, including visceral and subcutaneous fat measured by CT during the 6-month of PD, which is not related to glucose absorption. In terms of prognostic value of body composition in PD patients, LBM is shown to be more critical than fat mass.

PROTEIN–ENERGY WASTING IN PATIENTS ON PERITONEAL DIALYSIS

Similar to nondialyzed CKD and HD patients, PEW is often correlated to disease condition per se and comorbidities in patients undergoing PD, which lead to adverse outcomes. As compared to HD, PD patients have some specific conditions which exert protective or harmful effects on metabolic balance. These factors will be discussed in detail below.

Metabolic Acidosis

The extent of metabolic acidosis is known to contribute to PEW by increasing muscle protein catabolism and stimulating the oxidation of essential amino acids. Because PD modality is a continuous renal replacement therapy, patients on PD generally have better acid–base balance. In a large study of 10,400 PD patients, serum bicarbonate levels greater than 22 mmol per L, the recommended threshold for best nutrition state, was observed in 75% of PD patients versus 60% of HD patients.

Residual Renal Function

PD therapy is considered as a more suitable modality for the preservation of residual renal function (RRF). RRF is an independent risk factor for adverse outcomes, including cardiovascular events and mortality. From a nutritional viewpoint, numerous studies have shown that RRF plays important role in determining nutritional status. Patients with preserved RRF have comparatively reduced resting energy expenditure, less systemic inflammation, and higher removal of uremic toxins, which are likely to induce less decreased protein catabolism compared to HD patients without RRF. It should be noted that for those having large amounts of urinary protein loss because of nephrotic range proteinuria, the existence of RRF may contribute to the aggravation of protein catabolism.

Psychosocial Stress and Quality of Life

Psychosocial issues such as depression are known to contribute to decreased appetite and a decline in nutrition status, and also play an important role in quality of life and clinical outcomes of patients on maintenance dialysis. Previous studies indicated that PD therapy has less influence on the psychologic status and physical well-being, and PD patients are reported to have better quality of life as compared to HD patients.

Volume Status

Volume overload leads to a higher risk for cardiovascular death and all-cause death in patients on maintenance dialysis. One study in 1,092 prevalent patients from 135 centers worldwide indicated that the majority of patients starting on PD are overhydrated. Volume overload is reported to be more prevalent in PD patients as compared to HD patients. The difficulties of volume control in PD patients are mainly related to the poor compliance to sodium and fluid intake, which may be caused by a stronger feeling of thirst and less frequent doctor–patient contact. For those with long duration of dialysis and multiple episodes of peritonitis, ultrafiltration failure is also a contributor to volume overload.

Volume overload leads to immunoactivation and increased cytokine production via bacterial or endotoxin translocation that could result in persistent systemic inflammation. In a cross-sectional study, volume overload was shown to correlate with markers of malnutrition, inflammation, and atherosclerosis in PD patients. A longitudinal study showed that improvements in fluid status are associated with improvements in subjective global assessment (SGA), whereas deterioration in fluid status is associated with the decreased handgrip strength as well as higher prevalence of malnutrition by SGA.

Appetite and Gastric Emptying

Gastrointestinal symptoms are prevalent in patients on PD. Early satiety, reduced appetite, and delayed gastric emptying are the most common complaints. PD patients are reported to have lower peak hunger, less change in fullness rating around mealtimes, and lower nutrient intake as compared to healthy controls. Apart from common physiologic basis for these symptoms in patients on ESRD, there are several potential causes specific for PD patients. Peritoneal cavity, as the main media of PD therapy, is filled with glucose-containing fluids. The estimated caloric load from glucose-based exchange can range from 200 to 1,000 kcal and contribute 30% of the total daily energy intake of a patient undergoing PD. This continuous intraperitoneal glucose exposure decrease plasma levels of ghrelin, an appetite stimulator from endocrine cells in the stomach. Therefore, patients undergoing PD could be regarded as continuous "eater." In addition, the increased intra-abdominal pressure may lead to the sensation of fullness and disturbances of gastrointestinal motility. Gastric emptying half-time was negatively correlated with LBM and body mass index in a small study in PD patients. After administration of promotility agents in patients with delayed gastric emptying, nutrition status is demonstrated to improve.

Protein and Amino Acid Losses

Although uremic toxins, potassium, and phosphorus are removed from the peritoneal capillaries in the process of PD, protein, amino acids, and a range of vitamins are also lost into the dialysate. The average of total protein loss in PD patients is around 5 g per day. The variation of protein loss is dependent on patient- and treatment-related factors. Patients with large body surface area, high transport rate, local or systemic inflammation, and endothelial function have higher protein losses. Longer dwell time, higher dialysis dose, and ultrafiltration can also lead to more protein losses into the dialysate.

PREVENTION AND TREATMENT OF PROTEIN–ENERGY WASTING IN PATIENTS ON PERITONEAL DIALYSIS

Protein and Energy Intake

The International Society of Renal Nutrition and Metabolism (ISRNM) recommended the target of protein and energy intake for PD patients as at least 1.2 g per kg of ideal body weight per day and 30 to 35 kcal per kg of ideal body weight per day, respectively, and at least 50% of the protein intake should be of high-biologic value. The British Dietetic Association suggests a lower target, 1.0 to 1.2 g per kg of ideal body weight per day in conjunction with an adequate energy intake. European guidelines suggest a protein intake ≥1.0 g/kg/d for maintenance dialysis patients in general.

Dietary Counseling

Dietary counseling is always the first step to help patients to enhance their nutrient intake. There is a paucity of studies investigating the effects of dietary counseling on nutrients intake. One small randomized clinical trial (RCT) indicated that two separate methods of dietary interventions failed to modify intake or parameters of nutrition over 4 months in PD patients.

Of note, dialysis dietary regimen is among the most restrictive diets, and these restrictions may render many patients frustrated and lead to suboptimal adherence and compliance. During the dietary counseling, we should always keep the balance between nutrition status and restrictions. For example, although phosphate intake would be inevitably increased while protein intake improved, we do not recommend patients with hyperphosphatemia to reduce protein intake inappropriately. Specific attention should be paid on the phosphorus content of the specific protein sources (dietary phosphorus to protein ratios) and restriction of phosphorus-containing additives/preservatives, especially from processed foods. Dietary sodium intake is parallel with nutrient intake. There are no convincing data from interventional studies to suggest that more dietary sodium restriction in dialysis patients has any bearing on outcomes, especially in PD patients. In view of that, restriction of dietary sodium at the expense of severely limiting overall dietary nutrient intake is not encouraged. Clearly, a patient-specific diet should be developed, especially in ones with underlying risks for salt retention such as ultrafiltration failure and heart disease.

Nutrition Supplements

If daily protein and energy requirements are not being met despite dietary counseling, nutritional supplementation should be considered. These include oral supplements and enteral nutrition via nasogastric feeding tubes. Oral supplement is a simple and cheap method that can be attempted first. One RCT indicated that the egg albumin-based supplement significantly improved several of general nutritional parameters during the 6-month follow-up in PD patients, whereas two separate RCTs only showed modest or no effect on nutrition status, as examined by serum albumin or normalized protein catabolic rate. Of note, the benefit of nutrition supplementation is dependent on the compliance of patients and gastrointestinal function. For those with poor appetite or refusing the flavor or taste of supplements, enteral feeding via a nasogastric tube may be tried, although the efficacy is unproven. Percutaneous endoscopic gastrostomy feeding is not advisable in PD patients because the incidence of peritonitis is extremely high.

Amino Acid-Based Dialysate
As a viable option to provide the nutrients, amino acid dialysate (AAD) could help PD patients to improve their nutrition status, especially for those whom cannot tolerate oral or enteral nutrition supplements. A 6-hour dwell time with a 1.1% amino acid solution enables approximately 16 g (72% to 78%) of amino acids to be absorbed, which is greater than the peritoneal loss of amino acids using conventional glucose solutions.

Three short-term studies have indicated the beneficial effects of AAD on net protein balance. Long-term RCTs did not show a conclusive efficacy of AAD in PD patients with PEW. Inadequate sample size, imprecise nutritional indices, and inconsistent dietary monitoring are limitations of these RCTs.

Dialysis Adequacy
It has been long suggested that adequate dialysis is to ameliorate uremic symptoms. This cause–effect relationship between dose of dialysis and nutrition is only observed in those newly starting PD or in patients being under dialyzed. The ADEMEX (ADEquacy of PD in MEXico) trial did not show an additional improvement in nutritional markers in subjects randomized to high peritoneal creatinine clearance, that is, 60 L/wk/1.73 m^2.

Biocompatible Peritoneal Dialysis Solutions
Numerous studies have been performed to the potential benefits of biocompatible dialysate in PD, showing no consistent results. Three biocompatible PD fluids (a neutral-pH, low-glucose degradation product [GDP], 1.5% glucose solution; a solution with 1.1% amino acid; and a fluid with 7.5% icodextrin) have had no effect on systemic inflammatory response. An RCT performed in a relatively large sample of 152 patients observed that low-GDP PD fluids significantly lower the levels of endothelial dysfunction markers, but not that of C-reactive protein (CRP) at 12-month follow-up. Overall, the nutritional benefits of biocompatible PD fluids are inconclusive.

Anti-Inflammatory Therapy
Anti-inflammatory agents may include antioxidative treatment, antiwasting treatment, drugs having pleiotrophic anti-inflammatory effects, and targeted anticytokine treatment. There are some encouraging findings from small-scale pilot studies in PD patients. An RCT over 8 weeks reported that oral N-acetylcysteine treatment reduced interleukin 6 (IL-6) levels in 15 patients. A 6-month RCT indicated that probiotics could significantly reduce the serum levels of endotoxin, pro-inflammatory cytokines (tumor necrosis factor α [TNF-α], IL-5, and IL-6) and increase that of anti-inflammatory cytokine (IL-10). In a double-blind, controlled and crossover trial, pravastatin significantly reduced serum levels of CRP with the decrease of total and low-density lipoprotein (LDL) cholesterol. Another RCT indicated that the therapy of rosuvastatin for 6 months significantly reduced serum CRP levels. A randomized crossover trial observed that 12-week pioglitazone therapy significantly reduced serum CRP with the decline of fasting blood glucose

and homeostatic model assessment of insulin resistance (HOMA-IR) index. A 24-week RCT found that diabetic patients receiving rosiglitazone combined with insulin had significantly lower CRP levels and insulin dosage than those receiving insulin only. Overall, there is reasonable evidence to suggest that inflammatory milieu can be improved in PD patients with several strategies, but the overall nutritional benefits of these interventions are to be determined.

Other Novel Treatment Options

The possible role of exogenous administration of hormones to reverse the protein catabolism has been investigated in PD patients. Recombinant human growth hormone (rhGH) and recombinant human IGF-1 (rh-IGF-1) are promising agents because both of them showed a protein anabolic effect in small, short-term studies. An RCT performed in malnourished HD and PD patients showed that the rhGH administered for 4 weeks significantly enhanced the body weight, daily protein intake with the increase in levels of serum IGF-1. A prospective, crossover trial indicated that patients self-administered rhGH for 7 days had a significant decrease in urea and dialysate nitrogen excretion rate and protein catabolic rate. Injections of rhIGF-1 in six malnourished PD patients also led to a strongly positive nitrogen balance within hours, and then the decrease in nitrogen output was sustained during the entire 20 day of treatment.

An RCT in clinically stable PD patients indicated that the androgen, nandrolone decanoate, given by intramuscular injections was associated with improvement in both anthropometric (weight, body mass index, triceps skinfold, mid-arm circumference [MAC], and mid-arm muscle circumference [MAMC]) and biochemical nutritional markers (serum total proteins, albumin, prealbumin, and transferrin) in 6 months. In this group, serum urea nitrogen, urea net excretion, and protein equivalent of nitrogen appearance significantly decreased. Moreover, there was a positive and significant correlation between the rise in IGF-1 concentrations and the increase in hemoglobin, hematocrit, MAC, and MAMC.

With regard to appetite stimulant, the efficacy of megestrol acetate has been investigated in PD patients. In one study of 32 patients undergoing PD, two-thirds of patients receiving megestrol lead to an increase in appetite, serum albumin, and weight gain without negative side effects. In another observational study, 26 hypoalbuminemic PD and HD patients who took megestrol acetate daily for 2 month got a significant increase in anthropometry and albumin concentration. Side effects, including hypogonadism, impotence, and increased risk of thromboembolism, should be closely observed when taking this medication.

Ghrelin is a potential therapeutic agent that could improve nutrition status. This hormone secreted by the stomach can improve nutrition status by stimulating appetite and suppressing the inflammatory response. In a randomized, double-blind, crossover study performed in nine malnourished PD patients, subcutaneous administration of single-dose ghrelin before a meal significantly increased the absolute energy intake as compared with placebo. There were no significant adverse events during the study. There are no long-term studies using ghrelin in maintenance dialysis patients.

METABOLIC SYNDROME

MS consists of a cluster of metabolic and hemodynamic abnormalities. The components of MS include obesity or abdominal obesity, hypertension, diabetes mellitus or insulin resistance, and dyslipidemia.

The prevalence of MS is remarkably high in patients with CKD and approximately one half to two-thirds of PD patients have MS. A prevalent cohort study showed that overall survival, cardiovascular survival, or technique survival did not differ between patients with and without MS, irrespective of the diagnostic criteria after adjustment for diabetes status. However, another study found that incident nondiabetic PD patients with MS had poorer patient survival compared to those without MS for both total and cardiovascular event-free patient survival.

Whether PD patients are more likely to develop the MS as compared to their HD counterparts is yet to be determined. The fat mass of PD is not necessarily higher than that of HD patients. Insulin resistance in nondiabetic PD patients is reported to be related to obesity rather than glucose load or peritoneal transport. Similarly, new-onset diabetes in PD patients was predicted by older age, obese, and inflammation rather than glucose absorption and peritoneal transport. These findings could explain that there is no extra risk for new-onset diabetes in PD patients as compared to HD patients.

Nevertheless, it is reasonable to use glucose-sparing strategies to minimize the glucose load as much as possible in PD patients. If glucose-based PD fluids are the only available products, we must limit the usage of high concentration of dialysate for the achievement of peritoneal ultrafiltration required to maintain euvolemia. This includes salt restriction and the usage of diuretics to a higher fluid and sodium removal via urine in patients with RRF. A weight management program involving dietary and exercise advice and monitoring, reduced body weight in 16% of obese patients, suggesting that improving physical conditioning is a viable strategy in PD patients.

Suggested Readings

Cheng LT, Tang W, Wang T. Strong association between volume status and nutritional status in peritoneal dialysis patients. *Am J Kidney Dis* 2005;45:891–902.

Dong J, Li YJ, Lu XH, et al. Correlations of lean body mass with nutritional indicators and mortality in patients on peritoneal dialysis. *Kidney Int* 2008;73:334–340.

Dong J, Li Y, Yang Z, et al. Low dietary sodium intake increases the death risk in peritoneal dialysis. *Clin J Am Soc Nephrol* 2010;5:240–247.

Ikizler TA, Cano NJ, Franch H, et al.; International Society of Renal & Metabolism. Prevention and treatment of protein energy wasting in chronic kidney disease patients: a consensus statement by the International Society of Renal Nutrition and Metabolism. *Kidney Int* 2013;84:1096–1107.

Kalantar-Zadeh K, Tortorici AR, Chen JL, et al. Dietary restrictions in dialysis patients: is there anything left to eat? *Semin Dialy* 2015;28:159–168.

Li FK, Chan LY, Woo JC, et al. A 3-year, prospective, randomized, controlled study on amino acid dialysate in patients on CAPD. *Am J Kidney Dis* 2003;42:173–183.

Mehrotra R, Duong U, Jiwakanon S, et al. Serum albumin as a predictor of mortality in peritoneal dialysis: comparisons with hemodialysis. *Am J Kidney Dis* 2011;58:418–428.

Sanchez-Villanueva R, Bajo A, Del Peso G, et al. Higher daily peritoneal protein clearance when initiating peritoneal dialysis is independently associated with peripheral arterial disease (PAD): a possible new marker of systemic endothelial dysfunction? *Nephrol Dialy Transplant* 2009;24:1009–1014.

Szeto CC, Kwan BC, Chow KM, et al. Metabolic syndrome in peritoneal dialysis patients: choice of diagnostic criteria and prognostic implications. *Clin J Am Soc Nephrol* 2014;9:779–787.

van Biesen W, Claes K, Covic A, et al. A multicentric, international matched pair analysis of body composition in peritoneal dialysis versus haemodialysis patients. *Nephrol Dialy Transplant* 2013;28:2620–2628.

Wang AY, Sea MM, Ip R, et al. Independent effects of residual renal function and dialysis adequacy on actual dietary protein, calorie, and other nutrient intake in patients on continuous ambulatory peritoneal dialysis. *J Am Soc Nephrol* 2001;12:2450–2457.

Wynne K, Giannitsopoulou K, Small CJ, et al. Subcutaneous ghrelin enhances acute food intake in malnourished patients who receive maintenance peritoneal dialysis: a randomized, placebo-controlled trial. *J Am Soc Nephrol* 2005;16:2111–2118.

14 Nutritional Management of Kidney Transplant Patients

Melissa B. Bleicher, Deirdre Sawinski, and Simin Goral

Successful kidney transplantation can be a liberating experience for the recipient. In addition to being freed from the rigors of maintenance dialysis, a recipient with advanced chronic kidney disease (CKD) is usually emancipated from the strict limitation of the "renal" diet. However, fewer dietary restrictions, along with an improved overall sense of well-being and improved appetite, can result in significant weight gain after transplantation. Additionally, the kidney transplant recipient faces a new set of dietary challenges, including posttransplant diabetes, potential new metabolic abnormalities, and nutritional requirements, which vary in the immediate- and long-term posttransplant period. Along with these challenges, some patients never achieve "normal" kidney function posttransplant, and most will eventually develop a decline in allograft function over time. In light of all of these dynamic factors, it behooves those caring for kidney transplant recipients to become knowledgeable in proper nutritional guidelines for this population.

OBESITY

Pretransplant Obesity

The prevalence of obesity among patients listed for a kidney transplant has increased significantly in recent years (the prevalence of mild obesity body mass index, [BMI] 30 to 35 kg per m^2 was 14% in 2006 and increased to 20% in 2011). In a registry-based analysis, it has been shown that the likelihood of receiving a kidney transplant progressively declined between 1995 and 2006 with increasing degrees of obesity. Similarly, in this particular study, the likelihood of being bypassed when an organ became available increased with each category of obesity. In another retrospective analysis of 702,456 incident patients with ESRD aged 18 to 70 years from the U.S. Renal Data System (USRDS), it was demonstrated that the association of BMI with access to transplantation varies between men and women, suggesting that obesity may contribute to the disparity in access to transplantation between men and women.

In the setting of a shortage of transplantable kidneys, it is incumbent upon the medical community to allocate this resource so as to maximize the benefit for society at large, and not just each individual or small cohort of individuals. There is conflicting data in the literature in regard to any adverse effect of BMI at the time of transplantation on patient and allograft outcomes, which makes decisions on treatment of obesity in patients with advanced CKD/ESRD quite difficult. Despite the limitations of retrospective design, large epidemiologic studies analyzing USRDS and Scientific Registry of Transplant Recipients databases support a survival benefit of transplantation over maintenance dialysis in the obese population. With respect to the allograft, although there is a higher incidence of delayed graft function (DGF), obese transplant recipients (BMI 30 to 40 kg per m^2) have only a slightly increased risk of graft loss and experience similar survival to recipients with normal BMI (18.5 to 24.9 kg per m^2). In subgroup analyses, transplantation from any donor source was reported to be associated with a survival benefit in obese patients ≥50 years, and diabetic patients, but the benefit was lower when a BMI was ≥40 kg per m^2 and a survival benefit was not demonstrated in the black patients with a BMI ≥40 kg per m^2. Patients with a BMI >40 kg per m^2 were reported to have nearly 3 times the odds of DGF as well as more postoperative wound complications. Results from a retrospective analysis of the United Network for Organ Sharing (UNOS) data set for super obese transplant recipients characterized by a BMI >50, were notable for a significant increase in length of hospital stay, increased incidence of DGF, and 4.6-fold increase in perioperative 30-day mortality compared to patients with a BMI <50, as well as worse patient and graft survival compared with transplanted patients within lower BMI subgroups. In a recent retrospective study, the impact of pretransplant BMI on long-term allograft outcomes after kidney transplantation was studied (Organ Procurement and Transplantation Network [OPTN] database from 2001 to 2009); in both unadjusted and adjusted models, increasing pretransplant levels of BMI were found to be independently associated with an increased cumulative incidence of allograft failure and all-cause graft loss. The authors could not identify a lower BMI to be independently associated with risk of allograft failure.

While many experts argue that BMI alone is not a perfect measure of risk related to body composition and adiposity, currently, many kidney transplant programs use a certain target BMI as a selection criterion for transplant candidacy. Although practice varies across centers, BMIs in the range of 35 to 45 kg per m^2 are usually the upper limit of acceptability for transplant candidates. In addition to BMI, parameters such as waist circumference, measurement of lean muscle mass, and weight distribution have also been suggested as metrics to guide the selection of transplant candidates, though not used in clinical practice at this time.

Obesity treatment with weight loss surgery (WLS) seems to be a feasible strategy for improving access to transplantation, though published studies are scarce at this time. A relatively small study identified 72 patients who had bariatric surgery prelisting and 29 while on the waitlist between 1991 and 2004; 69% of patients treated with bariatric surgery on the waitlist proceeded to transplant after surgery. However, although WLS may be an effective means of weight reduction in the pretransplant population, the nephrology community will need to clarify whether weight loss is to the benefit of these patients given the obesity paradox that exists within the dialysis population. More studies are needed to look at the effects of intentional pretransplant weight loss either through diet and exercise or WLS on transplant listing and outcomes.

Posttransplant Obesity

Weight gain is quite common in the posttransplant period. Mean weight gains seem to fall within the range of 8% ± 10% at 1 year and slightly greater thereafter. The impact of weight gain on patient and allograft survival remains unclear. A retrospective analysis revealed a correlation of poor weight gain and low BMI posttransplant with worse kidney function and a greater incidence of chronic allograft dysfunction. In contrast, two retrospective studies found that patients with better kidney function, measured by the Cockcroft–Gault equation, gained more weight posttransplant. Whether poor weight gain is a marker of other confounding factors associated with either an acute or a chronic inflammatory state and not a direct function of weight itself is unknown. Similarly, it is well established that weight gain is strongly associated with increased risk of an unfavorable metabolic milieu, including insulin resistance, diabetes, ischemic heart disease, reduced graft survival, hypertension, and hyperlipidemia, which are all highly prevalent posttransplantation. A prospective observational trial in 96 patients identified younger age, higher carbohydrate consumption, higher truncal fat percentage, and higher perception of mental health quality of life as pretransplant predictors of posttransplant weight gain; with the exception of age, the remaining are modifiable risk factors that could be studied as targeted interventions in the peritransplant period.

The stimulus for posttransplant weight gain is thought to be multifactorial (Table 14.1). Several studies demonstrated that weight gain might be more common in patients with younger age, female gender, lower income, pretransplant obesity, African-American ethnicity, absence of acute rejection, better recovery of kidney function, and living donor transplants. The impact of immunosuppressive therapy on posttransplant weight gain is of particular interest because this is one area in which a physician may intervene in an attempt to impact a change in weight. Over the past two decades, the majority of patients have been maintained on triple therapy, including low-dose prednisone, a calcineurin inhibitor (CNI), and an antiproliferative agent. Many in the transplant community believed that, based on the physiologic effects of excessive exogenous corticosteroid administration, chronic steroid therapy had an adverse effect on new-onset diabetes, hyperlipidemia, and weight gain posttransplant. A retrospective analysis evaluated the difference in posttransplant weight gain over the first 3 years posttransplant in 95 patients treated with standard triple immunosuppression versus those with either complete steroid avoidance or early steroid withdrawal. There was no significant difference among percentage of patients who gained weight after transplantation between groups ($p = 0.27$). In contrast, another retrospective analysis of the association between chronic steroid exposure and posttransplant weight gain, which included 328 patients, found that although all patients gained weight during the first posttransplant year, there was a significant difference between the steroid withdrawal and steroid maintenance groups. The results of a randomized, double-blind, placebo-controlled trial of 386 patients comparing outcomes with early corticosteroid withdrawal and chronic low-dose corticosteroid therapy were quite surprising: there were no differences observed for patients experiencing the primary end composite endpoint of death, graft loss, or moderate/severe rejection or renal function. There was a positive association between steroid withdrawal and lower serum triglycerides and a less posttransplant weight gain (5.1 vs. 7.7 kg, $p = 0.05$) but no difference in incidence of new onset diabetes after transplant. Similarly, either de novo or subsequent conversion from CNI to sirolimus was found to be associated with less posttransplant weight gain in a single-center retrospective analysis. Collectively these studies suggest that posttransplant weight gain is multifactorial. Moving beyond pharmacologic

TABLE 14.1   Contributors to Posttransplant Weight Gain

Loss of anorectic factors and improvement in taste of food
Loss of the dietary restrictions of CKD
Younger age
Female gender
Low-income status
Pretransplant obesity
African-American ethnicity
Transplantation from living donors
Effect of immunosuppressive agents

CKD, chronic kidney disease.

risk factors, a small study compared daily energy expenditure and its components (sleeping, basal and absorptive metabolic rates) in 19 nondiabetic kidney transplant recipients and nine healthy men matched for height, age, and lean body mass. The investigators found that while the weight gainers had less energy expenditure with a tendency toward higher energy intake, the nonweight gainers had an increased resting and sleeping energy expenditure that protected them from weight gain. They hypothesized that higher β-blocker consumption in the weight gaining group may account for some of this effect. Interestingly, these patients were not on steroids posttransplant.

The most common cause of allograft loss in the United States is currently death with a functioning graft secondary to cardiovascular diseases (CVDs). It is established within the general population that obesity and comorbidities related to increased adiposity increase the risk for CVD and death. While this has not been prospectively confirmed in the kidney transplant population, it is reasonable to speculate that minimizing all modifiable cardiovascular risk factors including obesity could improve both patient and allograft survival. Strategies to either maintain or lose weight posttransplant include lifestyle modification with caloric restriction and increased physical activity, pharmacotherapy, and surgery. A prospective study to assess the efficacy of a weight reduction program in motivated overweight, obese, and severely obese transplant recipients through lifestyle medication demonstrated less weight gain in the motivated group who met with a healthcare professional for 40 minutes, reviewed a detailed 3-day food diary, and had anthropometric measurements taken yet received no dietary recommendations. Although the group was too small to draw any conclusions, these encouraging findings suggest that simply making patients conscious of their dietary habits and making them aware of weight gain posttransplant without any further active intervention may have a significant impact.

Surgery, either in the form of gastric banding, sleeve gastrectomy, or gastric bypass, remains the most invasive option for weight loss. A meta-analysis by Hadjievangelou and colleagues studying WLS outcomes following 112 kidney transplant recipients found excess weight loss of 30% to 75% at 1 year postintervention. The wide variability is attributed to small sample size and use of different types of bariatric procedures. None of these studies (three prospective case series and one multicenter retrospective study) compared outcomes to nontransplant controls. There was one rejection episode within 30 days of surgery, which was concerning owing to the possible issues related to the bioavailability of immunosuppressive agents after WLS. Though in a study of five patients who underwent WLS, there was no need for dose alterations on immunosuppressive medications, in another study of eight patients, three required tacrolimus dose adjustments. In a retrospective single-center study of 10 patients who underwent laparoscopic sleeve gastrectomy, 2 patients had major complications which required revision. None of the patients suffered graft loss or death during follow-up, but half were lost to follow-up before the end of Year 1. In summary, currently, there is limited evidence that these procedures are reasonably safe and feasible after transplantation with variable but positive short-term outcomes. Long-term effects of WLS on graft and patient survival remain unknown. Patients undergoing WLS require a close follow-up and frequent measurement of CNI levels, especially in the early postoperative period and also until their weights are stabilized.

The issue of weight loss should be discussed in detail with all obese transplant candidates. Surgical techniques used for weight loss are evolving and improving rapidly. Obese candidates should be directed to weight loss programs when available. Timing of the transplant in obese patients depend on many factors, including transplant center's experience with such patients, use of living versus deceased donor kidneys, waiting time in the region, and availability of certain interventions to accomplish the planned target weight loss. Lifestyle modification with diet and exercise is crucial to achieve and support sustained weight loss after transplantation. It should be noted that high-protein intake (Ornish and Atkins) and high-fat intake (Atkins) diets may not be advisable in kidney transplant recipients. This topic merits further clinical investigation to drive best practice recommendations.

HYPERGLYCEMIA

Abnormalities in glucose metabolism following kidney transplantation have been recognized as common complications that may adversely affect long-term both allograft and patient outcomes. Transplant-associated hyperglycemia (TAH) has been proposed as terminology that encompasses new-onset diabetes mellitus (NODM), impaired fasting glucose, and impaired glucose tolerance. The incidence of NODM posttransplantation falls within the range of 2% to 53%. While prospective randomized controlled interventional trials are absent in the posttransplant population, ample evidence exists within the general population supporting the benefit of aggressive glycemic control on limiting microvascular and possibly cardiovascular events.

The pathogenesis of TAH is complex and multifactorial. In brief, TAH is the end result of an imbalance between insufficient insulin secretion, increased insulin metabolism, and insulin resistance by target organs. Often, some degree of impaired glucose tolerance may be present but unrecognized in the pretransplant setting, because the kidney contributes to insulin degradation and loss of kidney function results in decreased insulin metabolism; the well-functioning allograft will restore normal insulin metabolism and unmask this imbalance. Using an insulin sensitivity index calculated from insulin and glucose levels measured while fasting and during a glucose tolerance test, it was demonstrated that insulin sensitivity worsened after transplantation suggesting that insulin sensitivity has a major role in TAH. The incidence of TAH is highest in the early months following transplantation, when steroid and CNI dosages are usually highest. Nonmodifiable risk factors for TAH include advanced age, male gender, nonwhite ethnicity, family history, and polycystic kidney disease. Modifiable risk factors include hepatitis C (HCV) infection, obesity, physical inactivity, weight gain, and immunosuppressive regimens (Table 14.2).

Screening strategies for impaired glucose metabolism vary across transplant centers. Screening should begin during the initial transplant evaluation through taking a thorough medical and family history along with assessment of fasting plasma glucose. Those with normal fasting plasma glucose (glucose <100 mg per dL) or impaired fasting glucose (100 < glucose < 126 mg per dL) should have follow-up screening by an oral glucose tolerance test (OGTT) either annually or biannually while waiting for a transplant. Screening by OGTT will identify those with isolated postprandial hyperglycemia and those

TABLE 14.2	Contributors to Transplant-Associated Hyperglycemia
Nonmodifiable Risk Factors	**Modifiable Risk Factors**
Advanced age	Hepatitis C infection
Male gender	Obesity
Nonwhite ethnicity	Physical inactivity
Family history	Weight gain
Polycystic kidney disease	Immunosuppressive medications

with diabetes mellitus, which is masked by decreased insulin metabolism secondary to advanced CKD. These newly diagnosed diabetics or prediabetics should then be referred to a diabetologist for intensive education and initiation of treatment. Pretransplant evaluation will also identify HCV-positive patients, and in the era of highly efficacious, direct acting antivirals for HCV therapy it is hoped that HCV eradication after renal transplantation will reduce the risk of TAH.

Hyperglycemia is very common in the immediate posttransplant setting. Most patients receive some form of induction therapy, which includes high-dose corticosteroids, and this along with the stress of surgery is implicated as the main contributors to impaired glycemic control during the first posttransplant week. Monoclonal antibodies against CD25, the interleukin 2 receptor, used for induction immunosuppression have been associated with a greater incidence of TAH. Within 1 week of surgery the dose of steroids is tapered or completely withdrawn, making it less of a contributor to hyperglycemia.

Maintenance immunosuppression, which often includes low-dose prednisone, a CNI, an antiproliferative agent, or rapamycin, is yet another contributor to TAH. Inferences from the transplantation literature seem to suggest that low-dose maintenance glucocorticoid therapy has minimal if any effect on long-term glucose metabolism. A large prospective randomized controlled trial that compared the glycemic influence of cyclosporine and tacrolimus showed that tacrolimus was associated with a significant increased risk of TAH and impaired fasting glucose at 6 months posttransplant without any difference in efficacy between the two agents. Sirolimus has been reported to be more diabetogenic than cyclosporine, making conversion to sirolimus a less attractive option to the transplant physician seeking to minimize modifiable risk factors for TAH.

Diabetic education should begin prior to discharge from the hospital, and each patient with hyperglycemia should monitor both fasting and 2 hours' postprandial glucose concentrations. As always, treatment should include intensive education for lifestyle modifications including daily moderate exercise such as walking for at least 30 minutes daily, weight loss mediated by caloric restriction and increased energy expenditure, and dietary modification. The currently recommended diet should limit the daily carbohydrate intake to 130 to 180 g as part of a 1,800 to 2,000 kcal diet, with complete avoidance of concentrated sweets. Along with lifestyle modification, pharmacologic therapy might be necessary as well. In the immediate posttransplant period, exogenous insulin remains the treatment of choice; when both dosing of glucocorticoids and daily caloric intake varies from day to day, glycemic management is most safely and quickly attained with "sliding scale" dosing of rapid-acting insulin every 6 hours. Once postoperative stress subsides and the patient's diet and steroid dosing begins to stabilize, the cumulative insulin requirement is calculated and administered as a combination of basal and bolus insulin. Usually, one-third to one-half of the daily insulin requirement is administered as basal long-acting insulin, whereas the remaining insulin is administered as rapid-acting insulin immediately before each meal. When the 24-hour insulin requirement falls below 20 units per day, one can then consider transitioning the patient to oral agents. Because glycemic management is complex and dynamic in the early posttransplant period, a time when transplant recipients find themselves taking many new medications, collaboration with an endocrinologist would be helpful to achieve safe and effective glycemic control and any opportunity to begin this education and the associated lifestyle changes pretransplant could be helpful.

Kidney transplant recipients are felt to remain at increased risk for TAH throughout the life span of their allograft and therefore, continued diabetic screening is recommended in this population. For those patients who are not hyperglycemic on discharge from the hospital, international consensus guidelines recommend weekly assessment of fasting plasma glucose for the first posttransplant month and then every 3 months thereafter. Long-term management of TAH is similar to management in the general population. Minimizing exposure to diabetogenic maintenance immunosuppressive agents like glucocorticoids, CNI, and sirolimus may improve glycemic control. The adjunctive use of mycophenolic acid to spare tacrolimus exposure may reduce the incidence of TAH. Pharmacologic options in the long-term kidney transplant recipient are similar to that of the CKD population, with occasional dose adjustment necessary with deteriorating kidney function. Sulfonylureas directly stimulate insulin secretion from β-cells of the pancreas, thereby improving both fasting and postprandial glycemic control. Glipizide, a second-generation sulfonylurea, is predominantly metabolized by the liver and as such can be used with advanced kidney disease. However, such patients remain at increased risk for hypoglycemic events in the setting of a failing allograft and consequently will often require a dose adjustment. Thiazolidinediones, such as rosiglitazone and pioglitazone, which increase insulin sensitivity, and meglitinides, such as repaglinide and nateglinide, which potentiate insulin secretion, are quite effective oral agents. They do not have any apparent interaction with CNI metabolism and are considered both safe and effective for treatment in the kidney transplant recipients. Metformin is cleared by renal tubular secretion, and there are case reports of lactic acidosis in the setting of advanced renal impairment, limiting use of this agent in the setting of severe allograft dysfunction glucagon-like peptide 1 (GLP1) receptor agonists, such as exenatide, stimulate insulin secretion in a glucose-dependent manner with minimal hypoglycemic potential. Additionally, they slow gastric emptying thereby suppressing appetite. Immunosuppressive drug levels should be monitored closely with initiation of therapy. Sodium-glucose co-transporter 2 inhibitors, such as canagliflozin and dapagliflozin, block the glucose reabsorption in the kidney, increase glucose excretion, and lower blood glucose levels. Unfortunately, vaginal yeast infections and urinary tract infections are common side effects of these new drugs. Transplant patients must be monitored very closely when they are on these medications because there is no data on safety of this class of medications in kidney transplant recipients.

HYPERLIPIDEMIA

Hyperlipidemia after transplantation is multifactorial resulting from genetic and environmental factors. Dyslipidemia and long-standing vascular disease from preexisting hyperlipidemia, prolonged dialytic support, or diabetes mellitus are nonmodifiable factors in contrast to immunosuppressive therapy, diet, posttransplant proteinuria, chronic allograft dysfunction, and weight gain posttransplantation. The prevalence of dyslipidemia is reported to be within the range of 16% to 60% after kidney transplantation. Whereas hypertriglyceridemia is the more common abnormality in lipid metabolism among patients undergoing dialysis, transplantation is associated with an elevation in total and low-density lipoprotein (LDL) cholesterol. A strong family history of dyslipidemia among first-degree relatives as well as apolipoprotein E polymorphisms are predictive of dyslipidemia posttransplantation and perhaps may be useful to preemptively identify patients at increased risk.

Exposure to different immunosuppressive agents, such as steroids, CNIs, and sirolimus, appears to influence the incidence and severity of dyslipidemia posttransplant. The antimetabolite immunosuppressive drugs, such as mycophenolate mofetil and azathioprine, are not associated with the development of dyslipidemias.

| TABLE 14.3 | Treatment of Posttransplant Hyperlipidemia |

Diet
Total fat intake only 30%–25% of calories
Saturated fats <7% of total calories
Dietary cholesterol <200 mg/d
LDL lowering options
25–30 g/d soluble fiber
2 g/d plant stanol/sterol
   Statins if needed
Weight loss
Increased physical activity

LDL, low-density lipoprotein.

The Kidney Disease Outcomes Quality Initiative (KDIGO) published an extensive guideline in 2004 addressing dyslipidemias in the kidney transplant recipient. These recommendations were later endorsed by the KDIGO 2013 clinical practice guideline for care of the kidney transplant recipient. These guidelines classified transplant recipients in the highest cardiovascular risk category, and both lipid monitoring and treatment of dyslipidemia with a combination of lifestyle modification and pharmacotherapy were recommended to achieve a target LDL <100 mg per dL (Table 14.3).

Many small prospective observational studies have assessed the effect of dietary modification on hyperlipidemia in the kidney recipient with limited success. Currently, the recommended posttransplant diet should contain wholegrain, high fiber (25 to 30 g per day), low glycemic index carbohydrates, and monounsaturated fat. Total fat intake should contribute only 30% to 35% of daily calories. Dietary management of hyperlipidemia has been studied in a single-center fashion in the kidney transplant population. One study randomized patients to modified Mediterranean-style diet compared to a standard Central European low-fat diet. Patients in the intervention arm were encouraged to eat fresh vegetables with each meal and limit animal protein to <50 g per day. After 6 months of follow-up, patients in the treatment arm had decrease in total cholesterol and triglycerides, whereas no change was observed in the control group. Another study assessed the effectiveness of a modified American Heart Association (AHA) Step One diet in lowering serum lipids in stable kidney transplant patients; after 12 weeks on the diet, there was a reduction in total cholesterol, LDL, and triglycerides.

Fish oils, which contain ω-3 polyunsaturated fatty acids including α-linolenic acid, eicosapentaenoic acid, and docosahexaenoic acid, have been found to be beneficial in preventing CVD in the general population. A meta-analysis of 15 studies of fish oil treatment on 733 kidney transplant recipients on CNI therapy found that fish oil did not significantly affect patient or graft survival, acute rejection rates, or CNI toxicity when compared to placebo. There was a beneficial effect on diastolic blood pressure and HDL cholesterol. The effect on lipids was not significantly different than low-dose statins. Fish oil use was not associated with any difference in patient or allograft survival, acute rejection, or CNI toxicity. Currently, the available data is insufficient to globally recommend routine use in kidney transplant recipients.

The results of the large Assessment of Lescol in Renal Transplantation trial demonstrated that statin use, fluvastatin, was both safe and effective in this patient population. The study was underpowered for a primary prevention study to detect a significant reduction in cardiac events, but they demonstrated a 35% reduction in the secondary endpoints of cardiac death and nonfatal myocardial infarction with statin therapy. Further post hoc analysis demonstrated the greatest benefit with early initiation of therapy. A recent meta-analysis of 22 studies which included 3,465 participants on statin use in transplant recipients demonstrated that statins may reduce major cardiovascular events and cardiovascular mortality but had uncertain effects on all-cause mortality. Statin treatment also had uncertain effects on stroke, kidney function, and toxicity outcomes in kidney transplant recipients. Owing to heterogeneity in comparisons, they could not analyze the data directly comparing differing statin regimens. The cumulative benefits of statin therapy may extend beyond that of lipid lowering and may include decreases in interstitial fibrosis, proteinuria, and inflammatory response, which require further studies. Acute kidney injury, doubling of serum creatinine, and proteinuria are reported with rosuvastatin, a newer statin, especially when higher doses were used. Currently, despite limited evidence, the KDIGO guideline suggests use of statins for kidney transplant recipients older than 30 years of age. Regarding the use of fibrates, there have been reports of elevated serum creatinine as well as increased risk of rhabdomyolysis because of concurrent use of statins and fibrates. Furthermore, fenofibrate is contraindicated in patients with estimated glomerular filtration rate (eGFR) <30 mL/min/1.73 m^2. Additional studies are needed regarding the use of fibrates in transplant patients with elevated triglycerides. Bile acid sequestrants, such as cholestyramine or colesevelam, are generally not recommended in transplant recipients because they can interfere with the absorption of immunosuppressive medications. Ezetimibe is another alternative in patients who are intolerant to statins. Owing to the significant potential interactions between CNIs and statins by slowing their metabolism via the cytochrome P450 system, transplant recipients should be started on low-dose statin with cautious dose increase depending on the lipid profile and symptoms.

PROTEIN METABOLISM

The immediate posttransplant period is associated with a negative nitrogen balance secondary, in part, to the stress of surgery, increased requirements for wound healing, and increased hepatic gluconeogenesis stimulated by pulse dose steroids used for induction immunosuppression. Investigators have shown that one can prevent the generation of a negative nitrogen balance by increasing a patient's dietary protein intake, especially in the first 4 weeks after transplantation. The current recommended postoperative protein intake falls within the range of 1.3 to 1.5 g per kg ideal body weight. In the case of a patient with apparent pretransplant protein–energy wasting, it would be prudent to adjust his or her dietary intake to the upper range. Daily caloric intake must be sufficient for the protein to be utilized for anabolic needs as opposed to gluconeogenesis. The caloric requirement of the average patient is within the range of 35 kcal per kg ideal body weight for the first several weeks following transplantation. Obese patients may benefit from caloric restriction to the range of 25 to 30 kcal per kg ideal body weight in an attempt to avoid excessive posttransplant weight gain. Adequate protein intake during administration of high-dose glucocorticoids has been shown to minimize some steroid-induced side effects, including a cushingoid appearance and steroid-induced myopathy.

While increased protein intake is beneficial in the immediate posttransplant period, optimal long-term dietary protein intake is less well established. The relatively low doses of steroid use are not felt to strongly impact protein catabolism. The knowledge of a high-protein diet causing glomerular hyperfiltration and chronic allograft dysfunction centering around nephron underdosing and chronic hyperfiltration injury has led some to believe that protein restriction to be beneficial in prolonging allograft function. One study, which compared stable kidney transplant recipients who were adherent with a diet containing protein (0.8 g/kg/d), sodium (3 g per day), and fat (<30% caloric intake) with those who were nonadherent, found a decline in allograft function in the nonadherent group as measured by creatinine clearance and renal scintigraphy. In the setting of a lack for evidence to support any specific recommendation, dietary protein intake is recommended in the range of 1 g/kg/d, similar to patients with Stages 2 and 3 CKD.

BONE AND MINERAL METABOLISM

CKD is associated with a spectrum of bone disease, ranging from high-bone turnover osteitis fibrosa, low-bone turnover including osteomalacia and adynamic bone disease, and mixed uremic osteodystrophy. Secondary hyperparathyroidism has also been implicated in vascular and soft tissue calcifications, increased cardiovascular mortality, and neurologic issues in patients with CKD. It is not surprising that the spectrum of posttransplant bone disease is variable as well, due to preexisting pretransplant bone disease along with posttransplant factors. Diagnosis of a particular pathologic process is challenging, because bone biopsy still remains the gold standard. In a review characterizing the pathology of bone biopsies in transplant recipients, high-turnover bone disease was the most prevalent, with 47% of patients having mild or moderate osteitis fibrosa; approximately 12% having mixed bone disease; 9% having low-turnover bone disease, either adynamic bone disease or osteomalacia; 23% had reduced bone mass in the absence of pathology associated with renal osteodystrophy; and only 9% having normal bone morphology. Bone disease is often assessed using the noninvasive dual energy x-ray absorptiometry (DEXA) scan. However, interpretation of this test is very difficult in the CKD and kidney transplant population because it does not provide any information on microarchitecture or the volume of either cortical or trabecular bone. Furthermore, interpretation of a standard DEXA of lumbar vertebrae is confounded by calcification of the overlying abdominal aorta, which will seemingly increase the mineralization score. Newer techniques, including micro-magnetic resonance imaging, are emerging as better noninvasive modalities of differentiating between high- and low-bone turnover diseases.

Alterations in bone metabolism posttransplant are attributed to a complex interplay of allograft function, the parathyroid gland, posttransplant immunosuppression, vitamin D synthesis as well as polymorphisms of the vitamin D receptor, along with calcium and phosphate metabolism. In general, because of better kidney function posttransplant, parathyroid hyperplasia would slowly regress, unless the patient has tertiary hyperparathyroidism. While serum calcium levels tend to fall within the lower end of the normal range pretransplant, it most often rises posttransplant, occasionally resulting in mild hypercalcemia and hypophosphatemia. This change is attributed to elevated parathyroid hormone (PTH) levels. Similarly, hypophosphatemia is common following kidney transplant, affecting up to 93% of patients in the early posttransplant period. While it usually resolves within the first few months posttransplant, hypophosphatemia may persist for many years in some patients. Initially, hypophosphatemia was attributed to elevated PTH levels as a consequence of secondary hyperparathyroidism and persistent hypophosphatemia attributed to tertiary hyperparathyroidism. Recent investigation has uncoupled this relationship, because renal phosphate wasting may be found in the absence of an elevated PTH. Other factors that support the uncoupling of this association is the concomitant finding of inappropriately low-serum calcitriol levels in the presence of normal allograft function and hypophosphatemia, a potent stimulus of calcitriol synthesis. FGF 23 is known to induce renal phosphate wasting and inhibit 1-α hydroxylation of 25-hydroxyvitamin D [25(OH)D]. A longitudinal study of 27 living donor kidney recipients confirmed the association between excess FGF 23 at the time of transplantation and both renal phosphate excretion and serum phosphate level posttransplant. Serum phosphate levels should be followed in the posttransplant period, and repletion should be considered for those with persistent hypophosphatemia despite adequate dietary intake. However, vigorous repletion may exacerbate existing secondary hyperparathyroidism, and therefore the minimal necessary supplemental dose should be administered.

How to best address hypercalcemia due to persistent hyperparathyroidism after kidney transplant has been the subject of intense debate. Although subtotal parathyroidectomy is the definitive therapeutic approach, patients are often reluctant to undergo another surgery, especially when cinacalcet, a calcium sensing receptor modulator, provides a therapeutic alternative. In a prospective study, 30 transplant recipients were randomized to subtotal parathyroidectomy versus cinacalcet therapy for persistent hypercalcemia. All of the parathyroidectomy patients and 66% of the cinacalcet patients achieved normal serum calcium levels by 12 months of follow-up. Importantly only subtotal parathyroidectomy was associated with an increase in femoral neck bone mineral density, and costs were similar if patients required cinacalcet therapy for 14 months or longer. Vascular calcifications remained unchanged in both the groups though. There have been some concerns about decreased renal function with both cinacalcet and parathyroidectomy in previous studies due to a renal hemodynamic mechanism. In this particular study, a 12-month GFR decline was seen in both the groups; although the change was greater in the cinacalcet group, the difference was not statistically significant.

The main concern regarding posttransplant bone disease centers around an increased risk of fracture compared with both the general population and the dialysis population. Therapeutic options for treating posttransplant osteodystrophy include the use of bisphosphonates, vitamin D analogues, calcitonin, and hormone replacement therapy. A Cochrane systematic review found that no individual intervention was associated with a reduction in fracture risk compared with placebo. Bisphosphonates had greater efficacy at minimizing loss of bone mineral density when compared with vitamin D supplementation. However, because these studies did not include bone biopsy and low-turnover bone disease is not uncommon in this population, many experts are hesitant about the use of bisphosphonates because the inhibitory effect of bisphosphonates on osteoclast-mediated bone resorption persists far beyond the duration of drug administration, and lack of loss of bone mineral density does not necessarily indicate the presence of structurally stable healthy bone.

Vitamin D deficiency after kidney transplantation is extremely common; in a prospective study, only 12% of incident renal transplant recipients had normal serum vitamin D levels and vitamin D deficiency was more common in African-American patients. Vitamin D deficiency in the renal transplant population is multifactorial; impaired renal function and increased FGF-23 levels reduce tubular 1α hydroxylase activity, immunosuppression increases vitamin D catabolism, and transplant physicians recommend strict sun avoidance to decrease skin cancer risk. Guidelines suggest that renal transplant recipients should take 1,000 to 1,500 mg per day of elemental calcium and 5 to 15 µg per day of vitamin D through either dietary sources or supplementation, unless they have significant hypercalcemia. Vitamin D-rich foods include oily fish, liver, eggs, and fortified milk, which may not be well represented in the average American diet and necessitate supplementation.

Vitamin D exerts potentially important effects in renal transplant recipients beyond skeletal maintenance; it is an important regulator of innate and adaptive immunity. Monocytes possess a vitamin D receptor and the 1α hydroxylase required to convert 25(OH)D to 1,25(OH)D. Vitamin D has been shown to inhibit CD4 and CD8 T cell activity and promote Treg differentiation, while modulating antigen presentation by dendritic cells and inflammatory chemokine production; these actions on the immune system may create a more favorable environment for the allograft. In clinical practice, vitamin D-deficiency posttransplant has been shown to be associated with an increased risk of DGF and acute rejection. Two prospective studies of vitamin D repletion in renal transplant recipients have been conducted: the Vitamin D Supplementation in Renal Transplant Recipients (VITALE) study randomized renal transplant recipients to low (12,000 IU) versus high (100,000 IU) dose vitamin D supplementation and will examine the development of diabetes, CVD, and cancer. The VITA-D study randomized patients to placebo versus 6,800 IU cholecalciferol daily and will assess allograft function, acute rejection rates, and infection. The forthcoming results of both studies will provide important insights as to whether repletion of Vitamin D can provide benefits beyond fracture prevention.

GUT MICROBIOTA AND KIDNEY

Microorganisms in the human gut permit breakdown and degradation of certain indigestible foods, synthesis of vitamins, as well as play a role in modulating our immune system to reduce allergic reactions. In patients with CKD, uremic toxins and bowel wall edema alter the composition of the gut ecosystem, leading to intestinal barrier dysfunction and translocation of endotoxins, live bacteria, and bacterial metabolites to the systemic circulation; this contributes to systemic inflammation and acceleration in CVDs. An imbalance between pathogenic and protective microorganisms called dysbiosis might transfer immune cells and signals to distant sites such as organ transplants. Use of antibiotics, exposure to alloantigens, immunosuppressive medications, and posttransplant CKD could significantly influence the composition of microbes in the gut of transplant recipients. Recently, there have been great interest in using prebiotics (nondigestible food ingredients that can induce the growth or activity of microorganisms, such as gum arabic fiber supplementation) and probiotics (living microorganisms), which may modify the bacterial composition of the intestines and maintain a well-balanced gut ecosystem. At present, this is an area of emerging research within the CKD and transplant population. In a study of 26 kidney transplant recipients, serial fecal specimens were collected during the first 3 months of transplantation to characterize the bacterial composition of the gut. Significant changes in the gut microbiota after kidney transplantation were demonstrated including an abundance of Enterococcus observed in transplant recipients with posttransplant Enterococcus UTI. Fecal microbiota transplantation (FMT) with donor stool (heterologous) or patient's own stool (autologous) administered by colonoscopy has been successful in recurrent *Clostridium difficile* infection seen in the general population. FMT has also been shown to be safe and efficacious in two solid organ transplant recipients, one lung and one renal transplant, with refractory *C. difficile* colitis. No infectious complications were observed. The safety of probiotic supplementation in immunosuppressed patients is not well established. In a cohort of hematopoietic cell transplant recipients, the use of probiotics was reported to cause bacteremia, though infrequently. A recent review of nine studies that involved 735 people on the

Recommended Nutritional Intake for Kidney Transplant Recipients

First Month after Transplantation and during Therapy for Acute Rejection

Protein	1.3–1.5 g/kg/d
Calories	30–35 kcal/kg/d

After First Month

Protein	1.0 g/kg/d
Calories	Sufficient to achieve and maintain optimal weight for height

At All Times

Carbohydrates	50% of calories
Fats	Not >30% of calories
Cholesterol	Not >300 mg/d
Calcium	1,000–1,500 mg/d
Vitamin D	5–15 µg/d
Exercise	At least 30 minutes, 5–6 times/wk

use of probiotics in patients susceptible to urinary tract infections did not demonstrate a significant benefit of probiotic use compared with placebo or no treatment. Until we have more research/data to understand the impact of gut microbiota changes on posttransplant outcomes along with data guiding the safety and value of any interventions in this high-risk patient population, we would not be able to provide any recommendations.

CONCLUSION

Recommended diets for the immediate posttransplant period and for long-term therapy are summarized in Table 14.4. A recurrent theme in the preceding discussion of nutritional and metabolic abnormalities in recipients of kidney transplants is the lack of prospective randomized interventional studies with long-term follow-up to assess the benefit of most treatments. We believe that all kidney transplant recipients should be educated and continuously encouraged and motivated to maintain a healthy lifestyle through adherence to a heart-healthy diet along with regular exercise.

Suggested Readings

Ahmad S, Bromberg JS. Current status of the microbiome in renal transplantation. *Curr Opin Nephrol Hypertens* 2016;25(6):570–576.

Bhan I, Shah A, Holmes J, et al. Post-transplant hypophosphatemia: tertiary 'hyperphosphatoninism'? *Kidney Int* 2006;70:1486–1494.

Bloom RD, Crutchlow MF. New-onset diabetes mellitus in the kidney recipient: diagnosis and management strategies. *Clin J Am Soc Nephrol* 2008;(Suppl 2):S38–S48.

Cashion AK, Hathaway DK, Stanfill A, et al. Pre-transplant predictors of one yr weight gain after kidney transplantation. *Clin Transplant* 2014;28(11):1271–1278.

Chadban S, Chan M, Fry K, et al. Caring for Australasians with Renal Impairment (CARI) guidelines: nutrition in kidney transplant recipients. Available at: http://cari.org.au/Transplantation/transplantation_guidelines.html.

Cruzado JM, Moreno P, Torregrosa JV, et al. A randomized study comparing parathyroidectomy with cinacalcet for treating hypercalcemia in kidney allograft recipients with hyperparathyroidism. *J Am Soc Nephrol* 2016;27(8):2487–2494.

Fellström B, Holdaas H, Jardine AG, et al. Effect of fluvastatin on renal end points in the Assessment of Lescol in Renal Transplant (ALERT) trial. *Kidney Int* 2004;66:1549–1555.

Gill JS, Lan J, Dong J, et al. The survival benefit of kidney transplantation in obese patients. *Am J Transplant* 2013;13(8):2083–2090.

Hadjievangelou N, Kulendran M, McGlone ER, et al. Is bariatric surgery in patients following renal transplantation safe and effective? A best evidence topic. *Int J Surg* 2016;28:191–195.

Heng AE, Montaurier C, Cano N, et al. Energy expenditure, spontaneous physical activity and with weight gain in kidney transplant recipients. *Clin Nutr* 2015;34(3):457–464.

Hill CJ, Courtney AE, Cardwell CR, et al. Recipient obesity and outcomes after kidney transplantation: a systematic review and meta-analysis. *Nephrol Dial Transplant* 2015;30(8):1403–1411.

Joss N, Staatz CE, Thomson AH, et al. Predictors of new onset diabetes after renal transplantation. *Clin Nephrol* 2007;21:136–143.

Lim AKH, Manley KJ, Roberts MA, et al. Fish oil for kidney transplant recipients. *Cochrane Database Syst Rev* 2016;18(8).

Modanlou KA, Muthyala U, Xiao H, et al. Bariatric surgery among kidney transplant candidates and recipients: analysis of the United States Renal Data System and literature review. *Transplantation* 2009;87(8):1167–1173.

Naik AS, Sakhuja A, Cibrik DM, et al. The impact of obesity on allograft failure after kidney transplantation: a competing risk analysis. *Transplantation* 2016;100(9):1963–1969.

Vaziri ND, Zhao YY, Pahl MV. Altered intestinal microbial flora and impaired epithelial barrier structure and function in CKD: the nature, mechanisms, consequences, and potential treatment. *Nephrol Dial Transplant* 2016;31(5):737–746.

Enteral and Parenteral Nutrition in Kidney Disease: Practical Applications

Denise Mafra

Protein–energy wasting (PEW) is a common feature in patients with chronic kidney disease (CKD) and can adversely affect their prognosis. Anorexia, acute or chronic diseases, mechanical impairments to food intake (e.g., lack of dentures), uremia per se, dialysis procedure, psychiatric illnesses, loss of amino acid into dialysis, and other factors that increase the catabolism or decrease the anabolism may all contribute to PEW in patients with CKD.

In addition, anorexia results in nutrients deprivation causing changes in the gut, which include impaired mucosal integrity and barrier function, reduction on mucin synthesis, alteration on epithelial cell proliferation, and modification on gut microbiota. All these complications compromise the immunologic system in patients with CKD and provoke inflammation that is linked to PEW.

When patients present PEW associated with low-dietary energy and protein intake, oral supplementation should be given. However, for patients who are unable to tolerate nutritional supplementation by mouth, enteral tube feeding can be considered to achieve intake recommendations. If the patient cannot tolerate enteral nutrition, the parenteral or even intradialytic parenteral nutrition can be offered to treat PEW.

Nevertheless, there is still no consensus by the clinical guidelines on the type, time of initiation, or duration of use of enteral nutrition or parenteral nutrition in patients with CKD who were diagnosed with PEW. In this chapter, we will consider the practical applications of enteral and parenteral nutrition for patients with CKD based in some studies and general guidelines.

ORAL NUTRITIONAL SUPPLEMENTATION

The oral nutritional supplementation is the first choice for patients with CKD presenting PEW. In dialysis patients, when spontaneous energy intake is <30 kcal/kg/d and protein intake <1.0 g/kg/d, a nutritional intervention should be started. Renal-specific supplements offer high energy density and protein for dialysis patients and, in addition, low sodium and potassium ($\cong$400 kcal and 16 g of protein in 200 mL) or even low amount of protein with high calories ($\cong$400 kcal and 8 g of protein in 200 mL) for nondialysis patients.

Several studies have reported that oral nutritional supplementation leads to improvements in inflammatory status and biomarkers, such as albumin, quality of life and physical functioning, and reduction on hospitalizations and death.

Oral nutritional supplementation requirement depends on nutritional status and patient comorbidities. It's also important to consider the dose, smell, taste, and duration of oral supplementation and, patients should keep eating meals. For better results, the oral nutritional supplementation should be given 2 to 3 times a day, preferably 1 hour after main meals, late evening, or during dialysis. In fact, providing intradialytic oral nutritional supplements to dialysis patients can be a good strategy to reduce PEW risk.

The interaction with the renal dietitian during the supplementation period is important to increase patients' adherence. When patients receive extra care, more visits, and encouragement from their healthcare professional, the compliance may be improved. In addition, small volumes of oral nutritional supplementation may improve compliance. Moreover, the healthcare professional should provide supplements that meet patients' needs in terms of taste, flavor, and texture preferences to improve compliance to the treatment. A potential barrier for many patients, mainly in developing countries, are the high costs of these supplements and, in this case, the renal dietitians can suggest healthy ways to add calories to their diet such as use olive oil, nuts in muffins and breads, egg white omelets using olive oil, butter, cakes, and cookies (Table 15.1). Intradialytic intake of protein-rich food or snacks can be also effective in increasing calories and protein intake.

For patients who are unable to meet their protein and energy requirements with food intake and oral nutritional supplementation and still present an inadequate oral intake for more than 10 days and also severe PEW, enteral tube feeding is considered the first line of nutritional therapy. It's important to emphasize that healthcare professionals cannot wait for patients to develop PEW.

According to Guidelines from Society of Critical Care Medicine and American Society for Parenteral and Enteral Nutrition, delivering early nutrition support therapy, by the enteral route, is a proactive therapeutic strategy that may favorably affect patient outcomes.

ENTERAL NUTRITION

Enteral nutrition can be defined as nutrients, either a special liquid formula or pureed food, that are delivered to a patient through a tube directly into the gastrointestinal tract, usually into the stomach or small intestine. Enteral nutrition is less expensive as compared with parenteral nutrition, presents low septic complications, allows the provision of complete nutrition in a minimal fluid volume, provides a balanced nutrient, and can promotes trophic effects in the gastrointestinal tract.

Indications

Studies in patients with non-CKD suggest that enteral nutrition should be indicated when patients have oral intake lower than 60% of their requirements during 10 days. According to the Kidney Disease Outcomes Quality Initiative guideline, the period of inadequate intake after which nutritional support should be instituted ranges from days to 2 weeks, depending on the severity of the patients' clinical condition, malnutrition, and inadequacy of their nutritional intake degree. If severe undernutrition hemodialysis (HD) patients present spontaneous intake less than 20 kcal/kg/d or have stress conditions, enteral nutrition should be instituted.

Therefore, the higher the severity of the patients' clinical condition (like catabolic acute conditions, unconscious patients, for example, in neurology, patients in nursing homes), the severity of PEW and the inadequacy of nutritional intake, faster enteral nutrition should be instituted.

Hospitalized patients may receive nasogastric feeding until the acute illness resolves. For that, before considering nutrition support, the patient should receive a complete nutritional assessment. Elderly patients with CKD may require special attention. However, the nutrient requirements and the need for nutritional support in elderly patients have not been studied, although the prevalence of uremic patients older than 75 years is increasing.

An interesting point to consider when prescribing enteral feeding is the patients' willingness to accept the nasogastric tube. Healthcare professionals

TABLE
15.1   Patient with CKD on HD

Male, 58 years old, 55 kg, 1.71 m (BMI: 18.8 kg/m^2)
Body fat and arm circumference: reduced. Albumin: 3.6 g/dL
Energy: 35 × 64 kg (ideal body weight) = 2,240 kcal/d
Protein: 1.3 × 64 g = 83.2 g/d

Portion	Foods	Energy (kcal)	Protein (g)
	Breakfast		
50 g	Bread (1 portion)	125	4
8 g	Butter (2 teaspoon)	60	0
100 mL	Coffee (½ cup)	0	0
100 mL	Whole milk	55	3.2
12 g	Sugar (1 teaspoon)	48	0
100 g	Fruit (1 portion)	58	0.8
60 g	Cheese (1 slice)	60	4.0
	Example: 1 bread with butter and cheese + coffee and milk with sugar + apple		
	Sum breakfast	406	12.0
	Snack		
100 g	Fruit (1 portion)	58	0.8
	Lunch[*]		
25 g	Green salad (1 saucer)	5.5	0.4
100 g	Braised mix vegetables (4 tablespoon)	30	1.4
20 mL	Olive oil (4 teaspoon)	170	0
150 g	Rice (5 soup spoon)	207	3.0
40 g	Black beans (½ scoop)	31	2.0
100 g	Protein (1 portion)	180	22.0
100 g	Fruit (1 portion)	58	0.8
10 mL	Oil for coction	90	0
	Example: Lettuce salad + braised pumpkin and carrot + rice + beans + steak + strawberries		
	Sum lunch	771.5	29.6
	Snack		
200 mL	Oral supplement	400	15
	Dinner[*]		
25 g	Green salad (1 saucer)	5.5	0.4
100 g	Braised mix vegetables (4 tablespoon)	30	1.4
20 mL	Olive oil (4 teaspoon)	170	0
150 g	Pasta (5 soup spoon)	207	3.0
100 g	Protein (1 portion)	180	22.0
100 g	Fruit (1 portion)	58	0.8
10 mL	Oil for coction	90	0
	Example: 1 broccoli and spinach saucer salad + cauliflower + Spaghetti Bolognese + 2 thin slices of pineapple		
	Sum dinner	740.5	27.6
	Sum all meals	2,376	85.0

[*]If the patient does not accept the full meal, offer another supplement late evening.
BMI, body mass index; CKD, chronic kidney disease; HD, hemodialysis.

should discuss how important and beneficial is this treatment, because commonly the patients perceive this option as a punishment.

Routes, Implementation, and Recommendations

Enteral nutrition can be delivered via nasogastric or nasojejunal tubes or via percutaneous-endoscopic gastrostomy.

In patients with CKD, the choice route for enteral nutrition is preferentially temporary nasogastric tubing. In patients with gastroparesis (occurring especially in patients with diabetic nephropathy) or those patients who are intolerant to gastric feeds or at high risk for aspiration, post-pyloric or deep jejunal feeding is preferable. Percutaneous access (gastrostomy or jejunostomy) should be considered for long-term tube feeding in selected cases (enteral nutrition for >4 weeks). Owing to an increased incidence of peritonitis, percutaneous access is contra-indicated in adult peritoneal dialysis patients.

First, to enteral nutrition implementation, patients should undergo formal nutrition assessment, including evaluation of inflammation, with development of a nutrition care plan. This step is very important to evaluate the degree of PEW and the inadequacy of oral intake. Moreover, the nutrition assessment will be the baseline for the nutrition follow-up.

For patients with acute kidney injury (AKI) on dialysis therapy, the protein intake should range between 1.2 and 2.0 g/kg/d, up to a maximum of 2.5 g/kg/d, using usual body weight for normal weight patients and ideal body weight for obese and critically ill patients and, energy intake of 25 to 30 kcal/kg/d. For patients with stable CKD on dialysis, the protein intake recommendation is between 1.2 and 1.3 g/kg/d and energy intake recommendation around 30 to 35 kcal/kg/d. By contrast, patients on conservative treatment need to receive a low-protein diet with 0.6 g/kg/d.

Formula

Oral nutritional supplementation formula can be used as enteral nutrition formulas. For dialysis patients, CKD-specific formula should be preferred for enteral nutrition by tube feeding and the formula content in phosphorus and potassium should be checked.

Whey protein does not contain phosphorous. Hence, a supplement with 100% whey protein may be preferred. According to the European Best Practice Guidelines (EBPG), vitamin A supplements are not recommended for patients with CKD because vitamin A plasma levels are usually elevated. Moreover, the EBPG also state that vitamin K supplementation is not necessary, except in patients receiving long-term antibiotic treatment or those with altered coagulant activity. Then, the ideal formula should have good protein (100% whey protein) and should preferably be phosphorus (P), vitamin A (A), and K (K), PAK—free formula. For dialysis peritoneal patients, formula with a higher protein but lower carbohydrate content should be preferred.

When patients need to use enteral nutrition for more than 5 days, CKD-specific formula should be preferred, and there are several ready-to-use formula adapted to the nutrient requirements of patients on dialysis available. These formulas have a higher protein content (of high-biologic value partly in the forms of oligopeptides and free amino acids) and high-specific energy content of 1.5 to 2.0 kcal per mL, which limit the volume intake. Routine evaluation of K, Mg, P and Ca, albumin, creatinine plasma levels, edema, blood pressure, physical and clinical status, and body mass index deserves attention.

Complications

As proposed in European Society for Clinical Nutrition and Metabolism (ESPEN) guidelines for critically ill patients (and that can be used in patients with CKD undergoing enteral nutrition), patients should also be monitored for tolerance of enteral nutrition (determined by patients complaints of pain and/or distension, physical exam, passage of flatus, and stool). These points are very important in nondialysis CKD because nearly all gastrointestinal functions can be compromised. Impaired gastric emptying and intestinal motility, disturbances of digestive and absorptive functions, of biliary and pancreatic secretions, alterations in intestinal bacterial flora, aspiration, fluid overload, reflux esophagitis, and adequacy of feeding (determined by percent of goal calories and protein delivered) are complications that can occur during enteral nutrition therapy and patients should be monitored for risk. Diarrhea is another common complication during enteral nutrition and the guidelines suggest that enteral nutrition should not be automatically interrupted by this complication, but first it should be made to distinguish infectious diarrhea from osmotic diarrhea.

Complications can be avoided through well-established nurse-driven enteral feeding protocols, good strategies for delivery by volume-based or top-down feeding. In addition, adequacy of nutrition therapy can be enhanced by minimizing interruptions, and eliminating the practice of gastric residual volumes.

The use of prokinetic agent, continuous infusion, chlorhexidine mouthwash, elevate the head of bed, and divert level of feeding in the gastrointestinal tract, control of diabetes and treatment of diabetic neuropathy can reduce risk of aspiration and improve tolerance to enteral nutrition. In addition, the use of a mixed fiber-containing formula may be beneficial to the patients. There is also a need to consider that inappropriate cessation of enteral nutrition should be avoided.

Although complications and insufficient data of enteral nutritional support in patient with CKD, published studies have showed that enteral nutrition improves patient outcome. In fact, HD patients receiving enteral feeding have an increase on protein and energy intake and improvement in the albumin plasma levels.

Enteral nutrition plays an important role in the management of nutritional status in patients with poor food intake. Whenever, enteral support is contra-indicated or fails to reach the required intake targets, parenteral nutrition should be indicated.

PARENTERAL NUTRITION

A positive nitrogen balance can be demonstrated in patients with CKD submitted to surgery using parenteral nutrition. However, because of the risk of electrolyte disturbances, monitoring of the electrolytes, especially during the first weeks of parenteral nutrition support, is recommended. In addition, parenteral nutrition is associated with increased infectious complications, and requires a greater fluid volume to meet the calorie and protein needs. Besides that, it is significantly more expensive than enteral nutrition.

It is important to emphasize that parenteral nutrition should be reserved only for those patients who are unable to receive enteral nutrients. The guidelines suggest that for critically ill patient the use of parenteral nutrition should be considered after 7 to 10 days if unable to meet >60% of energy and protein requirements by the enteral nutrition.

Intradialytic Parenteral Nutrition
Intradialytic parenteral nutrition is a parenteral provision of nutrient through the extracorporeal circuit during HD. Intradialytic parenteral nutrition is a "Three-in-one" solution containing glucose/dextrose, amino acids, and fat emulsion, but in many studies, only amino acid solutions have been administered as intradialytic parenteral nutrition.

Intradialytic parenteral nutrition seems to increase albumin synthesis and whole body fat-free mass in patients with CKD. However, the largest nutritional intervention study (French Intradialytic Nutrition Evaluation) in patients with PEW showed that oral nutritional supplementation presented the same effects on rates of hospitalization or death when compared to intradialytic parenteral nutrition. Although it is a safe and efficacious modality of nutritional support, it should be reserved only for patients in whom oral nutritional supplementation or enteral nutrition are not feasible.

ADJUNCTIVE THERAPY: GOOD OR BAD?

Glutamine

A recent meta-analysis showed that glutamine-enriched enteral feeding significantly decreased gut permeability, but had no significant effect on length of hospitalization. According to the guidelines, the addition of glutamine to enteral nutrition has not been recommended to critically ill patients. There is no study in patients with CKD.

Probiotic

Although probiotic supplementation is theoretically sound, there has not been a consistent outcome benefit demonstrated for the general intensive care unit patient population. In patients with CKD, intervention trials confirming the beneficial effects on probiotic supplementation is still lacking.

Prebiotic

Based on the guidelines, fermentable soluble fiber (e.g., fructooligossaccharides and inulin) should be considered for routine use in all hemodynamically stable patients (10 to 20 g per day).

Antioxidant Vitamins and Trace Minerals

They may improve patient outcome, especially in burns, trauma, and critical illness requiring mechanical ventilation. However, most issues of administration, such as dosage, frequency, duration, and route of therapy, have not been well standardized. In addition, according to the guidelines, renal function should be considered when supplementing vitamins and trace elements.

CONCLUSIONS

Overall, the body of evidence supporting those oral nutritional supplementation, enteral nutrition or parenteral nutrition interventions is able to improve patient with CKD outcomes, and patients with PEW should receive the most appropriate nutritional support (oral supplements or enteral/parenteral support). A "food first" approach should be the first-line treatment, and if the patients no longer meet their protein and energy requirements, oral nutritional supplementation should be used during approximately 10 days. After this period, patients who are unable to tolerate nutritional supplementation by mouth, enteral tube feeding can be considered to achieve intake recommendations. If patients present some complication or enteral nutrition fails to reach the required intake targets, parenteral or even intradialytic parenteral nutrition should be an option (see Fig. 15.1).

Reports in the literature regarding the use of enteral, parenteral, or even oral supplementation in patients with CKD are scarce. Studies and guidelines on the effect of nutritional support on kidney disease are warranted. The role of nutrition in the management of CKD is important and needs to be included in future guidelines.

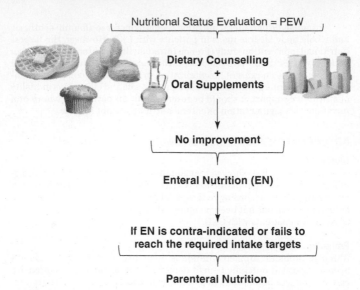

Nutritional Status Evaluation = PEW

Dietary Counselling
+
Oral Supplements

No improvement

Enteral Nutrition (EN)

If EN is contra-indicated or fails to reach the required intake targets

Parenteral Nutrition

FIGURE 15.1 Oral, enteral, and parenteral fluxogram. EN, enteral nutrition; PEW, protein–energy wasting.

Suggested Readings

Ash S, Campbell KL, Bogard J, et al. Nutrition prescription to achieve positive outcomes in chronic kidney disease: a systematic review. *Nutrients* 2014;6:416–451.

Brown RO, Compher C; American Society for Parenteral and Enteral Nutrition Board of Directors. A.S.P.E.N. clinical guidelines: nutrition support in adult acute and chronic renal failure. *JPEN J Parenter Enteral Nutr* 2010;34:366–377.

Cano NJ, Aparicio M, Brunori G, et al. ESPEN guidelines on parenteral nutrition: adult renal failure. *Clin Nutr* 2009;24:401–414.

Cano N, Fiaccadori E, Tesinsky P, et al. ESPEN guidelines on enteral nutrition: adult renal failure. *Clin Nutr* 2006;25:295–310.

Cano NJ, Fouque D, Roth H, et al; French Study Group for Nutrition in Dialysis. Intradialytic parenteral nutrition does not improve survival in malnourished hemodialysis patients: a 2-year multicenter, prospective, randomized study. *J Am Soc Nephrol* 2007;18:2583–2591.

Ikizler TA, Cano NJ, Franch H, et al. Prevention and treatment of protein energy wasting in chronic kidney disease patients: a consensus statement by the International Society of Renal Nutrition and Metabolism. *Kidney Int* 2013;84:1096–1107.

McClave SA, Taylor BE, Martindale RG, et al. Guidelines for the Provision and Assessment of Nutrition Support Therapy in the adult critically ill patient: Society of Critical Care Medicine (SCCM) and American Society for Parenteral and Enteral Nutrition (A.S.P.E.N.). *JPEN J Parenter Enteral Nutr* 2016;40:159–211.

Sabatino A, Regolisti G, Karupaiah T, et al. Protein-energy wasting and nutritional supplementation in patients with end-stage renal disease on hemodialysis. *Clin Nutr* 2016. doi:10.1016/j.clnu.2016.06.007.

Sezer S, Bal Z, Tutal E, et al. Long-term oral nutrition supplementation improves outcomes in malnourished patients with chronic kidney disease on hemodialysis. *JPEN J Parenter Enteral Nutr* 2014;38:960–965.

16

Trace Elements and Vitamins

Norio Hanafusa and Joel D. Kopple

TRACE ELEMENTS

Overview

The body burden and tissue concentrations of many trace elements are altered in chronic kidney disease (CKD) and kidney failure (Table 16.1). The following factors may contribute to these alterations:

1. Many trace elements are excreted primarily by the kidney, and with renal failure they may accumulate.
2. Dietary intake may be increased (e.g., aluminum or copper) or reduced (e.g., iron, zinc, and selenium).
3. Elements such as iron, zinc, and copper, which are protein bound, may be lost in excessive quantities with urinary protein losses as in the nephrotic syndrome.
4. Some medicines may bind trace elements in the intestinal tract which theoretically might decrease intestinal absorption. Sevelamer hydrochloride, for example, binds copper and zinc in vitro.
5. Some medicines that contain trace elements, when ingested, may increase intestinal absorption of those minerals. This has been shown, for example, for lanthanum and iron with the phosphate binders, lanthanum carbonate, ferric citrate, and sucroferric oxyhydroxide.
6. Excessive uptake or losses of trace elements may also occur during dialysis therapy depending on their relative concentrations in plasma and dialysate, the degree of binding to protein or red cells, and the quantity of protein lost into dialysate, as with peritoneal dialysis. Hemodialysis of copper, strontium, zinc, and lead should be minimal because they are largely bound to plasma proteins or red cells. Table 16.1 shows common abnormalities in trace elements in patients with chronic kidney failure (CKF).

Hemodialysis or hemodiafiltration may remove some trace elements if the dialysate concentrations are sufficiently low (e.g., bromide, iodine, lithium, rubidium, cesium, and zinc; Table 16.2). Because many trace elements are bound avidly to serum proteins, they may be taken up by blood against a concentration gradient when present in even small quantities in dialysate. In fact, therapeutic doses of trace elements may be administered through dialysis, as has been done for zinc. These observations provide part of the rationale for the intensive purification of dialysate used for maintenance dialysis (MD) patients. Data suggests that convection does not remove much additional trace elements, at least not if they are bound to protein in sera. Respiratory inhalation could result in increased intake of certain trace elements because it may occur in people exposed to certain industrial processes, fertilizers, insecticides, herbicides, or burning of fossil fuels.

Protein–energy wasting can be associated with decreased serum concentrations of proteins that bind trace elements; this can lower serum levels

Commonly Recognized Abnormalities in Trace Elements and Vitamins in Patients with Chronic Renal Failure*

Micronutrient	Effect of CKF[†]
Zinc	↓-N Serum[‡]; ↑ RBC; ↓ leukocyte in CKF and MHD; N in CPD
Selenium	↓ Serum in CKF, MHD, and CPD
Iron	↓-N Serum; ↓ tissue in CKF, MHD, and CPD
Aluminum	N-↑ Serum in CKF; ↑ serum and tissue in MHD and CPD
Copper	N-↑ Serum in CKF and MHD, N in CPD; ↓-N RBC
Thiamine	↓-N Serum in CKF, MHD, and CPD
Riboflavin	↓-N Serum in CKF, MHD, and CPD
Pyridoxine	↓-N Serum in CKF, MHD, and CPD; ↓ RBC in CKF and MHD
Cobalamin	↑ Serum in CKF; N serum in MHD and CPD
Folic acid	↓-N Serum and N-↑ RBC in CKF, MHD, and CPD
Ascorbic acid	↓-N Serum in CKF, MHD, and CPD
Vitamin A	↑ Serum in CKF, MHD, and CPD
Vitamin E	↓-N-↑ Serum in CKF, MHD, and CPD; ↓ RBC in MHD and CPD

*Refers to persons with CKF who are not receiving trace element or vitamin supplements.
[†]Serum levels of many trace elements and vitamins may be reduced in the nephrotic syndrome because of increased urinary losses and low serum levels of binding proteins.
[‡]Values ascribed to serum refer to serum or plasma.
↓, decreased compared to normal values; ↑, increased compared with normal values; CKF, chronic kidney failure; CPD, chronic peritoneal dialysis; MHD, maintenance hemodialysis; N, not different from normal values; RBC, erythrocytes.

of minerals including zinc, manganese, and nickel. Occupational exposure or pica can increase the burden of some trace elements. The effect of altered dietary intake of the patient with CKD on body pools of trace elements is unknown. Oral and, for MD patients, intravenous iron supplements or iron-containing intestinal phosphate binders are commonly provided to patients with CKD.

Assessment of the burden of trace element in patients with renal failure is often difficult because the serum concentrations of binding proteins may be decreased, thereby lowering serum levels of trace element, or the binding characteristics of these proteins may be altered in renal failure. This altered binding may change the relationship between serum levels and body burden of some trace elements. Red cell concentrations of trace elements may also not reflect pools in other tissues. In general, supplements of trace elements should be undertaken with caution, because impaired urinary excretion and the poor dialysance of trace elements, because of protein binding, increases the risk of overdosage. Dietary requirements for trace elements, excepting iron, have not been defined for patients with CKD because of the difficulties in conducting studies to determine nutritional requirements as well as the problems of identifying sensitive and reliable methods for determining deficiency or excess of trace elements.

Iron

Iron deficiency is common in patients with CKD, particularly in individuals undergoing maintenance hemodialysis (MHD). The causes for the frequent occurrence of iron deficiency in patients with advanced CKD are shown in Table 16.3. Iron requirements increase after starting erythropoietin therapy, especially when the hemoglobin is rising. Higher serum iron levels are also

TABLE 16.2	Summary of Serum, Plasma, or Tissue Concentrations of Other Trace Elements in Patients with Chronic Renal Failure and Patients Undergoing Maintenance Dialysis and Their Possible Clinical Consequences

	CKF	MHD	CPD	Dialysis Induced	Clinical Consequences*
Bromine	N	↓	↓	Yes	Altered sleep
Cadmium	↓ Kidney ↑ liver	↓ Kidney ↑ Liver	N		Growth retardation, hypertension, ↓ serum PTH
	N-↑ Serum ↓-↑ Blood	N-↑ Serum	N-↑ Serum		
Chromium	N	↑	↑	Yes	Carcinogenic
Cobalt	N	↑	↑	?	?
Lead	↑	↑	↑	No	Hypertension, gastrointestinal and neurologic diseases
Manganese	↓ - ↑	↓-N	↓-N	No	Anemia, impaired glucose tolerance
Molybdenum	N	↑	?	?	Arthropathy
Nickel	↑	↑-N-↓	?	Yes	Degeneration of heart muscle
Rubidium	N	↑-N-↓	N	Yes	Depression, central nervous system disturbances
Silicon	↑	↑	↑	Yes	↑ Serum silicon protects against aluminum toxicity
Strontium	↑	↑	↑	?	Osteomalacia
Tin	↓	↓↓	↓	?	
Vanadium	N - ↑	↑	?	No	Bone disease, hypoglycemia

*Adverse clinical effects that have been observed in the general population.
↓, decreased compared with normal; ↑, increased compared with normal; ?, unknown; CKF, chronic kidney failure; CPD, chronic peritoneal dialysis; MHD, maintenance hemodialysis; N, not different from normal; PTH, parathyroid hormone.

	Factors Leading to Iron Deficiency in Patients with Chronic Renal Failure or Patients Receiving Maintenance Dialysis

- Decreased iron uptake by intestinal mucosal cells and impaired intestinal iron absorption
- Gastrointestinal tract blood loss which may be clinically apparent or occult
- Blood drawing for testing
- Menstruation
- Massive proteinuria (caused by iron binding to urinary protein)
- Blood retention in hemodialyzer and blood lines at end of hemodialysis
- Binding of iron to dialyzer membranes and tubing
- Increased demand for iron during erythropoiesis stimulated by ESAs may deplete body's supply of non–hemoglobin iron
- Accidental blood loss from vascular access tubing, grafts, and fistulae

ESAs, erythropoiesis-stimulating agents.

associated with a greater response to erythropoietin. The management of blood hemoglobin levels in patients with CKD and especially MD patients (i.e., MHD and chronic peritoneal dialysis [CPD] patients) is the subject of a vast number of studies and clinical practice guidelines. Because the response to erythropoiesis-stimulating agents (ESAs) is dependent on the availability of iron, many of these studies and guidelines necessarily include protocols regarding iron intake. In general, these guidelines recommend that iron should be given if serum transferrin saturation (TSAT), which is usually estimated as the percent saturation of serum total iron-binding capacity, is ≤20% to 30% and serum ferritin is ≤100 to 200 ng per mL. Most guidelines do not clearly recommend a course of action if, of the two TSAT and ferritin criteria, only one is met. These are only guidelines, and in all cases, treatment should be based on good clinical judgement.

A small percentage of MD patients may maintain adequate serum iron with oral salts. Ferrous sulfate, 300 mg 3 times per day by mouth, one-half hour after meals may be tried. Some patients will develop anorexia, nausea, constipation, or abdominal pain; these individuals sometimes will tolerate other iron compounds, including ferrous fumarate, gluconate and sulfate, liposomal iron, and pyrophosphate and a polysaccharide-iron complex. Some iron salts are used to bind phosphate and decrease its absorption from the intestinal tract (e.g., sucroferric oxyhydroxide and ferric citrate). The iron in these latter salts may also be absorbed, may maintain serum TSAT or ferritin within the acceptable range in some MD patients receiving ESAs, and thereby reduce the need for intravenous iron treatment.

If adequate serum TSAT and ferritin levels are not achieved with oral iron or the patient does not tolerate oral formulations, the patient can be treated with intravenous iron. Intramuscular injections can cause pain and staining of skin, so intravenous iron, given as ferrous gluconate, ferrous sucrose, ferric gluconate, ferumoxytol, ferric carboxymaltose, iron isomaltoside, or iron dextran is generally the preferred method of administration. Iron dextran has a slightly greater risk of anaphylactic reactions, from 0.6% to 0.7%, and many physicians prefer to use other iron salts. Iron added to hemodialysate (e.g., ferric pyrophosphate citrate) can reduce iron losses during hemodialysis and possibly could be used to provide iron to iron-deficient patients. Although rare, iron overload can be treated by simply halting intake, by removal using deferoxamine (see below), or by injections of erythropoietin along with repeated phlebotomy.

Aluminum

In patients with Stage 5 CKD or those receiving MHD, increased aluminum has been implicated as a cause of a progressive dementia syndrome (particularly in patients receiving MHD), osteomalacia, weakness of the proximal muscles of the limbs, impaired immune function, and anemia. Although previously contamination of dialysate with aluminum was the major source of aluminum toxicity, the current methods of water treatment have removed virtually all aluminum from the dialysates. Instead, ingestion of aluminum binders of phosphate is probably the major cause of the excess burden of aluminum, and aluminum binders are now used sparingly if at all. Increased body burden and toxicity of iron or aluminum in patients receiving MHD or CPD may be reduced simply by eliminating intake or by infusion of deferoxamine (a dialyzable chelator of divalent cations). Care must be taken with the latter method because deferoxamine can promote loss of iron as well as certain serious infections, particularly mucormycosis.

Zinc

Although the zinc content of most tissues is normal in patients with CKF, serum and hair zinc levels are reported to be low, yet red cell zinc content is increased. Some reports indicate that dysgeusia (poor food intake) reduced peripheral nerve conduction velocities, abnormal serum cholesterol levels, low sperm counts, and impaired sexual function, and helper/suppressor T-cell (CD4/CD8) ratios may be improved in patients undergoing CKD and MHD by giving zinc supplements. Other studies have not confirmed these findings. Zinc deficiency in persons with non-CKD is manifested by Beau lines (transverse horizontal grooves in the fingernails), discolored nail plates, paronychia, and impaired growth in children. Intestinal absorption of zinc is not affected by administration of 1,25-dihydroxycholecalciferol.

The dietary requirement for zinc in patients with CKF and end-stage kidney disease (ESKD), especially in patients receiving MHD, is unclear. In nondialyzed patients with CKD, the fractional urinary excretion of zinc is increased. However, with a reduced glomerular filtration rate (GFR), urinary zinc excretion is decreased. Some data indicate that fecal losses of zinc may be increased, and this may raise the dietary zinc needs above the recommended dietary allowance (RDA). The problem in estimating zinc needs is compounded because the dietary zinc intake of many CKD, MHD, and CPD patients commonly is below the RDA for normal adults (i.e., generally 8 mg per day for women and 11 mg per day for men). It is probably both safe and clinically indicated to ensure that patients receiving CKD and MHD ingest this level of zinc. Zinc can be found in some multivitamin supplements. If the goal is to maintain normal serum zinc levels with zinc supplements, it may be prudent to monitor serum zinc. The relationship between dietary zinc supplements and serum zinc seems to be variable in MHD patients.

Selenium

Selenium is necessary for the selenium-dependent, glutathione peroxidases, and it participates in the defense against oxidative damage of tissues, an important problem for patients with renal failure. Selenium is largely protein-bound and binds to sulfur-containing amino acids as selenomethionine and selenocysteine. Generally, patients with CKF patients and patients receiving MD have low plasma or serum selenium levels; red cell selenium levels in patients with ESKD are conflicting. Impaired gastrointestinal absorption of selenium and selenium losses during dialysis are suggested as reasons for low serum selenium levels. Patients living in areas with higher soil selenium tend to have higher serum selenium. Changing from MHD treatment to hemodiafiltration does not seem to lower serum selenium (or zinc).

Low selenium values can contribute to the reduced plasma glutathione reductase activity found for patients undergoing MHD. Whether these abnormalities cause clinical disorders in patients with CKD and/or patients undergoing MHD or CPD is unknown. Selenium deficiency in adults without CKD can cause Keshan disease, which is associated with a cardiomyopathy. Interestingly, patients undergoing MHD who develop a cardiomyopathy have lower plasma and platelet selenium levels and low glutathione peroxidase activity as compared with patients undergoing MHD without cardiomyopathy. Low selenium levels in MHD patients are associated with a decrease in the red cell and platelet half-lives and altered thyroid status. Selenium deficiency and toxicity syndromes have not been identified in patients with CKD or ESKD. Therefore, routine selenium supplementation is not recommended.

Copper
Most patients with CKD and patients undergoing MHD are reported to have normal serum levels of copper and ceruloplasmin (although inflammation will elevate ceruloplasmin because it is an acute phase reactant). A high serum copper:zinc ratio has been associated with lower body mass index, serum albumin and serum creatinine, and evidence for oxidative stress, inflammation and impaired immune status in patients with CPD. Nutritional deficiency of copper is rare or absent in patients with CKD or patients undergoing MHD, unless there is an enteropathy or a requirement for total parenteral nutrition that does not provide copper.

Other Trace Elements
Plasma or tissue levels of other trace elements reported to be altered by CKD or dialysis are shown in Table 16.2. Notably, the evidence for clinical nutritional deficiencies or excesses of these elements in patients with CKD or patients undergoing MHD is very limited and probably is uncommon.

VITAMINS

Overview
Individuals with CKF and particularly MHD patients who do not receive vitamin supplements will have a high incidence of vitamin deficiencies. Table 16.1 shows the commonly occurring abnormalities in vitamins in patients with CKF. Deficiencies are caused by several factors:

1. 1,25-dihydroxycholecalciferol production by the diseased kidney is impaired.
2. Vitamin intake is often decreased in nondialyzed CKF, MHD, and CPD patients because of (i) anorexia and (ii) reduced food intake. (iii) Intercurrent illnesses, frequently present in patients with CKD and patients undergoing MHD also impair food intake. (iv) Many foods that are high in water-soluble vitamins or vitamin K are often restricted in nondialyzed CKF, CPD, and MHD patients because of the elevated protein or potassium content of such foods. For example, low levels of thiamine and, in some patients, thiamine and pyridoxine are more likely to occur in patients with CKD who are prescribed low-protein diets.
3. CKF appears to alter the absorption, metabolism, or activity of some vitamins. Animal studies indicate that intestinal transporters for thiamine and folate and intestinal absorption of riboflavin, folate, and vitamin D_3 are impaired in CKF. The metabolism of folate and pyridoxine can be abnormal in patients with CKF.
4. Certain medicines interfere with the intestinal absorption, metabolism, or actions of vitamins. Sevelamer HCl, for example, in vitro, absorbs vitamins C and K and folic acid, to a lesser extent vitamin B_6, but not B_{12}.

5. Water-soluble vitamins are removed by dialysis, and the high-flux/high-efficiency hemodialysis procedures can remove greater quantities of these water-soluble vitamins. MHD for >15 hours per week versus ≤15 hours per week was associated with lower blood levels of thiamine and vitamin C, higher blood pyridoxine (B_6), and no difference in vitamin B_{12} or folate. These results were observed even though about 31% and 46%, respectively, of patients receiving the shorter and longer weekly doses of MHD were prescribed multivitamins.

Deficiencies have been observed for 1,25-dihydroxycholecalciferol, folic acid, vitamin B_6 (pyridoxine), vitamin C, and, to a lesser extent, other water-soluble vitamins. Because a substantial proportion of patients with Stage 4 or 5 CKD and especially patients undergoing CPD or MHD appear to develop laboratory evidence for one or more vitamin deficiencies, intake of a multivitamin supplement is recommended in addition to the vitamins ingested in foods (Table 16.4). A retrospective Dialysis Outcomes and Practice Patterns Study analysis indicates that the adjusted mortality rate is lower in MHD patients who are prescribed multivitamin supplements.

Vitamin B₁ (Thiamine)

Decreased plasma or red blood cell thiamine levels have been reported in some but not in all studies of MHD patients who were not receiving vitamin supplements. But occasionally MHD patients developed syndromes suggestive of dementia or beriberi heart disease that improved when they were given large doses of thiamine. Both syndromes could have been due to causes independent of ESKD. To remove the possibility that thiamine deficiency will occur in patients with advanced CKD, we recommend a multivitamin supplement providing the recommended daily dose of thiamine for all patients with CKD 3b, 4, 5, nephrotic patients, and MHD and CPD patients (Table 16.4).

Vitamin B₆ (Pyridoxine HCl)

Low plasma and erythrocyte vitamin B_6 levels or altered red cell transaminase activities are not uncommonly found in advanced CKD, MHD, or CPD patients not receiving B_6 supplements. These can be normalized with pyridoxine HCl supplements. Some data suggest the presence of an inhibitor of vitamin B_6 in uremic sera that is removed by dialysis. Vitamin B_6 deficiency may impair immune function, and pyridoxine HCl supplements may also improve several measures of immune function including lymphoblast formation in white cells for MHD patients.

Plasma oxalate is often elevated in patients with advanced CKD. Increased plasma oxalate appears to be largely due to impaired urinary excretion. However, large doses of vitamin C (ascorbic acid), a precursor of oxalate, can increase oxalate production (see below). Glyoxylate, a metabolic precursor of oxalate, may be transaminated to form glycine, and this reaction is catalyzed by vitamin B_6. Vitamin B_6 deficiency can increase urinary oxalate excretion in rats with experimental renal insufficiency and in normal adults. In patients with CKD, large doses of pyridoxine HCl can decrease plasma oxalate levels but not to normal values. Large doses of one of the three forms of vitamin B_6, pyridoxamine, have been used to decrease serum advanced glycation products in patients with diabetic nephropathy. A preliminary report suggests that pyridoxamine may lower the rate of rise in serum creatinine in the patients.

Further, 5 mg per day of pyridoxine HCl normalizes the erythrocyte glutamate-pyruvate transaminase activation index in patients with clinically stable Stage 5 CKD, and 10 mg per day of pyridoxine HCl normalized this index in stable MHD patients as well as in patients with nondialyzed advanced CKD with superimposed infections.

Treatment with large doses of folic acid and/or pyridoxine HCl (some-times with vitamin B_{12}) can reduce the elevated plasma homocysteine levels which are commonly present in patients with advanced CKD, MD patients, and renal transplant recipients. High plasma homocysteine is a risk factor for adverse cardiovascular events in the general population. In MHD patients, the relation of elevated plasma homocysteine to adverse outcomes is less clear. Plasma homocysteine tends to be about 1.5 to 2.0 times the upper limit of normal in MHD patients. Clinical trials in both the general population and in patients with CKD or patients undergoing MHD (e.g., the Veterans Administration HOST Study) have failed to show a survival benefit of vitamin treatment of hyperhomocysteinemia, even though plasma or serum homo-cysteine levels decreased, often to normal, with supplements of folic acid, pyridoxine HCl, and vitamin B_{12} compared to placebo. The treatment group displayed a significant fall in serum homocysteine levels, but there was no reduction in cardiovascular or overall mortality. In clinical trials of subjects in the general population, adverse effects of megavitamin treatment of hy-perhomocysteinemic patients occur occasionally. Consequently, treatment of hyperhomocysteinemia with large doses of pyridoxine HCl, folic acid, and/or vitamin B_{12} is not recommended. Another study indicated that supplements of these three vitamins to patients with diabetic CKD was associated with a more rapid reduction in GFR and an increased incidence of a combination of adverse vascular events and all-cause mortality.

Vitamin C
MHD patients lose substantial amounts of vitamin C into dialysate. Hence, low plasma and leukocyte ascorbic acid concentrations can occur in patients receiving MHD who are not receiving supplemental vitamin C. Clinical signs suggestive of mild scurvy have been described in several patients undergoing MHD who have very low plasma ascorbic acid concentrations. Administration of ascorbic acid orally or into the dialysate can prevent negative vitamin C balance during hemodialysis. In MHD patients, oral vitamin C may enhance intestinal iron absorption. Vitamin C may facilitate release of iron from iron stores and from ferritin, increase transferrin iron saturation, blood hemo-globin, and reduce the needed erythropoietin doses. Some evidence, not definitive, indicates that vitamin C may decrease oxidative stress and also reduce restless leg syndrome. Large vitamin C doses (e.g., 500 mg per day) may increase plasma or, with functioning kidneys, urinary oxalate, which is very insoluble, and possibly lead to more rapid progression of CKD. Thus, we recommend about only supplementing patients with CKF and patients undergoing MD with an amount of vitamin C slightly less (70 mg per day) than the recommended daily allowance of vitamin C, that is, 75 mg per day for women and 90 mg per day for men (Table 16.4).

Folate
Blood folate concentrations are reported to be decreased in some MHD pa-tients who did not take folic acid supplements. Several investigators found hypersegmentation of polymorphonuclear leukocytes in such patients and reported that these abnormalities decreased with administration of folate supplements. The reticulocyte count and hematocrit can rise when patients undergoing MHD are given folic acid supplements. We have observed that serum folate concentrations are normal in virtually all patients undergoing MHD who received 1.0 mg per day of supplemental folic acid. Dietary folic acid requirements increase in patients with Stage 4 or 5 CKD when they com-mence erythropoietin therapy and undergo a major rise in their hemoglobin levels. Folate supplements can also improve abnormal vascular endothelial function, a risk for atherosclerosis risk factor in patients with ESKD. Folinic

TABLE 16.4 Recommended Daily Supplemental Vitamins for Persons with Chronic Kidney Disease and Those Undergoing Maintenance Hemodialysis or Chronic Peritoneal Dialysis*,†

Vitamin	RDA‡	Stages 3–5 CKD§	Maintenance Hemodialysis	Chronic Peritoneal Dialysis
Thiamine (mg/d)	1.2 for men 1.1 for women	1.2	1.2	1.2
Riboflavin (mg/d)	1.3 for men 1.1 for women	1.3	1.3	1.3
Pantothenic acid (AI‡, mg/d)	5	5	5	5
Niacin (mg/d)	16 for men 14 for women	16	16	16
Pyridoxine HCl (mg/d)‖	For 19–50 yr: 1.3 for both sexes For >51 yr: 1.7 for men; 1.5 for women	5	10	10
Vitamin B_{12} (μg/d)	2.4	2.4	2.4	2.4
Vitamin C¶ (mg/d)	90 for men 75 for women	70	70	70
Folic acid (mg/d)	0.4	1	1	1
Vitamin A (μg RAE‡/d)	900 for men 750 for women	No addition	No addition	No addition
Vitamin D (IU cholecalciferol [vitamin D_3]/d)	For 19–70 yr: 600 For >70 yr: 800	See text	See text	See text
Vitamin E (mg/d)	15	15	15	15
Vitamin K (μg/d)	120 for men (AI)‡ 90 for women (AI)‡	None	None	None

*These quantities are recommended in addition to the patient's daily intake of vitamins from foods ingested.
†The proposed supplemental daily vitamin intakes are based on the recommended daily requirements for normal adults. Because the recommended daily allowances may vary according to gender and age group in adults, the highest recommended level for nonpregnant, nonlactating adults was selected. Exceptions are made to this policy when evidence indicates that patients with CKD or patients receiving maintenance dialysis have an increased need or decreased tolerance for a given vitamin.
‡Abbreviations from the Food and Nutrition Board of the National Institute of Medicine for nonpregnant, nonlactating adults: AI, adequate intake; RAE, retinoic acid equivalents; RDA, recommended dietary allowances.
§CKD: patients with chronic kidney disease who are not receiving dialysis treatments.
‖10 mg of pyridoxine HCl is 8.21 mg of free pyridoxine.
¶Estimated average requirement of vitamin C: 75 mg/d for normal men and 60 mg/d for normal women.

acid is reported to improve endothelium-dependent vasodilation in the forearm in patients with ESKD. One study suggests that folic acid, 0.8 mg per day, with enalapril, 10 mg per day, may slow down the progression of CKD.

Niacin (Nicotinamide, Nicotinic Acid)

Low plasma niacin (i.e., nicotinic acid) concentrations have been reported in some patients undergoing MHD, but other reports have not confirmed this when patients received 7.5 mg per day of supplemental nicotinic acid. Nicotinamide, a metabolite of niacin, may in large oral doses (500 to 1,500 mg per day) suppress intestinal absorption of phosphate and reduce serum phosphorus by inhibiting the Na/Pi type IIb cotransporter in the intestinal brush border. These large doses of nicotinamide may also reduce body phosphorus burden by inhibiting renal tubular phosphorus resorption and increasing urinary phosphorus excretion in people with sufficient renal function. The clinical use of nicotinamide to prevent or treat hyperphosphatemia in patients with CKD is slowly increasing. Niacin (nicotinic acid) has been used in the general population to decrease serum low-density lipoprotein (LDL) cholesterol and triglycerides and to increase high-density lipoprotein cholesterol. Side effects of nicotinic acid include flushing, and side effects of nicotinamide include thrombocytopenia and hepatic toxicity.

Vitamin B_{12}

Deficiency of vitamin B_{12} is uncommon in patients with CKD because the daily requirement for this vitamin is very small (e.g., 2.4 μg per day for normal, nonpregnant, nonlactating adults). In addition, body storages of this vitamin are great, and little is removed during hemodialysis because vitamin B_{12} is largely protein bound and hence, poorly dialyzed. Nonetheless, one study reported low serum vitamin B_{12} concentrations in 19 of 60 MHD patients; the serum vitamin B_{12} concentrations tended to fall progressively over months of dialysis treatment. More interestingly, serum vitamin B_{12} levels were directly correlated with nerve conduction velocities, which improved with ingestion of large quantities of vitamin B_{12}. Occasionally, the hematocrit is reported to improve after patients received vitamin B_{12} injections. It is important to recognize that the average age of MD patients is similar to the age at which pernicious anemia is most likely to occur.

Other Water-Soluble Vitamins

Despite the water solubility of riboflavin, thiamine, pantothenic acid, and biotin, plasma concentrations of these vitamins are usually not decreased in MHD patients. It is possible that losses of these vitamins into hemodialysate or peritoneal dialysate are usually offset by the lack of urinary excretion.

Fat-Soluble Vitamins

Vitamin A

Serum retinol-binding protein and vitamin A are increased in patients with CKF. Even relatively small supplements of vitamin A, that is, 7,500 to 15,000 IU per day (about 1,500 to 3,000 retinal equivalents or μg per day), may be associated with bone toxicity and hypercalcemia in some individuals.

Vitamin D

Vitamin D is discussed in Chapter 5.

Vitamin E

Normal, low, and increased plasma or red cell vitamin E (α-tocopherol) levels have been described in patients with nondialyzed CKD and patients undergoing MHD. Vitamin E deficiency can lead to oxidative injury to tissues. One meta-analysis indicated that performing hemodialysis with vitamin E-coated dialyzers may decrease serum levels of oxidants and proinflammatory cytokines such as thiobarbituric acid reacting substances, oxidated LDL, C-reactive protein (CRP), and interleukin 6 with no change in total antioxidant status or superoxide dismutase. Another meta-analysis indicated that vitamin E-coated hemodialyzers may decrease erythropoietin resistance. In the placebo-controlled Secondary Prevention with Antioxidants of Cardiovascular Disease in Endstage Renal Disease (SPACE) trial, MHD patients at increased risk for adverse cardiovascular events exhibited less such events when given α-tocopherol 800 IU per day. In the general population, prospective randomized placebo-controlled clinical trials indicate that vitamin E, vitamin C, β-carotene, or combinations of these compounds do not significantly reduce total adverse cardiovascular events or cancer. Indeed, in the Heart and Outcomes Prevention Evaluation (HOPE) and HOPE-The Ongoing Outcomes (HOPE-TOO) trials conducted in patients at higher risk for cardiovascular disease, the majority of whom did not have CKD, a moderate dose of vitamin E (400 IU per day) given long term was associated with an increased risk of heart failure and hospitalization for heart failure. In a subset of these latter patients who had mild to moderate CKD, there was no reduction in the incidence of adverse cardiovascular events with 400 IU per day of vitamin E. The reasons for these discrepant responses in patients with CKD and patients undergoing MHD as compared to the general population are not known. It is possible that the greater oxidant stress of patients with CKD may enable them to benefit from vitamin E therapy.

Vitamin K
The most common dietary form of vitamin K is vitamin K_1 (phylloquinone). Vitamin K_2 (menaquinone) is also found in foods. Vitamin K is a cofactor for the enzyme γ-glutamyl carboxylase which activates a number of vitamin K-dependent proteins which inhibit vascular calcification (e.g., matrix Gla protein) and maintain bone health (osteocalcin). This process of activation includes carboxylation of these proteins. Vitamin K activates other proteins, at least partly by carboxylation; these include proteins involved with the clotting process. Vitamin K may contribute to other normal biologic processes as well. Measurement of vitamin K status by testing integrity of the blood coagulation process usually indicates that vitamin K deficiency is uncommon in patients with CKD and patients undergoing MD, unless they receive vitamin K antagonizing anticoagulants. However, in patients with CKD and patients undergoing MD, the high frequency of blood uncarboxylated and dephosphorylated matrix Gla proteins and uncarboxylated osteocalcin which decrease with vitamin K supplements indicates that vitamin K deficiency actually may be common in these individuals. Patients with CKD who do not eat foods containing vitamin K or receive antibiotics that suppress intestinal bacteria may be at increased risk for vitamin K deficiency. The daily dietary vitamin K needs in patients with CKD or ESKD are not well defined. The Dietary Reference Intakes of the U.S. Institute of Medicine state that the adequate intake of vitamin K is 120 μg per day for normal men and 90 μg per day for normal women. However, the recommended vitamin K intake for healthy adults varies widely among other institutions. A number of clinical trials are underway to examine whether vitamin K supplements will decrease the rate of calcification, usually of blood vessels or heart valves, in MD patients. Because evidence indicates that vitamin K deficiency may be hazardous in patients with CKD, some workers suggest that patients with Stage 3 or possibly Stage 4 CKD who need anticoagulation should be treated with the newer anticoagulants (e.g., dabigatran, rivaroxaban, and apixaban) that do not inhibit vitamin K activity. These newer anticoagulants appear to be as effective and safe as warfarin. There is not yet sufficient experience to recommend the newer anticoagulants for MD patients.

Some investigators suggest that patients undergoing MHD who do not receive vitamin supplementation can avoid developing signs of water-soluble vitamin deficiencies for months. These results suggest that vitamin supplements should not be prescribed routinely to patients receiving MD. This conclusion is supported by findings indicating the maintenance of normal plasma or blood cell levels of vitamins in patients undergoing MHD, even though they did not receive supplements for periods of less than 1 year. Still, the levels of water-soluble vitamins can fall to borderline low levels in several patients.

In patients undergoing CPD, the dietary intake of several vitamins, including vitamin A, vitamin C, vitamin B_1 (thiamine), vitamin B_6, vitamin B_{12}, and nicotinamide, is often lower than the recommended allowances for normal adults. Patients undergoing CPD who are not receiving supplements can have a high incidence of low or normal plasma folate levels, low vitamin B_1, and low vitamin B_6 and vitamin C. Reduced plasma vitamin E has been reported in 13% of patients undergoing CPD, whereas others found increased plasma vitamin E levels.

Overall, a low intake of several vitamins is still common in patients with renal failure, and many reports continue to show that substantial numbers of these patients show evidence for vitamin deficiencies. Because the water-soluble vitamin supplements are generally safe, we believe that it is wise to recommend them routinely until these issues are more completely resolved. What is missing? The nutritional requirements for most vitamins are not well defined for patients with renal failure. Besides the vitamins present in foods, the following daily supplements of vitamins will prevent or correct vitamin deficiency: pyridoxine HCl, 5 mg in nondialyzed patients with Stage 3 to 5 CKD and 10 mg for patients receiving MHD or CPD; folic acid, 1.0 mg; and for all other water-soluble vitamins. We recommend the daily allowance for normal nonpregnant, nonlactating adults. Because the recommended daily allowances may vary according to gender and age group in adults, the highest recommended level for nonpregnant, nonlactating adults should be selected. Based on the disappointing results arising from the treatment of hyperhomocysteinemia in patients with CKD and patients undergoing MHD, the large doses of vitamins B_6, vitamin B_{12}, and folic acid are not recommended. Of course, this negative recommendation does not apply to individuals who have the genetic forms of hyperhomocysteinemia, because this problem can be associated with severely elevated plasma homocysteine concentrations that might be treated with vitamins.

Supplemental vitamin C should probably be 70 mg per day, which is slightly less than the RDA: 75 mg per day for women and 90 mg per day for men, because ascorbic acid can be metabolized to oxalate. Large oral or intravenous doses of ascorbic acid were associated with an increase in plasma oxalate and the risk of deposition on tissue of renal failure patients. Oxalate is highly insoluble. The concern about high plasma oxalate concentrations could lead to precipitation in the kidney, possibly causing further impairment in renal function in the nondialyzed patient with renal insufficiency.

Supplemental vitamin A is not recommended because serum levels are increased, and there is a high risk of vitamin A toxicity with even relatively small supplements. Although some studies indicate that vitamin E supplements in patients undergoing MHD may be beneficial, it is still not certain that vitamin E supplements are necessary. Indeed, there are negative or adverse results resulting with long-term vitamin E supplementation in the general population. Additional vitamin K is not needed unless the patient is not eating and receives antibiotics that suppress intestinal bacteria that synthesize vitamin K. Recommendations for vitamin D intake are given in Chapter 5.

Suggested Readings

Boaz M, Smetana S, Weinstein T, et al. Secondary prevention with antioxidants of cardiovascular disease in endstage renal disease (SPACE): randomised placebo-controlled trial. *Lancet* 2000;356:1213–1238.

Boelaert JR, de Locht M, Van Cutsem J, et al. Mucormycosis during deferoxamine therapy as a siderophore-mediated infection—in vitro and in vivo animal studies. *J Clin Invest* 1993;91:1979.

Bovio G, Piazza V, Ronchi A, et al. Trace element levels in adult patients with protein-uria. *Minerva Gastroenterol Dietol* 2007;53:329–336.

Chazot C, Kopple JD. Vitamin metabolism and requirements in renal disease and renal failure. In: Kopple JD, Massry S, Kalantar-Zadeh K, eds. *Nutritional Management of Renal Disease*. 3rd ed. New York: Elsevier Inc; 2013:339–349.

Huang J, Yi B, Li AM, et al. Effects of vitamin E-coated dialysis membranes on anemia, nutrition and dyslipidemia status in hemodialysis patients: a meta-analysis. *Ren Fail* 2015;37:398–407.

Jamison RL, Hartigan P, Kaufman JS, et al; Veterans Affairs Site Investigators. Effect of homocysteine lowering on mortality and vascular disease in advanced chronic kidney disease and end-stage renal disease: a randomized controlled trial. *JAMA* 2007;298:1163–1170.

Kopple JD, Mercurio K, Blumenkrantz MJ, et al. Daily requirement for pyridoxine supplements in chronic renal failure. *Kidney Int* 1981;19:694–704.

Nanayakkara PW, van Guldener C, ter Wee PM, et al. Effect of a treatment strategy consisting of pravastatin, vitamin E, and homocysteine lowering on carotid intima-media thickness, endothelial function, and renal function in patients with mild to moderate chronic kidney disease: results from the Anti-Oxidant Therapy in Chronic Renal Insufficiency (ATIC) Study. *Arch Int Med* 2007;167:1262–1270.

Swaminathan S. Trace elements, toxic metals, and metalloids in kidney disease. In: Kopple JD, Massry S, Kalantar-Zadeh K, eds. *Nutritional Management of Renal Disease*. 3rd ed. New York: Elsevier Inc; 2013:351–382.

Tonelli M, Wiebe N, Hemmelgarn B, et al. Trace elements in hemodialysis patients: a systematic review and meta-analysis. *BMC Med* 2009;7:25.

Westenfeld R, Krueger T, Schlieper G, et al. Effect of vitamin K_2 supplementation on functional vitamin K deficiency in hemodialysis patients: a randomized trial. *Am J Kidney Dis* 2012;59:186–195.

Yang SK, Xiao L, Xu B, et al. Effects of vitamin E-coated dialyzer on oxidative stress and inflammation status in hemodialysis patients: a systematic review and meta-analysis. *Ren Fail* 2014;36:722–731.

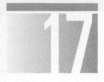

Dietary Salt Intake for Patients with Hypertension or Kidney Disease

Michael S. Lipkowitz and Christopher S. Wilcox

Our genes were selected to adapt us to life in the African continent where the climate is hot and dry, perspiration substantial, and dietary salt intake was low. At present, individuals living in rural African communities have very low levels of blood pressure until they migrate to an urban environment, where salt intake rises steeply and, with it, the incidence of hypertension. These observations suggest that we are adapted to retain, rather than eliminate, salt through a salt appetite and renal mechanisms for avid salt retention. Recent genetic analyses of populations around the world confirm this hypothesis because salt retaining forms of a number of genes were reported to be more prevalent in global regions where salt is scarce and hot temperatures promote salt loss. Despite these evolutionary adaptations, most normal subjects maintain an extracellular fluid volume that changes by less than 1 L (1 kg of body weight) and a blood pressure that changes by less than 10%, despite wide variations in daily salt intake. These subjects are termed "salt-resistant" and encompass the majority of healthy adolescents and young adults. However, a minority are unable to maintain a normal, low level of blood pressure in face of a steep rise in salt intake and are termed "salt-sensitive." Salt sensitivity precedes hypertension. It is a cardiovascular risk factor and complicates antihypertensive therapy. Moreover, it may contribute to progressive loss of kidney function in patients with chronic kidney disease (CKD), exacerbate proteinuria, and diminish the antiproteinuric response to drugs in those with renal disease. Thus, the evaluation and management of dietary salt intake is an important component of care for patients with high blood pressure, kidney disease, or cardiovascular risk. Some physicians erroneously believe that dietary salt intake does not require attention in the era of modern diuretics. This chapter will outline arguments for a more comprehensive assessment of dietary salt intake than is presently customary and provide goals and steps to appropriate management.

Most sodium is ingested as salt (NaCl). Moreover, the increase in blood pressure in salt-sensitive subjects fed salt is not apparent if an equivalent quantity of sodium is given with another anion. Specifically, intake of sodium bicarbonate does not normally raise the blood pressure. However, an intake is usually quantitated as sodium. A daily intake of 100 mmol of sodium chloride is equivalent to 5.8 g of salt or 2.3 g of sodium.

EPIDEMIOLOGY OF DIETARY SALT INTAKE

Daily sodium intake varies widely in modern Western societies but is generally between 80 and 250 mmol. A multinational INTERSALT study concluded that the mean level of blood pressure of individuals in a country increases with ambient salt intake. Because hypertension is the leading cause of cardiovascular disease and cardiovascular disease is the leading cause of death, any increase in population blood pressure is a cause for concern.

A reduction of salt intake in patients with pre- or established hypertension has been recommended by the World Health Organization and the Joint

National Commission on Prevention, Detection, Evaluation, and Treatment of High Blood Pressure. Clandestine promotion of high salt intake by food and beverage companies in the United States, for example, by the Salt Institute, has unfortunately been highly successful. Whereas prior to 1980s, the total sales of food salt and the prevalence of hypertension in the United States were decreasing, since then the use of salt has increased by as much as 90%. This has been accompanied by an increase in age-adjusted prevalence of high blood pressure in the U.S. population. The relationship between salt intake and blood pressure varies between individuals. This obscures the overall effect of dietary salt on blood pressure and cardiovascular disease and has complicated the public health case for salt restriction in food.

ASSESSMENT OF SALT SENSITIVITY

Salt sensitivity is defined arbitrarily as a greater than 10% increase in blood pressure on passing from a low to a high salt intake. Salt-sensitive individuals constitute approximately 30% of the young adult population. A shortened protocol to assess salt sensitivity has been developed whereby individuals are given dietary advice to achieve a 150 mmol per day sodium intake for 3 days. They then receive 2 L of 0.9% saline intravenously over 4 hours to provide high salt intake. The following day, they receive a salt-restricted diet of 10 mmol daily and three oral doses of 40 mg furosemide. The blood pressure is compared at the end of the high- and low salt periods. This shortened protocol is reproducible in defining salt-sensitive and salt resistant individuals. However, there is a normal distribution of salt-induced blood pressure. Therefore, a division into salt resistant and salt sensitive is arbitrary.

Unfortunately, this protocol is too cumbersome for routine clinical use. The proportion of salt-sensitive subjects is rather greater in African Americans than Caucasians, is associated with a low plasma renin activity, increases with age, and increases markedly with declining renal function. Salt sensitivity is more frequent in hypertensive than normotensive subjects. Therefore, elderly or African-American hypertensives, and especially those with CKD can reasonably be assumed to be salt sensitive. In practice, salt sensitivity often becomes apparent as a large fall in blood pressure with dietary salt restriction and thiazide diuretic therapy.

SALT INTAKE, BLOOD PRESSURE, AND CHRONIC KIDNEY DISEASE

The degree of salt sensitivity increases exponentially with declining kidney function. As patients approach end-stage renal disease, the great majority are salt sensitive. The exceptions are those with primary tubulointerstitial disease who typically do not retain NaCl and have normal blood pressure.

Because the level of blood pressure determines the progression of kidney disease in those with more than 1 to 3 g per 24 hours of protein excretion, attention to dietary salt and proper use of diuretics are essential in hypertensive patients with chronic proteinuric kidney disease. Moreover, a high level of dietary salt increases protein excretion in patients with proteinuric kidney disease, appears to enhance the progression of underlying CKD, and prevents the anti-proteinuric effect of angiotensin-converting enzyme (ACE) inhibitors. Therefore, dietary salt restriction and proper use of diuretics are important components of the management of the great majority of patients with CKD. Indeed, because proper management of blood pressure (often with a lower than normal blood pressure goal) is required for optimum control of progressive proteinuric kidney disease, control of salt intake and proper use of diuretics should be a part of the initial clinical management of these patients. This follows from the observations that salt intake determines blood pressure, whereas blood pressure determines not only the progression of CKD but also the rapidity and severity with which cardiovascular events develop in this high-risk population.

In addition to the clinic blood pressure, the diurnal variation of blood pressure, in particular the normal nocturnal dip in blood pressure, has significant prognostic importance. Thus, the nondipping status confers increased cardiovascular risk. Blood pressure in patients with CKD tends to remain stable or even rise at night rather than dip. There is emerging data that there is a link between salt sensitivity and high salt intake and nondipping status, and that normal dipping can be restored by salt restriction.

SALT INTAKE AND CARDIOVASCULAR DISEASE

Current estimates suggest that the high level of dietary salt in the United States presently could account for up to 15% of strokes and 8% of coronary artery disease. In countries such as Finland where national programs to reduce salt intake have been effective, there is a reduction in blood pressure and a greater than 70% decrease in stroke and coronary heart mortality in the population younger than 65 years.

PATHOPHYSIOLOGY

Normal Responses to Changes in Dietary Salt

A healthy individual whose daily dietary salt intake is changed abruptly from a low-level (e.g., 20 mmol) to a high-level (e.g., 200 mmol) achieves dietary salt balance within 2 to 3 days. During this nonequilibrium time, renal sodium excretion, although increasing, remains below the level of sodium intake, accounting for a net positive balance of approximately 150 mmol of sodium and chloride matched by an increase in body weight of approximately 1 kg. Thereafter, the high level of salt intake is matched by an equivalent level of sodium and chloride excretion (e.g., 200 mmol per day). Homeostasis is achieved by integrated changes in renal hemodynamics and tubular function, key hormones, the sympathetic nervous system, and cardiovascular function.

An increase in dietary salt intake in healthy subjects is accompanied by an initial increase in renal blood flow without a change in glomerular filtration rate (GFR). The accompanying reduction in filtration fraction reduces proximal tubular sodium chloride and fluid reabsorption. Because there is little or no increase in plasma sodium concentration or GFR, the increase in renal sodium excretion is related to a reduction in tubular sodium chloride reabsorption. The nephron segments responsible have been studied indirectly in human subjects from changes in the clearance of lithium, which is reabsorbed almost exclusively in the proximal tubule in parallel with sodium. Such techniques demonstrate a modest reduction in proximal sodium reabsorption accompanied by a larger fractional reduction in distal sodium reabsorption.

Within the first 1 to 2 days of increased dietary salt intake, there is a sharp decline in plasma renin activity, serum aldosterone concentration, and plasma catecholamine levels. Plasma levels of atrial natriuretic peptide (ANP) increase in response to an increase in central blood volume and stretch of cardiac atria. Because angiotensin II and α-adrenergic activation enhance reabsorption throughout most of the nephron and reabsorption in the collecting ducts is enhanced by aldosterone but reduced by ANP, these neurohumoral changes dictate appropriate changes in tubular sodium chloride reabsorption with dietary salt intake.

Because the changes in renal sodium and fluid excretion lag behind the changes in intake, an increase in dietary salt is associated with some increase in the extracellular and plasma fluid volumes. The ensuring increase in venous return enhances cardiac output. In salt-resistant subjects, this is offset by a reduction in peripheral resistance such that blood pressure changes little.

Similar studies in salt-sensitive patients document two linked abnormalities. First, most but not all studies indicate that salt-sensitive patients retain a slightly greater fraction of dietary NaCl during adaption to a high salt intake. Because infusion of saline into salt-resistant normotensive subjects leads to little or no increase in blood pressure, this by itself is insufficient to explain the rise in blood pressure in salt-sensitive individuals. The second difference is that salt-resistant subjects, although showing an early rise in cardiac output during salt loading, have a blunted or absent reduction in peripheral resistance, thereby leading to a rise in blood pressure. At present, the causes for the defective renal sodium and chloride elimination and the defective reduction in peripheral resistance with salt intake in salt-sensitive subjects are poorly understood.

Salt Intake and Elimination in Patients with Renal Disease

Patients with CKD have several differences in their response to a high dietary salt intake. First, the majority of such patients are salt sensitive and therefore have a rise in blood pressure with dietary salt. As the GFR declines, salt balance can only be achieved by a parallel reduction in the fraction of the filtered sodium reabsorbed. This restricts the capacity of the tubules for rapid and effective achievement of salt balance during large changes in salt intake. Accordingly, patients with moderate or advanced CKD are unable to change renal salt excretion as rapidly, or as effectively, during changes in salt intake as normal subjects. This results in greater gains of salt and body fluids during high salt intake and, especially in those with tubulointerstitial disease, greater losses of salt and body fluids during reductions in salt intake. Therefore, salt intake should be adjusted carefully and incrementally in patients with advanced CKD, and these patients must be carefully followed. Second, unlike normal individuals, patients with CKD typically experience reductions in GFR with low dietary salt and increases in GFR with high salt intake.

Patients with heavy proteinuria and the nephrotic syndrome respond poorly to an increase in salt intake. The underlying avid renal salt retention, together with the low plasma oncotic pressure, increases the body weight and the peripheral edema. Moreover, increases in dietary salt increase proteinuria and obviate the antiproteinuric effect of ACE inhibitors. Therefore, dietary salt restriction is especially important in patients with CKD with heavy proteinuria and the nephrotic syndrome. The exception may be some younger subjects with minimal change nephropathy in whom the plasma volume is already contracted and the edema due almost entirely to the low plasma oncotic pressure. These subjects respond poorly to salt restriction.

DIURETICS

Effects of Salt Intake on the Fluid Depleting and Antihypertensive Responses to Diuretics

Studies in normal human subjects given a daily dose of a loop diuretic such as 40 mg of furosemide show the anticipated sharp increase in sodium excretion after the diuretic that leads initially to a negative balance for sodium and fluid. However, because of the short duration of loop diuretics of 4 to 6 hours, this is followed by 18 to 20 hours during which renal function is no longer dictated by the direct effects of the diuretic on the kidney. During this postdiuretic period, dietary salt and fluid may be retained sufficiently to counteract the immediate effects of the diuretic on the kidney. Studies at a high daily level of dietary salt intake (e.g., 300 mmol) demonstrate that this postdiuretic renal sodium retention is sufficient to prevent any negative loss of sodium or fluid over 24 hours. In contrast, studies at a low daily level of dietary salt intake (e.g., 20 mmol) show that negative salt balance is ensured because the diuretic-induced loss of salt is greater than the total daily intake. During dietary salt restriction, sodium balance is achieved by a declining natriuretic response to the drug (tolerance).

Salt restriction in normal subjects to a level of 100 to 120 mmol per day is required to ensure a sustained loss of body salt and fluid. Thiazide and distal potassium-sparing diuretics generally have longer durations of action than loop diuretic. This restricts the capacity of the kidney to restore salt loss with once daily diuretic dosing. This likely accounts for the greater effectiveness of thiazide and distal diuretics, compared with loop diuretics, as antihypertensives. Thus, some dietary salt restriction is required to ensure negative salt balance, especially with the short-acting loop diuretics despite their extreme acute natriuretic potency.

All antihypertensive agents, with the possible exception of calcium channel blockers, are less effective in reducing the blood pressure during high dietary salt intake. Dietary salt restriction is especially important for patients receiving diuretics and drugs that inhibit the renin–angiotensin–aldosterone system.

Drug-resistant hypertension is defined as sustained hypertension despite the use of three or more antihypertensive agents including a diuretic. Almost invariably, drug-resistant hypertension can be ascribed to inappropriate, ongoing high levels of salt intake and insufficient use of diuretics.

ACEIs and angiotensin receptor blockers are widely used to reduce protein excretion in patients with proteinuric kidney disease. This antiproteinuric action is lost during high levels of dietary salt intake, whereas a reduction in dietary salt itself produces a fall in protein excretion.

These observations lead to the proposal that dietary salt intake requires assessment and attention in all patients with more than the most modest levels of hypertension or CKD and any with heavy proteinuria.

GOALS OF DIETARY SALT RESTRICTION

The aim of salt restriction is to combat salt-sensitive hypertension, enhance antihypertensive drug responsiveness, achieve an appropriate level of blood pressure, prevent progressive loss of kidney function, limit proteinuria, and reduce cardiovascular risk. The level of salt intake required to achieve these goals varies with the clinical circumstance and the severity of the underlying condition.

An ideal daily level of dietary sodium intake for healthy, normotensive individuals is not clearly established but is likely about 150 mmol. The first step in antihypertensive therapy, and the only step presently recognized for patients with prehypertension, is nonpharmacologic therapy of which dietary salt restriction is a key component. The goal daily salt intake for these individuals should be about 100 to 120 mmol. Patients with drug-resistant hypertension and those with edema, nephrotic syndrome, or heavy protein-uria require a greater degree of dietary salt restriction. In practice, a goal of 80 mmol of sodium daily is often chosen. However, patients who are able to achieve lower levels of salt intake often have a further reduction in blood pressure or protein excretion. Therefore, more severe levels of salt restriction may be encouraged in those willing and able to comply. This requires a careful monitoring because patients with CKD not infrequently experience an initial reduction in GFR as salt intake is reduced. This reduction in GFR should reverse within weeks. Indeed, salt restriction should slow the progressive loss of GFR over time. However, these goals have not been extensively tested in clinical trials comparing different degrees of salt restriction. There is conflicting data from observational studies some of which show a linear relation of salt intake with outcomes, but others that show no benefit to restrictions of Na^+ intake to less than 100 mmol, and some even suggesting harm for sodium intake less than 100 mmol.

ASSESSMENT OF DIETARY SALT INTAKE

A dietary history, even with the help of a skilled nutritionist, provides only an approximate insight into salt intake. This is in large part owing to the large amounts of salt in prepared food that vary significantly by manufacturer. Because greater than 95% of sodium ingested normally is excreted by the kidneys, a properly collected 24-hour urine for sodium excretion is the best indication of sodium intake. Patients should be instructed in how to undertake a 24-hour collection and cautioned against changes in dietary intake or diuretic therapy in the week preceding the collection. The completeness of collection should be assessed from measurements of creatinine excretion, which should be 14 to 22 mg per kg for women and 20 to 25 mg per kg for men (with allowance for body size and muscle mass). Subjects with fever, a strenuous aerobic exercise program, diarrhea, and especially those with an ileostomy have significant extrarenal sodium losses. Renal sodium excretion in these subjects is not an accurate measure of sodium intake. Because sodium excretion fluctuates widely during the day in response to meals, a spot urine collection for sodium/creatinine ratio is a poor indication of dietary salt intake, although many recent studies have used data extrapolated from spot urines to link salt intake to renal and cardiovascular outcomes owing to the simplicity of the collection. A 24-hour urine collection also provides an opportunity to assess creatinine clearance, microalbumin or protein excretion, and the excretion of other food constituents such as potassium and calcium, which can also contribute to the level of blood pressure.

During accommodation to diuretic therapy in a subject without edema, there is initially a loss of body fluids resulting in approximately a 1 kg weight loss that is complete within 1 to 3 days. However, a negative sodium and fluid balance in patients with edema may persist for days or weeks during diuretic therapy. Dietary salt intake reflects renal sodium excretion in patients on diuretics only during the steady state. Therefore, patients should be provided adequate time to accommodate to diuretic therapy. Their body weight should be stabilized for some days before the 24-hour urine collection is undertaken. Because restriction of dietary salt is recommended even for patients with prehypertension and for most patients with CKD, especially those with proteinuria, a 24-hour urine collection for sodium excretion is an important initial assessment in all such subjects. If the level of sodium excretion is above goal, the 24-hour urine collection should be repeated about 1 month after providing dietary advice to assess compliance. A 24-hour urine collection for sodium excretion is important in patients with drug-resistant hypertension and those accumulating edema, because inappropriate salt intake is a frequent contribution to these problems.

SALT CONTENT OF FOODS

Unfortunately, more than 80% of the salt ingested presently in the United States is already added to food prior to serving. Therefore, abolition of table salt cannot make more than a modest contribution to reducing salt intake. There are current initiatives to entice commercial food providers to reduce the sodium content in prepared foods, but this has met with resistance because of changes in taste and shelf life of the products. Similar programs have been very effective in several European countries in reducing salt consumption. At present, reductions in dietary salt require changes in food intake and in eating habits. Dietary salt restriction is most effective in those individuals who can consume their meals in their own home from foods prepared in the household from fresh ingredients. These subjects should be able to reduce salt intake to recommended goals. The use of low salt-containing flour and other ingredients can reduce daily salt intake to less than 50 mmol in subject eating home-prepared foods. Unfortunately, most individuals eat food that is already prepared for them in restaurants or fast-food outlets or prepared from processed or tinned foods in the home. These sources usually contain much higher levels of dietary salt, which may not be acknowledged explicitly by the food provider. Individuals eating in this manner have a much harder task to restrict dietary salt, because even lower salt versions of these foods may have a very high sodium content. They may require advice from a nutritionist or insight from reading nutritional pamphlets or books.

A critical component of success in dietary salt restriction is the motivation of the physician to assess salt intake regularly from 24-hour sodium excretion and to encourage patients as their salt intake improves or identify problem areas of salt intake in those in whom sodium excretion is not falling to goal levels. Obese subjects who have an excessive intake of food almost invariably have an excessive intake of salt. Such subjects are unlikely to be successful with salt restriction unless this is matched by restriction of calorie intake as part of a weight reduction program.

The body salt burden can also be reduced modestly by regular aerobic exercise with perspiration. A regimen of 30 minutes of daily aerobic exercise is an important component of nonpharmacologic therapy for patients with hypertension and may also reduce progression of CKD, although this has been less well studied. Therefore, diet and exercise should be considered together and exercise adjusted appropriately within a subject's capacity.

Subjects accustomed to a high level of dietary salt intake may experience salt craving as they adapt to a lower salt intake. This salt-seeking behavior normally adjusts after 1 to 2 weeks to meet the new level of salt intake. Therefore, advice about a low-salt diet should contain a warning that the subject may experience a salt-seeking drive in the first few weeks but that this will abate with time. Salt can be substituted in the food by potassium chloride, provided there is no hyperkalemia or advanced CKD, or by a highly spiced diet. Nevertheless, most patients require advice about what foods contain an intrinsically high level of salt and must be avoided or their consumption restricted.

A National Institutes of Health–funded controlled study of dietary advice to stop hypertension (DASH) demonstrated that over a relatively short period of months, a healthy diet with a high intake of fruits, vegetables, nuts, and skimmed mild products with fish and white meat but little processed foods and red meat led to a remarkable reduction in blood pressure in normotensive and mildly hypertensive subjects. This DASH diet is an excellent basis for a healthy dietary intake but is not very low in salt. Therefore, it may need to be combined with advice on salt restriction for those with severe hypertension. Studies have shown that the blood pressure lowering effect of the DASH diet and of salt restriction are additive.

RECOMMENDATIONS

The management of dietary salt intake starts with setting appropriate goals for blood pressure, sodium, and sometimes potassium intakes (Fig. 17.1). Blood pressure should be assessed prior to changing the diet. The blood

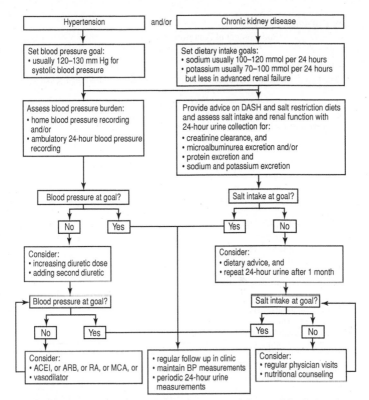

FIGURE 17.1 A proposed algorithm for the management of dietary salt intake in patients with hypertension or chronic kidney disease. ACEI, angiotensin-converting enzyme inhibitor; ARB, angiotensin receptor blocker; DASH, dietary advice to stop hypertension; MCA, mineralocorticoid antagonist; RA, renin antagonist.

pressure burden is best assessed by home blood pressure recordings or ambulatory 24-hour blood pressure recordings. Dietary advice then should be given. This can include advice about the DASH diet, together with referral to appropriate literature sources on the DASH diet or foods to avoid because of high salt content (Table 17.1). The effectiveness of this advice should be assessed by a 24-hour urine collection for sodium excretion, which can be combined with creatinine clearance and excretion of microalbumin and other minerals. If salt intake and blood pressure are at goal, regular follow-up in the clinic can be scheduled with measurements of blood pressure and periodic measurements of 24-hour sodium excretion to assess long-term compliance. Where sodium excretion is not at goal, especially if blood pressure remains elevated, patients require further dietary advice and repeated 24-hour urine collection after approximately 1 month. Persistent failure to achieve goal sodium excretion requires regular physician visits and a nutritional consult.

Salt Content of Common Foods

Food that contain *much* salt:
- Constituents of fast food, especially hamburgers,* pizza,* Thai,* and Mexican food*
- Olives in brine,* salted nuts,* and potato chips*
- Canned beans,* corn,* and peas*
- Sauerkraut,* tomato ketchup,* or tomato puree*
- Peanut butter
- Corn flakes
- Bread,* crackers,* donuts, muffins, pies, pretzels,* and scones*
- Cheese (especially Roquefort,* processed cheese,* and camembert*)
- Bacon,* ham, pate,* sausages,* and salami*
- Pickled, smoked, or canned fish
- Sardines

Foods that contain *little* salt:
- Fruits and fruit juices
- Vegetables and salads
- Unsalted nuts
- Grains and pasta
- Eggs, milk, yogurt, and ice cream
- Chocolate
- Most fresh meats, fish, and shellfish
- Cottage cheese
- Carbonated drinks and alcoholic beverages

*Food especially rich in salt.

Sources of Dietary Advice for Patients

Mattes RD, Donnelly D. Relative contributions of dietary sodium sources. *J Am Coll Nutr* 1991;10:383–393.

Moore T, Svetkey L, Lin P-H, et al. *The DASH Diet for Hypertension: Lower Your Blood Pressure in 14 Days Without Drugs.* New York: The Free Press; 2001.

U.S. Department of Health and Human Services, NIH, NHLBI. NIH Publication No. 06-4082, 2006. *Your Guide to Lowering Your Blood Pressure with DASH Eating Plan.* Bethesda, MD: NIH, NHLBI.

Willett WC. *Eat, Drink and Be Healthy: The Harvard Medical School Guide to Healthy Eating.* New York: The Free Press; 2001.

Suggested Readings

Cappuccio FP. Salt and cardiovascular disease. *Br Med J* 2007;334:859–860.

Cobb LK, Anderson CA, Elliott P, et al. Methodological issues in cohort studies that relate sodium intake to cardiovascular disease outcomes: a science advisory from the American Heart Association, American Heart Association Council on Lifestyle and Metabolic Health. *Circulation* 2014;129:1173–1186.

Esnault VL, Ekhlas A, Delcroix C, et al. Diuretic and enhanced sodium restriction results in improved antiproteinuric response to RAS blocking agents. *J Am Soc Nephrol* 2005;16:474–481.

Franco V, Oparil S. Salt sensitivity, a determinant of blood pressure, cardiovascular disease and survival. *J Am Coll Nutr* 2006;25:247S–255S.

Fukuda M, Kimura G. Salt sensitivity and nondippers in chronic kidney disease. *Curr Hypertens Rep* 2012;14:382–387.

Graudal N, Jürgens G, Baslund B, et al. Compared with usual sodium intake, low- and excessive-sodium diets are associated with increased mortality: a meta-analysis. *Hypertension* 2014;27:1129–1137.

He FJ, MacGregor GA. Effect of modest salt reduction on blood pressure: a meta-analysis of randomized trials. Implications for public health. *J Hum Hypertens* 2002;16:761–770.

Institute of Medicine. *Sodium Intake in Population.* Washington, DC: National Academies Press; 2013.

Kelly RA, Wilcox CS, Mitch WE, et al. Response of the kidney to furosemide: II. Effect of captopril on sodium balance. *Kidney Int* 1983;24:233–239.

Mills KT, Chen J, Yang W, et al. sodium excretion and the risk of cardiovascular disease in patients with chronic kidney disease. Chronic Renal Insufficiency Cohort (CRIC) Study Investigators. *JAMA* 2016;315:2200–2210.

Ritz E. Lowering salt intake—an important strategy in the management of renal disease. *Nat Clin Pract Nephrol* 2007;3:360–361.

Sacks FM, Svetkey LP, Vollmer WM, et al. Effects on blood pressure of reduced dietary sodium and the Dietary Approaches to Stop Hypertension (DASH) diet. DASH-Sodium Collaborative Research Group. *N Engl J Med* 2001;344:3–10.

Schmidlin O, Forman A, Sebastian A, et al. What initiates the pressor effect of salt in salt-sensitive humans? Observations in normotensive Blacks. *Hypertension* 2007;49:1032–1039.

Young JH, Chang YPC, Kim JD, et al. Differential susceptibility to hypertension is due to selection during the out-of-Africa expansion. *PLoS Genet* 2005;1(6):e82.

18 Nutritional Aspects of Kidney Stones

John C. Lieske

The lifetime risk of kidney stones varies from 1% to 5% in Asia, 5% to 9% in Europe, 10% to 15% in the United States, and 20% to 25% in the Middle East, and is thus the third most common urologic disease worldwide among both males and females, with renal colic accounting for 1% of hospital admissions internationally. In the United States, the prevalence of kidney stones has increased by 70% over the last 15 years. Recurrence rates are approximately 20% for the 5 years after the first stone, and increase with subsequent kidney stone events. Owing to its high prevalence, over $10 billion is spent annually in the United States for treatment of stones.

Consequently, efforts to prevent stone formation are essential. Tailored dietary recommendations to prevent stone recurrence should be offered to every patient and based on a metabolic evaluation. In many patients, medications will be necessary to reduce stone risk, but use of medications does not obviate the need for an effective dietary and fluid prescription.

Most data on the relation between diet and stone disease come from observational and physiologic studies rather than randomized trials. There is not yet a consensus on the specifics of dietary modification, but several important concepts should be kept in mind when designing a therapeutic regimen. First, short-term intervention studies examining changes in urine composition are of interest, but ideally clinical regimens should be based on studies using actual stone formation as the desired outcome. This is because stone formation cannot be perfectly predicted by urinary composition, and it is likely that many factors influence urinary supersaturation but are not identified by the computer algorithm (EQUIL2) used to calculate supersaturation (e.g., phytate). Second, it is important to individualize recommendations based on stone type and urinary composition (derived from one or more 24-hour urine collections obtained at least 4 weeks after a stone episode are required for the initial evaluation). For example, dietary oxalate restriction is not helpful for individuals with pure uric acid or cystine stones. Third, the impact of dietary risk factors varies by age, sex, and body mass index. Fourth, patients must provide follow-up 24-hour urine collections to evaluate the impact of dietary recommendations. If the urine composition does not change in response to a dietary change, then alternative approaches should be tried. Finally, it is important to distinguish stone passage from new stone formation. If a patient implements dietary changes and then passes a preexisting stone, this does not indicate treatment failure.

DIETARY RISK FACTORS FOR CALCIUM STONE DISEASE

The majority (more than 80%) of kidney stones contain calcium, often a mixture of calcium oxalate and calcium phosphate (in the form of hydroxy-apatite), and are often termed "idiopathic calcium oxalate stones" (referred to as calcium oxalate stones in this chapter). Consequently, the majority of studies have focused on the prevention of these common calcium oxalate stones. Dietary factors purported to be associated with increased or decreased

TABLE 18.1	Putative Dietary Factors Associated that May Increase or Decrease Idiopathic Calcium Oxalate Kidney Stones*
Dietary Factor	**Proposed Mechanism(s)**
Increase Risk	
Oxalate	Increased urinary oxalate excretion
Sodium	Increased urinary calcium excretion
Animal protein	Increased urinary calcium and uric acid excretion; reduced urinary citrate excretion
Vitamin C	Increased oxalate generation and excretion
Carbohydrates	Increased urinary calcium excretion
Decrease Risk	
Dietary calcium	Binding of dietary oxalate in gut
Potassium	Increased urinary citrate excretion; reduced urinary calcium excretion
Phytate	Inhibition of calcium oxalate crystal formation
Magnesium	Reduced dietary oxalate absorption; inhibition of calcium oxalate crystal formation
Vitamin B_6	Vitamin B_6 deficiency may increase oxalate production and oxaluria

*Phosphorus and n-3 fatty acids are discussed in the text.

risk of calcium oxalate stone are listed in Table 18.1. Less common types of stones include pure calcium phosphate, uric acid, struvite, and cystine. Dietary recommendations, and the importance of diet for their prevention, differ in certain respects for each of these other stone types.

Calcium

In the past, a high calcium intake was incorrectly believed to increase the risk of stone formation. This was primarily based on the observation that approximately 20% of ingested calcium is absorbed, and that this proportion increases in individuals with idiopathic hypercalciuria. However, substantial evidence demonstrates that a higher calcium diet is associated with a *reduced* risk of stone formation. One potential mechanism to explain this apparent paradox is that the higher calcium intake will bind dietary oxalate in the gut, thereby reducing oxalate absorption and urinary excretion. It is also possible that dairy products (the major source of dietary calcium) may contain factors that inhibit stone formation.

Several large prospective observational studies in men and women consistently support a reduced risk of stone formation with increasing dietary calcium intake. Compared to individuals in the lowest quintile of dietary calcium intake, those in the highest quintile had more than a 30% lower risk of forming a stone. These results were adjusted for multiple factors, including age, body mass index, total fluid intake, the use of thiazide diuretics, and the intake of nutrients such as animal protein, magnesium, phosphorous, sodium, and potassium. The risk of stone formation associated with calcium intake is an example of how the impact of a risk factor can vary by age: there was no association between dietary calcium and stone formation in men aged 60 years or older.

These observational findings were subsequently confirmed by a 5-year randomized, controlled clinical trial which compared stone recurrence in individuals with a history of calcium oxalate nephrolithiasis and idiopathic hypercalciuria assigned to a diet low in calcium (400 mg per day) or to a diet with "normal" calcium content (1,200 mg per day) plus lower amounts of animal protein and sodium. The risk of developing a recurrent stone on the higher calcium diet was 51% lower than for the low-calcium diet. Because both dietary sodium and animal protein can contribute to the formation of calcium stones, these results, although suggestive, did not directly address the independent role of dietary calcium in the pathogenesis of kidney stones. Nonetheless, there is overwhelming evidence that dietary calcium should not be restricted; such a diet increases the risk of stone formation and may be harmful to bone health by inducing negative calcium balance.

The impact of supplemental calcium on stone risk differs from the influence of dietary calcium. In an observational study of older women, calcium supplement users were 20% more likely to form a stone than women who did not take supplements. The Women's Health Initiative randomized trial also found an increased risk with calcium supplementation, though in this case, the supplements also contained vitamin D. In observational studies of younger women and men, there was no association between calcium supplement use and the risk of stone formation. This discrepancy between the risks from dietary calcium versus calcium supplements may be due to the timing of calcium intake. Calcium supplements are not typically taken with meals, which would diminish the binding of dietary oxalate.

It must be noted that in these studies the absolute risk of forming a first kidney stone is only slightly increased among calcium supplement users (1.2 cases/1,000 women per year) compared to those not taking them (1.0/1,000 per year), indicating that supplement use is not a major contributor to stone risk. However, for an individual who has had a stone, the impact of calcium supplementation on urine composition should be evaluated before recommending calcium supplement use. It has also been suggested in a smaller study that timing of calcium supplement intake with meals may have a net neutral effect on urinary supersaturation owing to a rise in urine calcium but fall in urine oxalate excretion, whereas taking them on a fasting stomach increases both urinary calcium and supersaturation. In all cases, it is important to balance bone risk with kidney stone risk for any given patient. If a patient cannot get sufficient calcium from dairy sources, and morbidity of bone disease is of concern, use of supplements timed with meals may be the best approach. The net effect on a subsequent 24-hour urine calcium excretion and overall supersaturation may also help to judge the net effect of this on future stone risk.

Oxalate

Urine oxalate concentration is clearly an important risk factor for calcium oxalate stone formation, but the role of dietary oxalate in the pathogenesis of calcium oxalate nephrolithiasis is less clear. First, the proportion of urinary oxalate derived from dietary oxalate is controversial, with estimates ranging from 10% to 50%. Thus, a substantial proportion of urinary oxalate is derived from endogenous production (metabolism of glycine, glycolate, and hydroxyproline). Second, other dietary factors influence excretion of oxalate in urine. For example, vitamin C supplementation appears to be an important contributor because it can be metabolized to oxalate. Third, much of the oxalate in food may not be readily absorbed owing to low bioavailability. Finally, there is significant variation in the gastrointestinal (GI) tract absorption of oxalate. For instance, up to one-third of patients who have calcium oxalate nephrolithiasis may experience increased absorption of dietary oxalate. Those colonized with *Oxalobacter formigenes*, an intestinal bacterium that degrades oxalate, may have reduced oxalate available for absorption from food. Emerging evidence suggests that other components of the gastrointestinal microbiome may also influence oxalate bioavailability and absorption. Overall, the role of the intestinal microbiome in kidney stone risk remains an area of great interest.

Older lists of the oxalate content in food may be unreliable owing to measurement issues related to the quality of the assay procedure, as well as the variability in oxalate content of different foods. More reliable assays for the direct determination of the oxalate content of foods, including ion chromatography and capillary electrophoresis have been developed, and subsequent large prospective cohort studies in men and women of the relationship between dietary oxalate and kidney stone formation revealed that the impact of dietary oxalate was minimal in men and older women and not associated with stone formation in younger women.

In general, the emphasis on dietary oxalate should be tailored to the individual patient. If urine oxalate excretion is low, it may be adequate to avoid large quantities of high-oxalate foods (e.g., certain nuts including almonds, peanuts, cashews, walnuts, and pecans; certain vegetables including beets and spinach; wheat bran and rice bran). Most types of chocolate are not high in oxalate. A list of the oxalate content of several hundred food items can be found at https://regepi.bwh.harvard.edu/health/Oxalate/files, which can be a useful resource for patients since (unlike calcium or sodium) oxalate content is not listed on food labels.

Sodium

Higher sodium intakes result in decreased proximal sodium reabsorption and greater distal delivery. This results in faster flow past key sites of calcium reabsorption in the thick ascending limb and thus less efficient calcium reabsorption and relative hypercalciuriu. In u prospective randomized study, there was a powerful effect of concomitant dietary sodium and animal protein restriction to reduce urinary calcium excretion. Observational studies reveal a positive, independent association between sodium consumption and new kidney stone formation in women but not men. Urine sodium excretion in a 24-hour collection, a direct reflection of dietary sodium intake, appeared to be associated with an increased risk in men but not consistently in women. Thus, there appears to be differences in the impact by age and gender. While the importance of sodium restriction to <2.5 g per day is clear for lowering of blood pressure (justifying the recommendation to limit sodium intake for the general population), its role in calcium stone formation requires further study.

Potassium

Dietary potassium restriction can increase urinary calcium excretion. In addition, hypokalemia stimulates citrate reabsorption, decreasing the urinary excretion of citrate, an important inhibitor of calcium oxalate stone formation. Potassium in food also accompanies organic anions such as citrate that are metabolized to bicarbonate. Thus, the consumption of potassium-containing foods such as fruits and vegetables represents an alkali load that increases the urinary excretion of citrate. A high potassium intake is inversely associated with kidney stones in men and older women, but not younger women.

Animal Protein

From a metabolic standpoint, animal protein should be divided into dairy (e.g., milk, yogurt) and nondairy (meat, chicken, seafood) sources. The metabolism of sulfur-containing amino acids in animal flesh generates sulfuric acid so nondairy animal protein provides an acid load that may increase urinary calcium excretion and reduce urinary citrate excretion. Nondairy animal protein can also increase calcitriol production. A positive association between total animal protein consumption and new kidney stone formation was noted in men but not women, however these studies did not explicitly look at the two separate sources of animal protein. As the amount of dietary calcium is inversely associated with stone formation, and dairy foods are a major source of dietary calcium, it is likely that dairy protein would be inversely associated with risk. Therefore, restriction of nondairy animal protein, but not dairy protein, may be beneficial.

Phytate
Dietary phytate (inositol hexaphosphate) may play a role in preventing the formation of calcium-containing stones. Phytate is found in many foods high in fiber, such as cereals, legumes, and vegetables and it binds strongly to calcium in the intestine. Phytate is also absorbed from the GI tract and is excreted in the urine where it inhibits urinary crystallization of calcium salts. This is relevant because urinary levels of phytate in some calcium oxalate stone formers appear to be low. Observational data from younger women showed that dietary phytate was inversely associated with incident kidney stone formation, but there was no similar relationship in men.

Magnesium
Magnesium may reduce oxalate absorption in the gastrointestinal tract and can form soluble complexes with oxalate in the urine, potentially decreasing calcium oxalate supersaturation. The few randomized trials studying the effect of magnesium supplementation on stone recurrence yielded inconclusive results, because magnesium was given in combination with other compounds (e.g., thiazide diuretic or potassium citrate) and patient dropout rates were high. In observational studies, higher dietary magnesium was associated with a 30% lower risk of stone formation in men, but not in women.

Carbohydrates
Carefully performed physiologic studies demonstrated that carbohydrate ingestion can increase urinary calcium excretion, an effect that may be at least partially mediated by insulin. A positive association between sucrose intake and new kidney stone formation has been shown to occur in women but not men. Higher fructose intake also increases the risk of stone formation in men and women, although no specific association with urinary composition has been demonstrated.

Vitamin C
Vitamin C (ascorbic acid) can be metabolized to form oxalate. In one study, vitamin C (1,000 mg twice daily) increased urinary oxalate excretion by 22%. In a large cohort, there was a 40% higher risk of stone formation in men who consumed 1,000 mg or more per day of vitamin C compared to men who consumed less than 90 mg per day (the recommended dietary allowance). This relationship was observed only after adjusting for dietary potassium. It seems reasonable to *not* recommend restricting *dietary* vitamin C (as foods high in vitamin C are also high in inhibitory factors such as potassium), but a calcium stone former should be instructed to limit any vitamin C supplements to less than 1,000 mg per day.

Vitamin D
The role of vitamin D in stone formation is also unclear. While very high intakes of vitamin D and calcium can increase urine calcium excretion, the impact of usual levels of intake is uncertain. In the Women's Health Initiative Study, the increase in stone risk was ~20% higher in women who were given calcium supplements (1,000 mg per day) that also contained vitamin D_3 (400 IU per day), so it is ultimately unclear if the increase in risk was due to the calcium supplement (most likely), the vitamin D (less likely), or the combination of both. In a recent analysis, vitamin D intake was not associated with the risk of incident kidney stones in men or younger women, but the risk was higher

in older women who ingested greater than 1,000 IU per day. Although not statistically significant, the adjusted hazard ratio (HR) for incident stones among men taking > 1,000 IU (HR 1.23) was similar to that of the older women (HR 1.38). Despite these concerns, recent studies in small numbers of stone formers did not demonstrate that replacing 25(OH) vitamin D stores with 6 weeks of oral ergocalciferol (50,000 IU per week) worsened hypercalciuria. Given the high prevalence of vitamin D deficiency in the United States, even among healthy individuals, and the adverse impact on bone health, it is reasonable to measure plasma 25(OH) vitamin D and replete it in deficient individuals, even if they have high urine calcium. Taking higher daily doses of vitamin D (>1,000 IU) should, however, be avoided.

Vitamin B$_6$

Vitamin B$_6$ is a cofactor in oxalate metabolism, and thus vitamin B$_6$ deficiency increases oxalate production and oxaluria. Although a very high dose of vitamin B$_6$ can reduce urine oxalate in selected patients with a very specific genetic disorder (a subgroup of type 1 primary hyperoxaluria), the use of vitamin B$_6$ in other settings remains unclear. While substantial vitamin B$_6$ supplements may reduce the risk of kidney stone formation in women, this relationship was not found in men.

Phosphorus

Higher levels of dietary phosphate will decrease intestinal absorption of dietary calcium. One of the challenges for studying independent associations of dietary phosphate with kidney stone formation is its high correlation with calcium in the diet. For patients who have calcium phosphate stones, there is a theoretical benefit to reducing phosphate intake to reduce phosphate excretion, but there are no data documenting benefits in stone formation.

n-3 Fatty Acids

It has been proposed that dietary fatty acids can modulate the urinary excretion of calcium and oxalate, and that fish oil supplementation will lower urinary calcium and oxalate. However, a prospective study found no association between the intake of n-3 fatty acids and the risk of kidney stone formation in men or women.

Calories

There are no data on the direct relation between total caloric intake and stone risk. However, higher body weight, a larger waist circumference, and a higher body mass index plus weight gain are associated with an increased risk of kidney stone formation, independent of diet. Although there are no available data to support weight loss as a preventive treatment for stone disease, stone formers should be encouraged to exercise and modulate their intake of calories to maintain a healthy weight.

BEVERAGES AND CALCIUM STONES

Total Fluid

Nephrolithiasis is a disease arising from increased concentration of the urine and its constituents. Even if the total amounts of lithogenic substances excreted in the urine are reasonable, a low urine volume can raise the concentrations leading to stone formation. Thus, modifying the concentration of the lithogenic factors is the focus of stone prevention and fluid intake, the main determinant of urine volume, is a critical component of stone prevention. Observational studies and a randomized, controlled trial have demonstrated that a higher fluid intake reduces the risk of stone formation.

A recent meta-analysis confirmed the utility of increased water intake as being effective to reduce kidney stone risk. A short-term study that used a vasopressin type 2 inhibitor to increase urinary dilution (and hence fluid intake) confirmed that increased urine flows do not increase excretion of lithogenic substances, and thus dramatically decreases urinary supersaturation for calcium oxalate, calcium phosphate, and uric acid. Given these results, patients must be given specific advice on how much to drink to form at least 2 L of urine per day. In addition to fluid intake, other factors such as insensible losses and the water contained in foods influence urine volume. Rather than arbitrarily specifying a certain amount of fluid intake (e.g., eight glasses of water per day), the recommendation should be tailored based on the total volume of 24-hour urine collections of each individual patient. For example, if an individual produces 1.5 L of urine per day, consuming an additional two 8-ounce (240 mL) glasses of water would raise their output to the target of 2 L. Patients should be reminded that consistency of fluid intake is important: producing 3 L of urine on one day will not cancel out the crystal-forming potential from 1 L of output on the previous day. While some clinicians suggest that a patient should drink enough fluids to wake up at least once per night, there are no data to support such guidelines and the desire to have constantly diluted urine needs to be balanced against the harm of sleep disruption.

Individual Beverages

When advised to increase to their fluid intake, patients often want to know what they should and should not drink. The associations of specific beverages, beyond fluid intake, with kidney stone formation are presented in Table 18.2. Despite previous beliefs to the contrary, alcoholic beverages, coffee, and tea do not increase the risk of stone formation. In fact, observational studies have found that coffee, tea, beer, and wine *reduce* the risk of stone formation. The mechanism for this protective association is likely related to the impact on antidiuretic hormone (ADH) in the kidney by caffeine, and the inhibition of ADH secretion by alcohol. The role of tea deserves special mention. There is a widespread belief that tea is high in oxalate and should be avoided. A cup of tea contains 14 mg of oxalate. While this is not insignificant, the bioavailability does not appear to be high, and when tested there was a negligible impact on urinary oxalate. Citrus juices, such as orange and grapefruit juice theoretically could reduce the risk of stone formation by increasing urine citrate, but prospective studies found no association with orange juice. In fact, grapefruit juice intake was associated with a 40% higher risk of stone formation. Grapefruit juice can affect a number of intestinal enzymes, but

Beverage Type	Risk	Proposed Mechanism(s)
Coffee and tea	Decreased	Caffeine interferes with anti-diuretic hormone action, leading to decreased urinary concentration
Alcohol	Decreased	Alcohol inhibits secretion of anti-diuretic hormone, leading to decreased urinary concentration
Milk	Decreased	Binding of dietary oxalate in gut
Grapefruit juice	Increased	Possible increased oxalate production

TABLE 18.2 Select Beverages, Risk, and Mechanism for Idiopathic Calcium Oxalate Stone Formation*

*Orange juice and soda are discussed in the text.

the mechanism for the observed increased risk is unknown. One prospective study found that grapefruit consumption did increase urine citrate, but also substantially increased urine oxalate.

The relation between soda ("soft drink") consumption and stone risk is complicated. Dietary patterns associated with sweetened soda consumption were found to increase the risk of stone formation. As sweetened sodas contain fructose which increases the risk of stone formation, these beverages should be avoided.

Dietary Patterns

Beyond specific nutrient information, some patients prefer to receive advice about an overall dietary approach. The Dietary Approaches to Stop Hypertension Study (DASH) found that a diet rich in fruits, vegetables, nuts, legumes plus low-fat dairy and low sodium substantially reduces blood pressure. While this pattern theoretically should reduce the risk of stone formation (in addition to lowering blood pressure), there are no published studies that have specifically examined this question. However, in a prospective study, individuals with self-selected diets that more closely mirrored a DASH diet had a lower risk of incident stones. In contrast, high animal protein diets promoted to cause weight loss may increase the risk of stone formation, but this has not been formally tested.

PREVENTION OF STONE RECURRENCE—OTHER STONE TYPES

For the less common types of stones, there are few data supporting specific dietary manipulations. The following recommendations, therefore, are based largely on pathophysiology.

Uric Acid Stones

The two driving forces for uric acid crystal formation are the uric acid concentration and urine pH (the solubility of uric acid increases substantially as the urine pH increases from 5.0 to 6.5). Decreasing the consumption of meat, chicken, and seafood will decrease purine intake and, therefore, uric acid production; it may also increase urinary pH. Higher intake of fruits and vegetables should raise the urine pH and reduce the risk of uric acid crystal formation.

Cystine Stones

Patients with cystine stone disease nearly always require medications but dietary modification may also help. Restricting sodium intake appears to strongly reduce the urinary excretion of cystine, and the solubility of cystine increases as urinary pH rises. Thus, greater fruit and vegetable consumption may be beneficial. Urinary cystine excretion also correlates with urinary urea nitrogen excretion, a marker of protein intake. However, there is no evidence that severely restricting intake of proteins high in cystine reduces stone formation, though moderately reducing animal protein intake may be beneficial by decreasing cystine excretion and increasing urine pH.

Calcium Phosphate Stones

Information on dietary factors related to calcium phosphate stone formation is limited. Because patients with type 1 renal tubular acidosis and stone disease may benefit from alkali supplementation, generally as potassium citrate, they may also benefit from a diet high in fruits and vegetables. It should be noted, however, that an increase in urinary pH can increase the risk of calcium phosphate crystal formation. Dietary maneuvers directed at decreasing urinary calcium excretion (see Table 18.3) and urinary phosphate excretion would be expected to decrease calcium phosphate stone recurrence.

TABLE 18.3	Dietary Recommendations for Idiopathic Calcium Oxalate Stone Prevention According to Urinary Risk Factor
Urinary Abnormality	**Dietary Changes**
High calcium	Adequate dietary calcium intake
	Reduce nondairy animal protein intake (5–7 servings of meat, fish, or poultry/wk)
	Reduce sodium intake to <2.5 g/d
	Reduce sucrose intake
High oxalate	Avoid high-oxalate foods
	Avoid vitamin C supplements
	Adequate dietary calcium intake
Low citrate	Increase fruit and vegetable intake
	Reduce nondairy animal protein intake
Low volume	Increase total fluid intake to maintain urine volume ≥2 L/d

Calcium Oxalate Stones Associated with Enteric Hyperoxaluria

Any gastrointestinal disorder that causes fat malabsorption can lead to over-absorption of oxalate from the diet, termed enteric hyperoxaluria. Since the majority of oxalate is absorbed in the colon, enteric hyperoxaluria is only observed in patients with an intact colon. Common causes include inflammatory bowel disease, pancreatic insufficiency, and malabsorptive bariatric surgical procedures (most commonly Roux-en Y Gastric Bypass). Strict dietary regimens are essential in this patient group including low oxalate and fat intake, and ample dietary calcium. Calcium supplements are also useful to act as oxalate binders.

CONCLUSIONS

Dietary factors play an important role in kidney stone formation, and dietary modification can reduce the risk of stone recurrence. Because stone recurrence rates may be as high as 30% to 50% after 5 to 10 years, individualized dietary intervention to prevent stone recurrence should be offered to every patient willing to participate in a diagnostic workup and to adhere to treatment recommendations. The necessity of prescribing medications does not obviate the need for an effective dietary and/or fluid prescription. Dietary interventions and subsequent evaluations of therapeutic efficacy can most easily be based on results of repeated 24-hour urine collections, since certain urinary excretions reflect key dietary intakes (Table 18.4). Adequate fluid intake and appropriate dietary modifications based on the increasingly available

TABLE 18.4	Clues to Dietary Intake from the 24-hour Urine Composition
Diet Intake	**Urine Component**
Sodium	Sodium, chloride
Animal Protein	Sulfate, urine urea nitrogen
Fluid	Volume, osmolality
Fruits and vegetables	Potassium, citrate, pH
Oxalate	Oxalate[*]

[*]In the absence of a genetic cause of hyperoxaluria.

scientific evidence may substantially reduce the morbidity and costs that are associated with recurrent nephrolithiasis.

Suggested Readings

Borghi L, Schianchi T, Meschi T, et al. Comparison of two diets for the prevention of recurrent stones in idiopathic hypercalciuria. *N Engl J Med* 2002;346(2):77–84.

Cheungpasitporn W, Erickson SB, Rule AD, et al. Short-term tolvaptan increases water intake and effectively decreases urinary calcium oxalate, calcium phosphate and uric acid supersaturations. *J Urol* 2016;195(5):1476–1481.

Cheungpasitporn W, Rossetti S, Friend K, et al. Treatment effect, adherence, and safety of high fluid intake for the prevention of incident and recurrent kidney stones: a systematic review and meta-analysis. *J Nephrol* 2016;29(2):211–219.

Curhan GC, Willett WC, Knight EL, et al. Dietary factors and the risk of incident kidney stones in younger women: Nurses' Health Study II. *Arch Intern Med* 2004;164(8):885–891.

Curhan GC, Willett WC, Rimm EB, et al. A prospective study of dietary calcium and other nutrients and the risk of symptomatic kidney stones [see comments]. *N Engl J Med* 1993;328:833–838.

Curhan GC, Willett WC, Speizer FE, et al. Comparison of dietary calcium with supplemental calcium and other nutrients as factors affecting the risk for kidney stones in women. *Ann Intern Med* 1997;266(7):497–504.

Ferraro PM, Taylor EN, Gambaro G, et al. Vitamin D intake and the risk of incident kidney stones. *J Urol* 2017;197(2):405–410.

Jackson RD, LaCroix AZ, Gass M, et al. Calcium plus vitamin D supplementation and the risk of fractures. *N Engl J Med* 2006;354(7):669–683.

Lemann JJ, Piering WF, Lennon EJ. Possible role of carbohydrate-induced calciuria in calcium oxalate stone formation. *N Engl J Med* 1969;280:232–237.

Lieske JC, Rule AD, Krambeck AE, et al. Stone composition as a function of age and sex. *Clin J Am Soc Nephrol* 2014;9(12):2141–2146.

Rule AD, Lieske JC, Li X, et al. The ROKS nomogram for predicting a second symptomatic stone episode. *J Am Soc Nephrol* 2014;25(12):2878–2886.

Siener R, Bangen U, Sidhu H, et al. The role of Oxalobacter formigenes colonization in calcium oxalate stone disease. *Kidney Int* 2013;83(6):1144–1149.

Taylor EN, Curhan GC. Dietary calcium from dairy and nondairy sources, and risk of symptomatic kidney stones. *J Urol* 2013;190(4):1255–1259.

Taylor EN, Curhan GC. Fructose consumption and the risk of kidney stones. *Kidney Int* 2008;73(2):207–212.

Taylor EN, Stampfer MJ, Curhan GC. Dietary factors and the risk of incident kidney stones in men: new insights after 14 years of follow-up. *J Am Soc Nephrol* 2004;15(12):3225–3232.

Practical Aspects of Dealing
with the Gut Microbiome in
Patients with Kidney Disease

Pieter Evenepoel and Björn Meijers

INTRODUCTION

Composition and Activity of the Gut Microbiota

The human intestinal tract, and predominantly the large intestine, is colonized by trillions of microbes, which collectively possess hundreds of times as many genes as coded for by the human genome. The combined genetic repertoire of the endogenous flora is referred to as the "microbiome." The microbiome codes for a complex web of unique metabolic capacities, encompassing synthesis of several vitamins and fermentation of carbohydrates, lipids, proteins, and bile acids.

The composition and activity of the gut microbiota co-develop with the host from birth and are subject to a complex interplay between host genome, nutrition, and extrinsic environmental and lifestyle factors (Fig. 19.1). Nutrition is one of the key regulators of intestinal microbial composition and microbial metabolism. Amounts of nutrients entering the colon mainly depend on dietary intake(s) and on the efficiency of the assimilation process in the small intestine. Dietary fiber, being resistant to digestion in the small intestine, is the main supply of carbohydrates to the colon. These carbohydrates are fermented to short-chain fatty acids (SCFAs). SCFAs play an important role in maintaining energy homeostasis and gut epithelial integrity. Nitrogen is provided to the large intestine by dietary proteins escaping digestion in the upper gut, by endogenous proteins (pancreatic and intestinal secretions, sloughed epithelial cells), and by blood urea diffusing in intestinal contents. The fate of colonic α-amino nitrogen (amino acids and intermediates) is dependent on the amount of energy (mainly carbohydrates) available for bacterial growth and cell division. In case of adequate carbohydrate supply, α-amino nitrogen will predominantly be incorporated in the bacterial biomass. In case of carbohydrate deprivation, conversely, α-amino nitrogen will be predominantly fermented to phenols, indoles, amines, among other co-metabolites. Dietary fat is believed not to reach the colonic microbiota in significant amounts as it is mostly digested and absorbed in the small intestine. Dietary fat can have an indirect effect on the colonic microenvironment as bile acids, which are excreted in the small intestine to aid digestion of fat, and can reach the colon and be converted by the microbiota. Foods rich in fats are moreover often rich in the dietary nutrients phosphatidylcholine (lecithin), choline, and carnitine. Gut microbiota can use these nutrients as a carbon fuel source. While mammals do not have the enzyme, gut microbes have trimethylamine (TMA) lyases, which can cleave the C–N bond of these nutrients, releasing the TMA moiety as a waste product (Fig. 19.2).

From an evolutionary point of view, the anatomy of the human colon is well adapted to an energy-poor/high-fiber diet (leaves, fruits, seeds, nuts), as our ancestors used to consume. Indeed, fermentation allows the extraction of energy out of dietary fiber and other nutrients that escape digestion and adsorption in the small intestine and thereby helps to maintain energy homeostasis. The anatomy of the human colon, conversely, is not well adapted

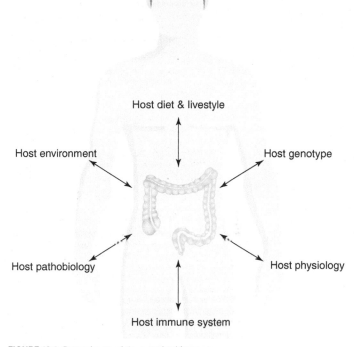

Host diet & livestyle

Host environment

Host genotype

Host pathobiology

Host physiology

Host immune system

FIGURE 19.1 Determinants of the gut microbiome.

to a low-fiber/high-protein and -fat diet (i.e., a Western diet). This mismatch between anatomy and diet causes a shift from beneficial carbohydrate fermentation toward potentially harmful protein and choline fermentation.

Another important and potentially modifiable determinant of colonic microbiota composition and activity is transit time. Slowing down colonic transit time induces an upstream expansion of proteolytic species, as a larger part of the colon becomes carbohydrate deprived, resulting in an increased generation and uptake of end-products of bacterial protein fermentation.

Bidirectional Crosstalk between Host and Microbiota in CKD

Host–microbe interactions are essential to many aspects of normal mammalian physiology, ranging from nutrition to immune homeostasis. A disturbed gut microbial composition and metabolism, coined as "gut dysbiosis," contributes to a multitude of ailments, from the obvious case of inflammatory bowel disease to complex diseases residing in organs outside the gut. Mounting evidence indicates that also in the setting of chronic kidney disease (CKD), there is intense bidirectional crosstalk between the intestinal microbiota and the host (Fig. 19.3).

On the one hand, mounting experimental and clinical evidence indicates that uremia per se or the uremic phenotype may fuel gut dysbiosis. The uremic phenotype is characterized by slow colonic transit (owing to sedentary lifestyle, polypharmacy, restricted intake of fluids, and dietary changes), high luminal pH (owing to increased ammonia concentrations), and low dietary

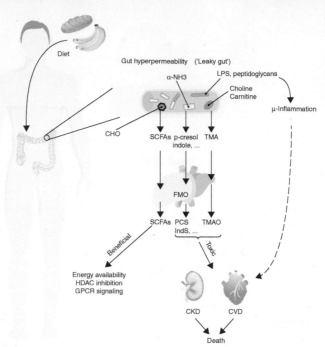

FIGURE 19.2 The diet–gut–kidney axis. Following dietary exposures of certain nutrients, gut microbiota can elicit both metabolism-dependent and metabolism-independent effects on the host. Metabolism-dependent effects include: (1) Microbial fermentation of dietary carbohydrates to generate short-chain fatty acids (SCFAs), which signal to the host to increase energy expenditure, inhibit histone deacetylase (HDAC) activity, and enhance G protein–coupled receptor (GPCR) signaling. (2) Microbial conversion of α-NH$_2$ nitrogen protein fermentation metabolites including phenols and indoles, which are subsequently metabolized in the colonocytes and liver to p-cresyl sulfate, indoxyl sulfate among others. (3) Microbial conversion of choline and L-carnitine to trimethylamine (TMA). TMA is subsequently converted by the host flavin monooxygenase (FMO) enzyme family to trimethylamine-N-oxide (TMAO) in the liver. SCFAs confer health benefits, while protein fermentation metabolites and TMAO exert multiple toxic effects, contributing to cardiovascular and progressive renal disease, ultimately culminating in premature death. Metabolism-independent effects include gut hyperpermeability (leaky gut), allowing bacterial cell wall products such as lipopolysaccharide (LPS) and peptidoglycans to enter the bloodstream. Low circulating levels of these bacterial components collectively activate macrophages, which can reduce reverse cholesterol transport and increase insulin resistance, hyperlipidemia, and vascular inflammation. LPS and peptidoglycans contribute to a micro-inflammatory state. CHO, carbohydrates; CKD, chronic kidney disease; CVD, chronic vascular disease; PCS, P-cresol sulfate.

fiber intake. Indeed, because of fear of hyperkalemia and hyperphosphatemia, consumption of fruit and vegetables, both rich in dietary fiber, is often restricted in patients with advanced CKD.

On the other hand, gut dysbiosis in CKD may increase the exposure to uremic toxins originating from microbial metabolism. Important representatives of this group of uremic toxins include p-cresyl sulfate, indoxyl sulfate, phenyl acetyl glutamine, and trimethylamine-N-oxide (TMAO). These toxins contribute to renal disease progression and the high cardiovascular disease

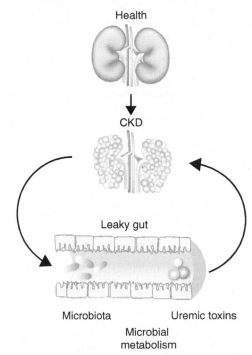

FIGURE 19.3 Bidirectional crosstalk between host and gut microbiota. CKD, chronic kidney disease.

burden in patients with CKD. Of note, many of these toxins are strongly protein-bound and thus difficult to remove by conventional dialysis. Gut dysbiosis, in addition, may induce a disruption of the epithelial barrier, ultimately resulting in an increased exposure to endotoxins (lipopolysaccharides). A leaky gut may represent an underappreciated cause of micro-inflammation and in the long run may trigger the phenomenon of "endotoxin tolerance," which may explain the concomitant acquired immunodeficiency of CKD.

DIETARY AND GASTROINTESTINAL INTERVENTIONS TARGETING GUT DYSBIOSIS IN CKD

The knowledge that gut dysbiosis significantly contributes to the uremic syndrome and that many of the uremic toxins originating from microbial metabolism are hard to remove by conventional dialysis techniques regained the interest in dietary and gastrointestinal interventions as adjuvant approaches.

Dietary Interventions

Given the central role of the diet in modulating the microbiome, dietary restrictions and supplements (nutriceuticals) are a logical strategy to reestablish microbial balance in CKD.

Dietary Protein Restriction

Low-protein diets have been advocated for many decades in the treatment of CKD, both for the attenuation of uremic symptoms and disease progression.

The latter has been subject to intense controversy. Recent insights, however, both from RCT and meta-analyses, reinforce the thesis that limiting protein, especially protein of animal origin, may slow the progression of CKD and the development of its complications. Underlying mechanisms are complex, multiple, and only partly understood. Besides improved glomerular hemo-dynamics and lower alimentary load of phosphate, hydrogen, salt, and uric acid precursors, a lower exposure to toxic co-metabolites (p-cresyl sulfate, indoxyl sulfate, phenylacetylglutamine, TMAO) may be in the causal pathway between a diet low in animal protein and improved outcomes. In line with this thesis, data from observational and intervention studies have shown a direct relationship between protein intake and circulating levels and/or generation rates of protein fermentation metabolites.

Balancing of protein intake is a complex process in CKD patients. Anorexia and other comorbid conditions may profoundly disturb eating patterns, rendering CKD patients at risk for protein energy malnutrition (PEM). PEM is common among patients with advanced CKD and is associated with poor outcome. Thus, the therapeutic window with regard to dietary protein intake is narrow in CKD.

Dietary Fiber Supplements

According to the European Union, dietary fiber means carbohydrate polymers with three or more monomeric units, which are neither digested nor absorbed in the human small intestine and belong to the following categories: (1) edible carbohydrate polymers naturally occurring in the food as consumed; (2) edible carbohydrate polymers which have been obtained from food raw material by physical, enzymatic, or chemical means and which have a beneficial physiologic effect demonstrated by generally accepted scientific evidence; and (3) edible synthetic carbohydrate polymers which have a beneficial physiologic effect demonstrated by generally accepted scientific evidence. Natural fiber is commonly found in fruits, vegetables, and whole grain, often as complex carbohydrates in plant cell walls (e.g., cereal fiber, inulin).

The physiologic effects of dietary fiber result from its chemical and physical properties such as fermentability, molecular weight, viscosity (gel-forming properties), and water-holding capacity (table). A multitude of beneficial effects have been attributed to dietary fiber. These include improved bowel function, reduced cholesterol levels, lower blood pressure, energy salvage, less inflammation, attenuation of postprandial blood glucose, and improved immune function. Dietary fiber may also suppress potentially harmful protein fermentation by (i) shortening of the colonic transit time, (ii) by lowering colonic pH (thereby limiting the protease activity), and (iii) by stimulating microbial growth and thus the incorporation of α-NH_2 nitrogen in the microbial biomass.

The dietary fiber intake by CKD patients averages 10 to 15 g per day. This is far below the 30 g per day recommended by current guidelines for the general population. This observation is not unexpected as food items rich in dietary fiber, such as fruits, vegetables, and whole wheat bread, are often restricted in advanced CKD to prevent or correct hyperkalemia and hyperphosphatemia. Importantly, fruits and vegetables differ in phosphate, potassium, and fiber content and density, so that a dietitian may help to make correct choices (Table 19.1). In a recent intervention study including CKD stage 3 to 4 patients, a fruit-and-vegetables-supplemented diet allowed to correct metabolic acidosis without inducing hyperkalemia. Moreover, recent epidemiologic evidence showed an inverse association between urinary potassium excretion (as a proxy of dietary potassium intake) and all-cause mortality in CKD patients, which is reassuring. With regard to phosphate, it should be emphasized that phosphate in grain, legumes, and nuts is largely

Potassium and Phosphate Content in Fiber-Rich Foods

Food	Portion size	Fiber (g)	Energy (kcal)	K (mg)	PO4 (mg)	g fiber/g K	g fiber/g PO₄
Black beans (boiled)	½ cup	7.5	114	305	120	25	63
Wheat bread	1 slice	1.2	77	51	43	24	28
Apple with skin	Large	5.4	191	239	25	23	216
Lentils (boiled with salt)	½ cup	7.8	115	365	178	21	44
Whole almonds	½ cup	8.9	414	524	344	17	26
Orange	Large	4.4	85	333	26	13	169
Green peas (boiled with salt)	1 cup	4.5	67	384	88	12	51
Broccoli (boiled with salt)	1 cup	5.1	55	457	105	11	49
Spinach (boiled with salt)	1 cup	4.3	41	839	101	5	43

Adapted from Sirich TL. Dietary protein and fiber in end-stage renal disease. *Semin Dial* 2015;28(1):75–80.

bound to phytate. Since humans lack the enzyme phytase, the bioavailability of phosphate in grain, legumes, and nuts is rather low. A vegetarian compared with meat dietary protein source thus may help to maintain phosphate homeostasis in CKD.

Preliminary intervention studies in CKD patients suggest that dietary fiber supplements could also have a beneficial impact on uremic toxin profiles and markers of oxidative stress and inflammation. Epidemiologic evidence shows lower levels of TMAO in individuals adhering to a Mediterranean diet as compared to a Western diet. Vegetarians and vegans, moreover, have lower circulating levels of TMAO, p-cresyl sulfate, and indoxyl sulfate than omnivores. Despite these promising results, large randomized controlled trials with hard endpoint studies assessing the role of dietary fiber supplements in CKD patients are not (yet) available.

Awaiting evidence-based guidelines for dietary fiber intake specifically in the CKD population, there is no reason why CKD patients should not comply with the dietary fiber intake guideline for the general population. Defining the optimal fiber composition is at present not possible, as this would require a much better understanding of the complex gut microbial ecosystem. From a theoretical point of view, a dietary fiber mix encompassing a broad spectrum of functionalities may be most beneficial.

The dose of dietary fiber supplement needs to be slowly titrated up as tolerated over the course of weeks to a target dose of 30 g of total dietary and supplementary fiber per day. Even when used judiciously, fiber can induce or exacerbate abdominal distension, flatulence, and diarrhea. When relying on naturally occurring fiber, potassium and phosphate levels need to be monitored, especially in high-risk patients such as diabetics. Finally, dietary fiber may increase the bioavailability of divalent cations, including magnesium and calcium, requiring vigilance in individuals consuming large doses.

Restricting Intake of Food Rich in (Phosphatidyl)Choline or Carnitine

Both choline and carnitine are essential nutrients, but when consumed in excess these nutrients may enter the large intestine and be converted to the toxic co-metabolite TMAO. Eggs, meat, poultry, fish, cruciferous vegetables, peanuts, and dairy products are especially rich in choline and/or carnitine. Another source of L-carnitine is dietary supplements. L-carnitine has been proposed as a treatment for a variety of metabolic abnormalities in end-stage renal disease (ESRD), including hypertriglyceridemia, hypercholesterolemia, and anemia. The debatable efficacy and proven link with TMAO and accelerated atherosclerosis warrant caution, if not a ban of oral supplements.

Gastrointestinal Interventions

Adsorbants

Similar to controlling serum phosphate and potassium, chelators or adsorbants may be considered as adjuvant therapy to control uremic retention molecules originating from microbial metabolism. AST-120 (Kremezin, Kureha Chemical Industry Co, Ltd) is an orally administered adsorbent consisting of spherical carbon particles 0.2 to 0.4 mm in diameter. AST-120 is capable of adsorbing significant amounts of various organic compounds in the large intestine, including indole, p-cresol, and food-derived advanced glycation end-products. The efficacy of AST-120 in decreasing circulating indoxyl sulfate levels and preventing renal, vascular, and bone damage has been demonstrated in numerous preclinical studies. Clinical studies have been less convincing, possibly owing to power issues and nonadherence related to high pill burden.

Interventions Accelerating Colonic Transit

Shortening the transit time is another means to limit protein fermentation and its detrimental consequences. Colonic transit times are prolonged in patients with end-stage renal disease, especially in patients on maintenance hemodialysis (HD) therapy, and constipation is common. Contributing factors include physical inactivity, phosphorus binders, dietary restrictions, low fluid intake, primary renal disease (e.g., polycystic renal disease), and comorbidity including diabetes, cerebrovascular disease, heart failure, and malnutrition.

Dietary fiber increases fecal volume and weight (bulking effect), improves stool consistency, decreases transit time, and increases stool frequency. The bulking effect is mainly owing to nonfermentable fiber, while fermentable fiber can increase the bacterial mass and thereby increase stool weight and frequency.

Drugs Interfering with Microbial or Human Metabolism

Probiotics and antimicrobials may also prove useful to reestablish microbial balance, but efficacy may be short-lasting and unpredictable. Probiotics have been defined as "viable organisms that, when ingested in sufficient amounts, exert positive health effects." Although numerous studies have evaluated the effects of probiotics, only a limited number have looked at their effects in kidney disease. Moreover, these studies only assessed biochemical endpoints. Preliminary data with host and bacterial enzyme inhibitors are promising and call for additional studies.

CLINICAL RECOMMENDATIONS

▪ Educate dietitians on health-promoting effects of dietary fiber and on dietary fiber content (absolute and relative to potassium and phosphate content) of common food items.

- Target a dietary fiber intake of 30 g per day either by allowing a more liberal intake of fruits and vegetables or by adding a fiber supplement to the diet. Practical tips for patients include:
  - Eat all the allowed servings of kidney-friendly fruits and vegetables suggested by your meal plan.
  - Eat peelings on fruit and vegetables when reasonable.
  - Snack on unsalted popcorn and raw vegetables.
  - Include a breakfast cereal with fiber (one that is approved by your dietitian).
  - Eat whole fruit instead of drinking juice.
- Start fiber supplement at low dose and titrate dose according to stool habits (one soft stool per day) and personal tolerance (borborygmi, flatulence).
- Monitor more closely potassium and phosphate serum concentrations in the initiation phase.
- Monitor calcium and magnesium serum concentrations when prescribing large doses of dietary fiber supplements.

RESEARCH RECOMMENDATIONS

- Benefits of dietary (and nondietary) therapies targeting the microbiome remain to be proven in adequately powered RCTs with hard or intermediate endpoints.
- Further studies are required to understand the complex gut microbial ecosystem. Does a "healthy" composition of the intestinal microbiota exist, and if so, how can this be achieved? As bacteria can rapidly adapt to their metabolic properties to different conditions, exploring gut dysbiosis should not only focus on microbiota composition. Gene expression profiles and gut microbial metabolism seem to be equally important.

Suggested Readings

Brown JM, Hazen SL. The gut microbial endocrine organ: bacterially derived signals driving cardiometabolic diseases. *Annu Rev Med* 2015;66:343–359.

Cummings JH, Hill MJ, Bone ES, et al. The effect of meat protein and dietary fiber on colonic function and metabolism. II. Bacterial metabolites in feces and urine. *Am J Clin Nutr* 1979;32(10):2094–2101.

Evenepoel P, Meijers BKI, Bammens BRM, et al. Uremic toxins originating from colonic microbial metabolism. *Kidney Int* 2009;76(S114):S12–S19.

Nicholson JK, Holmes E, Kinross J, et al. Host-gut microbiota metabolic interactions. *Science* 2012;336(6086):1262–1267.

Poesen R, Meijers B, Evenepoel P. The colon: an overlooked site for therapeutics in dialysis patients. *Semin Dial* 2013;26(3):323–332.

Ramezani A, Massy ZA, Meijers B, et al. Role of the gut microbiome in uremia: a potential therapeutic target. *Am J Kidney Dis* 2016;67(3):483–498.

Sirich TL. Dietary protein and fiber in end stage renal disease. *Semin Dial* 2015;28(1):75–80.

Zoetendal EG, de Vos WM. Effect of diet on the intestinal microbiota and its activity. *Curr Opin Gastroenterol* 2014;30(2):189–195.

Obesity in Kidney Disease

**Peter Stenvinkel, Maarit Korkeila,
Olof Heimbürger, and Bengt Lindholm**

Obesity, the epidemic of the 21st century, carries a markedly increased risk for comorbid complications, such as type 2 diabetes, cancer, hypertension, dyslipidemia, cardiovascular disease (CVD), sleep apnea, and chronic kidney disease (CKD). Among high-income countries, the United States has the highest body mass index (BMI). Abdominal obesity is, in addition to hyper-cholesterolemia, hypertension, and insulin resistance or glucose intolerance, one of the CVD precursors included in the metabolic syndrome (MS). The worldwide obesity epidemic carries not only a considerable increased risk for comorbid complications, such as type 2 diabetes, hypertension, nonalcoholic fatty liver, osteoarthritis, cancer, psychosocial complications, dyslipidemia, CVD, and sleep apnea, but also for CKD and its progression to end-stage renal disease (ESRD). Overweight and obesity share several risk factors together with diabetes, CVD, and CKD, and thus may all mutually contribute to the excess morbidity and mortality in patients suffering from these conditions. In CKD, the impact of overweight and obesity on morbidity and mortality differs depending on the CKD stage and treatment. Whereas obesity is a negative prognostic factor both for further progression of CKD and for morbidity and mortality during the earlier CKD stages, epidemiologic evidence suggests it becomes a *positive* prognostic factor in dialysis patients. In this chapter, we present an overview of clinically important aspects of overweight and obesity in patients with CKD.

MEASURES OF OBESITY IN PATIENTS WITH CHRONIC KIDNEY DISEASE

The most common method for defining obesity is based on BMI, that is, a person's weight (kg) divided by the square of his or her height (m). The World Health Organization considers a BMI between 20 and 25 kg per m^2 as normal weight, a BMI between 25 and 30 kg per m^2 as overweight, and >30 kg per m^2 as obese with increasing grading as BMI increases (Table 20.1). It should be emphasized that population norms of BMI could be different based on ethnic and racial background; that is, the proportion of Asian people with a high risk of type 2 diabetes and CVD is substantial at a lower BMI. Because BMI is a poor indicator of body composition, especially in patients with CKD with gross imbalance in hydration status, further studies should use methods, such as dual-energy x-ray absorptiometry (DEXA) and bioimped-ance, to better discriminate between different fat stores and lean body mass (LBM). Studies of body weight in patients with CKD are influenced by several confounding factors, such as the water balance before and after dialysis and muscle depletion because of protein–energy wasting (PEW). *Obese sarcopenia* is defined as a relative PEW and loss of LBM and has been shown to be common among patients with obese CKD and associated with both inflammation and poor outcome. Most of the studies on obesity in patients with CKD are based on BMI because other more specific measures of body composition are not ready available (Table 20.2). Many studies have indicated that the

TABLE 20.1 The International Classification of Adult Underweight, Overweight, and Obesity by Body Mass Index in Caucasians according to WHO*

Category	BMI (kg/m^2)
Underweight	<18.5
Normal weight	18.5–24.9
Overweight	25.0–29.9
Obese	≥30.0
Obese class I	30.0–34.9
Obese class II	35.0–39.9
Obese class III	≥40.0

*Other values apply to the Asian population.
BMI, body mass index; WHO, World Health Organization.

assessment of body composition (in particular LBM) is a more important prognostic determinant than BMI. Waist circumference (WC) and waist–hip ratio (WHR) have emerged as measures that better reflect *abdominal* or *central* obesity. The conicity index (an easy anthropometric estimate using WC, height, and weight to model the relative accumulation of abdominal fat without requiring the hip circumference) could be useful to identify patients with non–overweight CKD with an estimate of the wasting component. Many studies have concluded that compared with BMI, WC and/or WHR are better predictors of mortality both in the general population and in patients with CKD. A strong correlation has been observed between WHR and visceral fat mass assessed by computed tomography. Only a few systematic studies have compared the prognostic value of different measures of weight and body composition among patients with different stages of CKD

THE PATHOGENESIS OF OBESITY

Like most other chronic diseases that affect a large proportion of the population and are a public health priority, the pathophysiology of obesity is severely complex, including environmental changes, genetic predisposition, and individual preferences. More than 150 genetic loci are related with the development of obesity and type 2 diabetes. Because eating disorders are associated with altered neurotransmitter system function, it has been suggested that overeating could be regarded as a symptom and the host response to diverse nutrients commit to overeating and obesity. Thus, a much more complex sum of synchronized alterations, including neurocognitive factors, mutation of the uricase gene, psychosocial stress, changes in the epigenome gut dysbiosis, adenovirus infection, and metabolic changes triggered by specific nutrients may promote obesity (Fig. 20.1). Because the prevalence of obesity differs markedly between regions, nutritional factors are most certainly also of importance. It has been suggested that the markedly increased consumption of fructose in the United States (used as a soft drink sweetener) contribute to the increasing prevalence of obesity and cardiorenal disease in the United States. Many patients with CKD have a low physical activity because of decreased physical performance and increased tiredness because of CKD and comorbidity. In hemodialysis (HD) patients, the time needed for dialysis treatment and the common tiredness after an HD session may further contribute to physical inactivity. In patients treated with PD, the glucose absorption from the dialysate may represent a significant additional caloric load. Furthermore, many drugs commonly used in patients with CKD may contribute to obesity, such as steroids and insulin (Table 20.3).

TABLE 20.2 Different Methods for Estimating Weight and Body Composition in Patients with Chronic Kidney Disease

	BMI	WHR	Skinfold Thickness	Bio-impedance	Dual Energy x-ray Absorptiometry	Computed Tomography
Easy-to-use/cost	+++	+++	++	++	+	++
Reproducibility	+++	+++	+	+++	++	+++
Distinction fat mass vs. lean body mass	0	0	+	++	+++	+++

+++, excellent; ++, good; +, moderate; 0, poor; BMI, body mass index; WHR, waist–hip ratio.

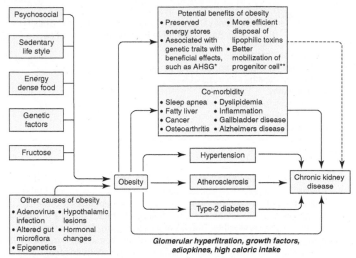

FIGURE 20.1 Relationships between obesity and chronic kidney disease. The pathophysiology of obesity is complex and includes both genetic (and epigenetic) and environmental factors associated with lifestyle. AHSG, Alpha2-HS glycoprotein. (Published with permission from Stenvinkel P, Zoccali C, Ikizler TA. Obesity in CKD—what should nephrologists know? *J Am Soc Nephrol* 2013;24(11):1727–1736.)
*A study shows that a common variant of α-Heremans—Schmid glycoprotein (AHSG) associated with lower fetuin levels is more common in learn than obese patients.
**A study shows that obesity promotes mobilization of progenitor cells.

List of Factors Known or Believed to Be Involved in the Pathogenesis of Obesity

- Increased caloric intake, especially rapid carbohydrates
- High fat intake
- Low physical activity/sedentary lifestyle
- Infectious complications, such as adenovirus infection
- Altered gut microbiota
- Epigenetic and genetics factors
- Hormonal changes, such as insulin resistance
- Psychosocial factors
- Drugs (such as steroids and insulin)

OBESITY-RELATED KIDNEY DISEASES

Obesity is an autonomous risk factor for development of CKD in the general population, which leads to hyperfiltration, enlarged glomeruli, and pathologic changes resembling diabetic nephropathy. Hyperinsulinemia, which commonly escort obesity, promote mesangial expansion, glomerular hyperfiltration, glomerular hypertrophy, and increased filtration fraction. These alterations may promote glomerulosclerosis and segmental glomerulosclerosis, that is, obesity glomerulopathy and are defined as the histopathologic changes resembling focal segmental glomerulosclerosis (FSGS). In addition, obesity-associated hyperleptinemia promotes renal fibrosis, oxidative stress, and activates the sympathetic nervous system, factors that increase risk of CKD.

	Chronic Kidney Diseases in which Overweight and Obesity Have Been Demonstrated to Be Independent Risk Factors

- Proteinuria of other causes
- Diabetic nephropathy/metabolic syndrome
- Ischemic nephropathy/nephrosclerosis
- IgA nephropathy
- Obesity-related focal segmental glomerulosclerosis
- Unilateral nephrectomy
- Chronic allograft nephropathy

IgA, immunoglobin A.

BMI independently predicted new-onset CKD, and European data showed that obesity increased the risk of microalbuminuria and loss of residual renal function after start of dialysis. Although weight loss decreases proteinuria in overweight patients, it is unclear if the histopathologic changes in obesity glomerulopathy are reversible. The risk of developing an obesity-related FSGS is considerable, and the glomerular lesions do differ from other types of FSGS. Both failing kidney function and microalbuminuria have been recognized as cardiovascular risk factors. Although microalbuminuria is considered as a marker for endothelial dysfunction leading to increased CVD morbidity, the exact mechanisms for such a relationship are unknown. Overweight increases the risk for progressive renal disease in immunoglobin A nephropathy, mainly through hypertension and increased proteinuria. It is likely that obesity glomerulopathy, hypertension, and proteinuria at obesity are unspecific prognostic factors for developing CKD at several glomerulopathies and after unilateral nephrectomy (Table 20.4).

ADIPOKINES

Adipose tissue is a hormonally active organ that releases a large number of bioactive proteins that regulate body weight, energy homeostasis, insulin resistance, dyslipidemia, inflammation, fibrinolysis, endothelial function, and coagulation. While the pluripotent role of fat is still not completely elucidated, it appears likely that a reduced renal clearance contributes to the accumulation of adipokines (such as leptin, adiponectin, and visfatin) originating in part or whole from the adipose tissue, offering novel pathways to explain the marked dysmetabolism that occur in uremia. Leptin was initially described as a modulator of feeding behavior and thus of fat mass. While leptin signaling is more complex in humans, there is no doubt that loss of kidney function leads to inappropriately elevated serum concentrations of leptin. Serum leptin levels are related to body fat mass and inflammation. Because most studies have demonstrated an association between inflammatory biomarkers and leptin in CKD, it has been suggested that leptin may play a role in uremic PEW. Indeed, because experimental uremic cachexia can be ameliorated by blockade of leptin signaling through the hypothalamic melanocortin-4 receptor, melanocortin receptor antagonism may provide a novel therapeutic strategy for inflammation-associated PEW. The fact that low leptin levels have been shown to predict poor outcome in dialysis patients probably reflects the detrimental effects of state of energy wasting and loss of fat mass on outcome in this patient group. Adiponectin is another adipokine that has attracted much interest because it improves insulin sensitivity in the liver and periphery, ameliorates endothelial dysfunction, and counteracts proinflammatory signaling. In contrast to other adipokines, increasing adipose tissue mass is inversely and paradoxically associated with low circulating levels of adiponectin. Low circulating adiponectin is generally found in populations at enhanced risk of CVD. Although plasma adiponectin levels are generally markedly elevated in patients with CKD, it has been reported that patients with CKD with relatively lower adiponectin levels have an increased risk of cardiovascular events. However, studies in larger patient materials have shown that a high, rather than a low, adiponectin level predicts mortality in both patients with CKD and congestive heart failure. Further studies are needed to study if the effects of adiponectin in the brain that decrease body weight can explain the paradoxic relationships between adiponectin and outcome. Emerging evidence suggests that adipose tissue is also a significant contributor to systemic inflammation. In fact, it has been estimated that adipose tissue (with resident macrophages) may contribute to about 20% to 30% of systemic interleukin 6 production. Other proinflammatory mediators, such as tumor necrosis factor, are also expressed in adipose tissue. Visceral adipose tissue releases more cytokines than subcutaneous fat.

EPIDEMIOLOGY OF OBESITY IN CHRONIC KIDNEY DISEASE

Overweight and Risk for Chronic Kidney Disease in Healthy Subjects

It is now generally accepted that obesity is a risk factor for developing CKD and for accelerating the rate of decline of glomerular filtration rate (GFR) in patients with early CKD stages. Thus, a high BMI correlates with higher cystatin C as a marker for kidney function in a healthy population without micro- or macroalbuminuria and estimated GFR >60 mL/min/1.73 m^2. Studies have shown that the risk for developing CKD (and eventually ESRD) increases linearly by increasing weight when adjusted for several confounders. Although part of this association is possibly mediated by the high prevalence of hypertension and MS among overweight subjects, the association has remained significant even after adjustment for blood pressure. Nondiabetic subjects with MS have a 50% higher risk for developing CKD over 9 subsequent years than those without MS. Thus, the likelihood of developing CKD is markedly increased in subjects with known MS. This could be because of several factors; for example, a variety of glomerular abnormalities have recently been described among extremely obese subjects without overt CKD. Moreover, the risk for developing proteinuria and CKD after unilateral nephrectomy is increased in obese subjects. However, it is most likely that the most important risk factors linking MS with increased risk of CKD are hypertension, insulin resistance, and hyperlipidemia.

Overweight and Obesity in Patients Receiving Hemodialysis

The observation that elevated BMI confers a survival advantage to patients with ESRD was first reported in 1999 and subsequently confirmed in several large U.S. cohorts. Residual confounding by PEW, inflammation, and competing mortality risk factors may in part explain this phenomenon. It should also be remembered that in these studies long-term mortality in the general population has been compared with short-term mortality in dialysis patients. Not all studies have confirmed that obesity is protective. One explanation for the discrepancy of the results might be the much higher prevalence of obesity in the United States compared with Europe, and the obesity paradox may be stronger in some ethnic subgroups, such as African Americans. The observations on this "obesity paradox" have led some to argue that weight gain should be promoted in maintenance dialysis patients regardless of the different body compartments, that is, fat or muscle mass. Obese and underweight patients receiving dialysis report poorer self-rated health status and physical function in particular, than normal weight or moderately overweight patients receiving HD. It should be emphasized that the "obesity paradox" has not been demonstrated in all studies compromising HD patients. There may be many reasons why obesity may be associated with a survival advantage paradox. Because an increase in BMI may reflect more LBM, the association between increased BMI and better outcome does not necessarily imply that the fat mass compartment is protective. However, it is likely that high BMI is a reflection of preserved energy stores and appetite. Because good appetite is associated with better outcome in HD and obese patients consume more energy dense food, this may indirectly explain the association between high BMI and better outcome. It should also be appreciated that increased fat mass besides detrimental metabolic effects, may also have beneficial effects in the toxic catabolic uremic milieu (Fig. 20.1). Besides indicating well-preserved energy stores, the presence of obesity may be associated with improved hemodynamic tolerance, better stem cell mobilization, less stress response as a result of neurohormonal alterations, and more efficient disposal of lipophilic uremic toxins. The obesity paradox is not only observed in ESRD but high BMI has been associated with better outcome in many other chronic debilitating disorders, such as congestive heart failure, rheumatoid arthritis, dementia, coronary heart disease, cancer, and diabetes. A recent study in 5,904 European HD patients confirmed that high BMI was associated with better survival. However, when inflammation was also taken into consideration, an interesting difference became evident. Whereas high BMI had a protective action and was linked to longer survival rates for chronically inflamed HD patients, no such protective effect of high BMI was found in uninflamed HD patients.

Overweight and Obesity in Patients Receiving Peritoneal Dialysis

Weight gain and accumulation of fat mass after starting peritoneal dialysis (PD) is a common clinical problem. Many PD patients have excessive weight gain mainly consisting of fat mass, and, in particular, intra-abdominal fat mass. Weight prior to PD, diabetes, female gender, genetics, comorbidity, and being a high transporter are the main determinants of weight gain and accumulation of fat mass during PD. Although the glucose load from PD solutions amounts to 100 to 200 g per day, most studies have not found any relation between the amount of absorbed glucose and gain in fat mass. However, an excessive glucose load in combination with obesity-predisposing gene polymorphisms may contribute to the excessive PD-related weight gain in some patients. Long-term body weight on PD treatment seems to be relatively stable, but studies on body composition show a relative increase of fat mass over time. Interestingly, PD patients who do not accumulate fat may risk losing LBM during PD. There is some evidence that patients with low-energy stores may benefit by PD as a dialysis modality because of possible weight gain after PD start. High BMI and preserved LBM in particular may be favorable for survival, because low body weight is also a bad prognostic sign in PD. The results on associations between overweight, obesity, and mortality in patients undergoing PD are conflicting. Whereas some studies report that the risk of death for obese patients receiving PD is equal or increased in comparison with patients receiving PD who have normal body weight, others reported a survival benefit for overweight and obese patients who are undergoing PD. Furthermore, obesity in patients undergoing PD has been reported to be associated with increased incidence of peritonitis, catheter loss, technique failure, and more rapid decline of residual renal function.

Obesity and Kidney Transplantation

Nephrologists need to know of the potential risks of obesity on renal graft function and its impact on postoperative complications. Obesity is an

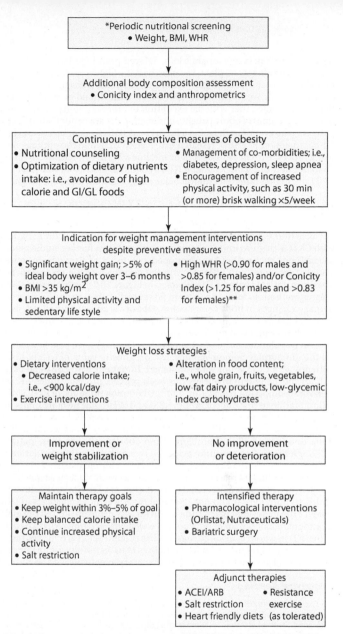

*Periodic nutritional screening
• Weight, BMI, WHR

Additional body composition assessment
• Conicity index and anthropometrics

Continuous preventive measures of obesity
• Nutritional counseling
• Optimization of dietary nutrients intake: i.e., avoidance of high calorie and GI/GL foods
• Management of co-morbidities; i.e., diabetes, depression, sleep apnea
• Enouragement of increased physical activity, such as 30 min (or more) brisk walking ×5/week

Indication for weight management interventions despite preventive measures
• Significant weight gain; >5% of ideal body weight over 3–6 months
• BMI >35 kg/m^2
• Limited physical activity and sedentary life style
• High WHR (>0.90 for males and >0.85 for females) and/or Conicity Index (>1.25 for males and >0.83 for females)**

Weight loss strategies
• Dietary interventions
  • Decreased calorie intake; i.e., <900 kcal/day
• Exercise interventions
• Alteration in food content; i.e., whole grain, fruits, vegetables, low-fat dairy products, low-glycemic index carbohydrates

Improvement or weight stabilization

No improvement or deterioration

Maintain therapy goals
• Keep weight within 3%–5% of goal
• Keep balanced calorie intake
• Continue increased physical activity
• Salt restriction

Intensified therapy
• Pharmacological interventions (Orlistat, Nutraceuticals)
• Bariatric surgery

Adjunct therapies
• ACEI/ARB
• Salt restriction
• Heart friendly diets
• Resistance exercise (as tolerated)

FIGURE 20.2 A proposed approach to management of obesity in patients with CKD. ACEI, angiotensin-converting enzyme inhibitor; ARB, angiotensin receptor blocker; BMI, body mass index; CKD, chronic kidney disease; GI, glycemic index; GL, glycemic load; WHR, waist–hip ratio. (Published with permission from Stenvinkel P, Zoccali C, Ikizler TA. Obesity in CKD—what should nephrologists know? *J Am Soc Nephrol* 2013;24(11):1727–1736.)
*Screening every 3–6 months is recommended.
**A study show that a conicity index of >1.25 predicted high coronary risk in men with a sensitivity and specificity of 73.9% and 74.9%, respectively. for women, a conicity index of >0.83 predicted high coronary risk with a sensitivity and specificity of 73.4% and 63.4%, respectively.

independent risk factor for graft loss, delayed graft function, and death in recipients of kidney transplant. Because there is a higher risk for postoperative complications and delayed graft function after renal transplantation (RTx), there is a controversy on which BMI cutoff level should be used. A recent debate concluded that with the exception of morbid obesity (BMI > 40 kg per m^2), outcomes of obese patients undergoing Rtx are better than in dialysis patients who are not undergoing RTx. Because BMI is a poor measure of body fat composition in ESRD, research are needed to define the optimal cutoff using more clear-cut fat assessment methods. WHR is an independent risk factor for new-onset diabetes after RTx, a condition associated with poor graft function, higher rates of cardiovascular complications, and poor prognosis.

PRACTICAL CONSEQUENCES OF OBESITY IN CHRONIC KIDNEY DISEASE

Because BMI is a poor indicator of body composition, especially in patients with CKD with gross imbalances in hydration status, further studies should use methods, such as DEXA and bioimpedance, to better discriminate between different fat stores and LBM. A proposed approach to the management of obesity in patients with CKD is depicted in Figure 20.2. Nephrologists should master methods to follow changes in fat mass distribution and know how to manage changes in body composition. Obesity is an established risk factor for developing CKD in the general population. In earlier CKD stages, obesity is a cardiovascular and metabolic risk factor comparable to that seen in the general population. Although decreased weight may have beneficial effects on the glomerular hemodynamics, the prognostic value of weight loss in patients with CKD is not yet established. In patient with ESRD, no excess risk for mortality due to obesity has been proven, probably much because of several competing risk factors and the common presence of PEW and/or inflammation in this patient group. LBM and WHR may be more important determinant for survival in CKD Stages 3 to 5 than BMI. Loss of LBM and inflammation occur in CKD Stages 3 to 5 regardless of body weight and are more dominating clinical problems than obesity per se in these patients. Although there is no scientific evidence to support a recommendation for decreasing weight in obese dialysis patients, nephrologists should aim for interventions that increase muscle mass and decrease visceral fat mass. High physical activity is recommended (see Chapter 21). Energy intake should be scaled to normal BMI and not to actual body weight in all stages of CDK. Despite the increasing magnitude of the obesity problem around the globe, treatment modalities for obesity are not well developed especially in patients with CKD in whom available drugs are either contraindicated or not tested. However, recent reports in limited numbers of patients indicate an improvement in renal parameters after bariatric surgery in patients with obese CKD.

Suggested Readings

Axelsson J, Qureshi AR, Suliman ME, et al. Truncal fat mass as a contributor to inflammation in end-stage renal disease. *Am J Clin Nutr* 2004;80:1222–1229.

Axelsson J, Stenvinkel P. Role of fat mass and adipokines in chronic kidney disease. *Curr Opin Nephrol Hypertens* 2008;17:25–31.

Elsayed EF, Tighiouart H, Weiner DE, et al. Waist-to-hip ratio and body mass index as risk factors for cardiovascular events in CKD. *Am J Kidney Dis* 2008;52:49–57.

Fouque D, Kalantar-Zadeh K, Kopple J, et al. A proposed nomenclature and diagnostic criteria for protein–energy wasting in acute and chronic kidney disease. *Kidney Int* 2008;73:391–398.

Johnson, RJ, Segal MS, Sautin Y, et al. Potential role of sugar (fructose) in the epidemic of hypertension, obesity and the metabolic syndrome, diabetes, kidney disease, and cardiovascular disease. *Am J Clin Nutr* 2007;86:899–906.

Sattar N, McConnachie A, Shaper AG, et al. Can metabolic syndrome usefully predict cardiovascular disease and diabetes? Outcome data from two prospective studies. *Lancet* 2008;371:1927–1935.

Stenvinkel P. Obesity—a disease with many etiologies disguised in the same over-sized phenotype: has the overeating theory failed? *Nephrol Dial Transplant* 2015;30:1656–1664.

Stenvinkel P, Gillespie IA, Tunks J, et al; ARO Steering Committee. Inflammation modi-fies the paradoxical association between body mass index and mortality in hemo-dialysis patients. *J Am Soc Nephrol* 2016;27(5):1479–1486.

Stenvinkel P, Zoccali C, Ikizler TA. Obesity in CKD—what should nephrologists know? *J Am Soc Nephrol* 2013;24:1727–1736.

Van Gaal LF, Mertens IL, De Block CE. Mechanism linking obesity with cardiovascular disease. *Nature* 2006;444:875–880.

Verani RR. Obesity-associated focal segmental glomerulosclerosis: pathological fea-tures of the lesion and relationship with cardiomegaly and hyperlipidemia. *Am J Kidney Dis* 1992;20:629–634.

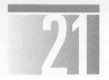

Exercise and Physical Function in Kidney Disease

Kirsten L. Johansen

There has been increasing recognition of the inextricable link between nutrition and physical activity. Recommendations about physical activity have been included in the last several editions of the *Dietary Guidelines for Americans*, a joint publication of the U.S. Department of Health and Human Services and the U.S. Department of Agriculture that is updated every 5 years, most recently in 2015, because physical activity is a major determinant of energy expenditure and a key component of energy balance. The *Dietary Guidelines for Americans* recommend that individuals consume a wide variety of foods to meet their nutrient needs. However, adequate nutrient intake must be achieved within calorie needs if neutral energy balance is to be maintained and weight gain to be avoided, and this can be difficult when energy expenditure is low. For these reasons and because of the recognition of the overall health benefits related to physical activity, the *Dietary Guidelines for Americans* contains an explicit recommendation to meet the *Physical Activity Guidelines for Americans*.

EXERCISE AND ITS BENEFITS IN THE GENERAL POPULATION

It may be helpful to review some general aspects of the terminology and physiology related to exercise and exercise training in the general population before applying these principles to chronic kidney disease (CKD) populations. Physical activity refers to any movement of the body that results in an increase in energy expenditure. Physical activity can include activities of daily living as well as home maintenance and occupational activities. In contrast, exercise generally refers to physical activity that is planned, structured, repetitive, and is often done with the objective of improving or maintaining one or more components of physical fitness (Table 21.1). Physical can be classified by its intensity, which can be characterized on an absolute or a relative scale. The most common way of classifying activity is as a function of energy expenditure, in units of metabolic equivalents (METs), where 1 MET is the energy expended (or oxygen consumed) at rest. In this classification, light activity constitutes activity that requires less than 4 METS (or less than three for older individuals), moderate activity requires 4 to 6 METs (or three to six for older individuals), and vigorous activity requires ≥ 6 METs (for specific examples of moderate and vigorous activities, see Table 21.2). Another way to categorize the intensity of physical activity is according to an individual's rating of perceived exertion. Moderate activities are those for which the perceived exertion is "somewhat hard," and vigorous activities are "hard" to "very hard."

Exercise can also be classified by type. Endurance (or aerobic) exercise and resistance (or strengthening) exercise are the most common types. Endurance exercise involves repetitive, dynamic, and rhythmic use of large muscles (e.g., walking, running, and bicycling) and is the major form of exercise that can improve cardiorespiratory fitness or maximal oxygen consumption (VO_2 max). Resistance exercise generally involves lifting weights or all or part of one's body weight, or moving the body against an externally

Glossary

Aerobic training—training that improves the efficiency of the aerobic energy-producing systems and that can improve cardiorespiratory endurance or fitness.

Body composition—A health-related component of physical fitness that relates to the relative amounts of muscle, fat, bone, and other vital parts of the body.

Cardiorespiratory endurance or fitness—A health-related component of physical fitness that relates to the ability of the circulatory and respiratory systems to supply oxygen during sustained physical activity.

Disability—The inability to perform or a limitation in the performance of actions, tasks, and activities usually expected in specific social roles that are customary for the individual or expected for the person's status or role in a specific physical environment.

Endurance training—Repetitive, aerobic use of large muscles (e.g., walking, bicycling, and swimming).

Exercise—Planned, structured, and repetitive bodily movement done to improve or maintain one or more components of physical fitness.

Flexibility—A health-related component of physical fitness that relates to the range of motion available at a joint.

Functional limitation—A deficit in the ability to perform a discrete task, such as stair climbing.

Maximal heart rate—The highest heart rate value attainable during an all-out effort to the point of exhaustion (often estimated as 220-age).

VO$_2$ max—The maximal capacity for oxygen consumption by the body during maximal exertion. Also known as aerobic power, maximal oxygen uptake, and cardiorespiratory endurance capacity.

MET—A unit used to estimate the metabolic cost (oxygen consumption) of physical activity. One MET equals the resting metabolic rate of approximately 3.5 mL O$_2$/kg/min.

Moderate physical activity—Activity that causes some increase in breathing or heart rate and is perceived as light to somewhat hard (e.g., brisk walking).

Muscle fatigue—The decline in ability of a muscle to generate force as a result of prolonged or repetitive contraction.

Muscular endurance—The ability of the muscle to continue to perform without fatigue.

Physical activity—Bodily movement that is produced by the contraction of skeletal muscle that increases energy expenditure above basal levels.

Physical fitness—A set of attributes that people have or achieve that relates to the ability to perform physical activity.

Physical function or functioning—A fundamental component of health status describing the state of those sensory and motor skills necessary for usual daily activities.

Physical performance—The execution or accomplishment of specific physical tasks (e.g., walking and stair climbing).

RPE—A person's subjective assessment of how hard he or she is working. The Borg RPE scale is a numerical scale for rating perceived exertion.

Resistance training—Training designed to increase strength, power, and muscular endurance.

Strength—The ability of the muscle to exert force.

Vigorous physical activity—Activity that causes a large increase in breathing or heart rate and is perceived as hard or very hard.

MET, metabolic equivalent; RPE, rating of perceived exertion; VO$_2$ max, maximal oxygen consumption.

TABLE 21.2   Examples of Moderate and Vigorous Physical Activities

Setting	Moderate	Vigorous
Exercise and leisure	Walking briskly, dancing, leisurely bicycling, or roller skating, horseback riding, canoeing, yoga	Jogging or running, fast bicycling, aerobic dance, martial arts, jump rope, swimming, step climbing
Sports	Volleyball, golfing, softball, baseball, badminton, doubles tennis, downhill skiing	Soccer, field hockey or ice hockey, lacrosse, singles tennis, racquetball, basketball, cross-country skiing
Home activities	Mowing the lawn with a push power mower, general lawn and garden maintenance, scrubbing floors or washing windows, vacuuming, sweeping	Mowing the lawn with a hand mower, shoveling, carrying and hauling, masonry, carpentry, moving or pushing furniture
Occupational activity	Walking and lifting as part of work, general carpentry	Heavy manual labor (e.g., digging ditches and carrying heavy loads)

imposed resistance (e.g., using a strength training machine or stretching elastic bands). There is overwhelming evidence that both types of exercise have large health benefits in the general population, including prevention of disease and disability as well as improvement in symptoms or management of chronic disease or disability. Higher levels of physical activity have been linked to lower risk of overall and cardiovascular mortality as well as lower risk of outcomes such as cardiovascular events and development of diabetes mellitus, hypertension, colon cancer, and depression. In addition, regular physical activity can improve the control of hypertension and diabetes among those with established disease; increase bone density and improve symptoms of arthritis; and improve physical functioning and psychological well-being among those with limitations. In 1996, the U.S. Surgeon General developed a report on physical activity and health, which concluded that "sedentary living habits clearly constitute a major public health problem." This landmark report contained several conclusions and recommendations that still underlie current exercise guidelines:

- People of all ages, both male and female, benefit from regular physical activity.
- Significant health benefits can be obtained by including a moderate amount of physical activity (e.g., 30 minutes of brisk walking or raking leaves, 15 minutes of running, or 45 minutes of playing volleyball) on most, if not all, days of the week. Through a modest increase in daily activity, most Americans can improve their health and quality of life.
- Additional health benefits can be gained through greater amounts of physical activity. Physical activity reduces the risk of premature mortality in general and of coronary heart disease, hypertension, colon cancer, and diabetes mellitus in particular. Physical activity also improves mental health and is important for the health of muscles, bones, and joints.

The report also included some discussion of the dose–response relationship between physical activity and health benefits, and it was noted that there "appears not to be a lower threshold [to the dose-response relationship], thereby indicating that any activity is better than none." However, this finding was not highlighted, nor were specific recommendations given for implementation of increased physical activity among elderly individuals or those with chronic diseases.

The American College of Sports Medicine and the American Heart Association issued joint guidelines for physical activity for older adults and individuals with chronic disease in 2007. They noted that the goals of exercise appropriate to younger adults, such as prevention of cardiovascular disease, cancer, and diabetes, and increases in life expectancy, should perhaps be replaced in the oldest adults with a new set of goals, which include minimizing biologic changes of aging, reversing disuse syndromes, the control of chronic diseases, maximizing psychologic health, increasing mobility and function, and assisting with rehabilitation from acute and chronic illnesses. In addition, these guidelines highlighted the importance of defining the intensity of physical activity on a relative rather than an absolute scale. In other words, what would be light activity to a younger, healthier individual might well qualify as moderate intensity activity for an elderly individual or an individual with "clinically significant chronic conditions and/or functional limitations" (such as CKD).

POTENTIAL BENEFITS OF INCREASED PHYSICAL ACTIVITY AMONG PATIENTS WITH CHRONIC KIDNEY DISEASE

As a group, patients with end-stage renal disease (ESRD) on maintenance hemodialysis (MHD) are extremely inactive, and inactivity is associated with lower survival in this population. In one study of 286 patients on MHD, 59% of participants reported that they were doing no physical activity beyond that needed for activities of daily living, and only 12% reported doing 30 minutes of physical activity on 3 or more days per week. A more recent study characterized physical activity among 1,547 ambulatory patients new to dialysis and found that physical activity was extremely low with scores for all ages and gender categories below the 5th percentile of healthy individuals.

Not only is physical inactivity prevalent in the ESRD population, but it has also been shown to be associated with loss of muscle mass, reduced physical functioning, and higher 1- and 4-year mortality among patients beginning maintenance dialysis. Low cardiorespiratory fitness (peak oxygen consumption) is usually associated with inactivity and is typically seen in patients with advanced CKD. Patients undergoing maintenance dialysis have peak oxygen consumption that is usually about 50% to 60% of age-predicted norms, patients with Stages 3 and 4 CKD are similarly low, and transplant patients are about 70% of age-predicted values. Low cardiorespiratory fitness has been shown to be associated with higher mortality among patients with ESRD on MHD as well as in the general population. Several studies have reported that exercise training can improve peak oxygen consumption among patients with advanced CKD and ESRD treated both with dialysis and transplantation.

Although peak oxygen consumption is an important physiologic variable directly linked to the level of physical activity and relevant to physical functioning and survival, it is problematic in the CKD population. First, many patients are so limited that they cannot perform the maximal treadmill testing or bicycle ergometry needed to measure exercise capacity in this way, limiting participation in studies to those who are healthy and active enough to perform maximal exercise testing. Second, the impact of improvements in peak oxygen consumption on patients' functioning is difficult to quantify.

Therefore, it is important to consider other aspects of physical functioning, such as self-reported functioning, physical performance, and physical frailty, which are more closely related to quality of life.

Patients on maintenance dialysis report poor physical functioning when asked about their level of difficulty in performing various tasks, and they perform poorly when asked to do such things as walk a short or longer distance, rise repeatedly from a chair, or climb a flight of stairs. Both self-reported functioning and physical performance are correlated with physical activity as measured by recall questionnaires and by accelerometry. Inactivity-associated muscle atrophy and muscle weakness have also been observed among patients with CKD and contribute to poor physical performance. These aspects of poor physical functioning have been associated with lower health-related quality of life, with higher mortality in the dialysis population, and with worse outcomes following kidney transplantation. Fortunately, several recent studies have shown that both aerobic exercise training and resistance exercise training interventions can improve self-reported physical functioning among patients on dialysis, and that resistance exercise training can increase muscle mass and strength.

Recently, the concept of physical frailty has been operationalized to allow its impact to be investigated among elderly community-dwelling individuals, where frailty has been associated with higher risk of disability, hospitalization, institutionalization, and death. Low physical activity is one of the five key components of this definition of frailty, and two of the others are related to poor physical performance (weak grip strength and slow gait speed). The final two components are weight loss and exhaustion, with a total of three or more of these marking a person as frail. Both frailty and its components have been associated with kidney function. In the Cardiovascular Health Study (CHS), patients with CKD, defined as serum creatinine greater than 1.3 mg per dL in women or 1.5 mg per dL in men, were almost 3 times as likely to be frail as individuals with normal kidney function. After adjusting for demographic characteristics, comorbidity, and laboratory parameters such as hemoglobin and C-reactive protein, persons with CKD remained 1.5 times more likely to be frail than others. Furthermore, some aspects of the frailty phenotype, in particular tests of physical performance, have been shown to correlate with cystatin C-based estimates of glomerular filtration rate (GFR), even at levels of GFR above 60 mL/min/1.73 m^2, with worse kidney function associated with worse physical performance. Carrying this into the dialysis arena, 30% of patients receiving dialysis were found to be frail by the same definition (compared to 6.9% of community-dwelling elders in the CHS), despite the fact that the dialysis cohort was not restricted to older individuals, and frailty was linked to higher mortality.

In addition to the physical sequelae of inactivity, patients on dialysis, as well as those with earlier stages of CKD and kidney transplant recipients, suffer from a great burden of other chronic conditions that are potentially modifiable by exercise participation, including hypertension, dyslipidemia, coronary heart disease, diabetes, and depression. There is little data specific to patients with CKD on whether exercise actually improves most of these conditions. However, there are studies to suggest that blood pressure control and symptoms of depression are improved by exercise training among patients on MHD, and the evidence in the general population is quite convincing.

Thus, CKD is associated with a host of conditions that are associated with physical inactivity and potentially modifiable by increasing activity. In some cases, particularly in the arena of exercise capacity and physical functioning, exercise has been shown to result in significant improvement among patients with CKD, but we must extrapolate from studies in healthy individuals when considering such benefits as reduced cardiovascular events

TABLE 21.3   Kidney Disease Outcomes Quality Initiative Guidelines about Physical Activity[*]

- All dialysis patients should be counseled and regularly encouraged by nephrology and dialysis staff to increase their level of physical activity.
  - Unique challenges to exercise in dialysis patients need to be identified to refer patients appropriately (e.g., to physical therapy or cardiac rehabilitation) and to enable the patients to follow regimens successfully. Such challenges include orthopedic/musculoskeletal limitations, cardiovascular concerns, and motivational issues.

- Measurement of physical functioning:
  - Evaluation of physical functioning and reevaluation of the physical activity program should be done at least every 6 mo.
  - Physical functioning can be measured using physical performance testing or questionnaires (e.g., SF-36).
  - Potential barriers to participation in physical activity should be assessed in every patient.

- Physical activity recommendations:
  - Many dialysis patients are severely deconditioned and therefore may need a referral for physical therapy to increase strength and endurance to the point where they are able to adopt the recommended levels of physical activity.
  - Patients who qualify for cardiac rehabilitation should be referred to a specialist
  - The goal for activity should be for cardiovascular exercise at a moderate intensity for 30 min most, if not all, days per week. Patients who are not currently physically active should start at very low levels and durations and gradually progress to this recommended level.

- Follow-up:
  - Physical functioning assessment and encouragement for participation in physical activity should be part of the routine patient care plan. Regular review should include assessment of changes in activity and physical functioning.

[*]Available at http://www2.kidney.org/professionals/kdoqi/guidelines_cvd/.

and increased survival. Nevertheless, the Kidney Disease Outcomes Quality Initiative (K/DOQI) Clinical Practice Guidelines for Cardiovascular Disease in Dialysis Patients included a set of guidelines related to physical activity (Table 21.3). Specifically, guideline 14.2 states that, "All dialysis patients should be encouraged by nephrology and dialysis staff to increase their level of physical activity."

RISK OF PHYSICAL ACTIVITY

It is important to consider the potential risks of increasing physical activity, particularly in the CKD population where physical functioning is generally poor and the risk of cardiovascular events is high relative to the general population. The two types of risks to consider are musculoskeletal injury and cardiovascular events. Regular physical activity is associated with a higher incidence of activity-related injury, particularly in the case of vigorous exercise and sports activities. However, there is some evidence that moderate physical activity may confer some protection against injuries, possibly through gains in neuromuscular control, balance, and muscle strength. A study using data from the 2000 to 2002 National Health Interview Survey examined this question. Respondents were asked about their level of physical activity, which investigators classified as inactive, insufficiently active, or active. They were also asked about any injuries that occurred in the last 3 months and about the setting in which the injuries occurred. Not surprisingly, there was a dose–response relationship between leisure-time physical activity level and incidence of injury episodes related to sports or leisure-time activities. Conversely, inactive individuals had the greatest incidence of non-sport or nonleisure-time activity injury episodes, and leisure-time physical activity level was not associated with the odds of reporting any injury after adjusting for age, sex, education, and race/ethnicity. The higher incidence of injuries related to leisure-time activity was offset by fewer nonleisure-time activity-related injuries.

As with musculoskeletal injuries, the risk of cardiovascular events such as myocardial infarction or cardiac arrest increases during vigorous physical exertion, and this is especially true for persons who are sedentary and who have coronary disease, either documented or undiagnosed. The higher risk of an event occurring during exercise compared with during a period of inactivity is greater with higher intensity exercise and with lower habitual physical activity level. In other words, compared with sedentary people who suddenly begin exercising vigorously, persons who exercise regularly have a lower risk of exercise-related sudden death, although even this group has a transient elevation of risk during and immediately after vigorous exercise. However, physically active or physically fit individuals have a 25% to 50% lower overall risk of developing cardiovascular disease, an important consideration for patients with earlier stages of CKD.

Patients with CKD have the potential to be at higher risk for both of these complications of exercise than the general population. Musculoskeletal risk may be higher as a result of hyperparathyroidism and bone disease, which may place patients at greater risk for fracture and spontaneous tendon ruptures. Overall, most musculoskeletal injuries related to physical activity are preventable by gradually working up to a desired level of activity and by avoiding excessive amounts of activity. Similarly, it is likely that the risk of cardiac events is higher among patients with CKD because of the high prevalence of known cardiac disease and risk factors for cardiac disease. Therefore, it is important to take steps to minimize these risks (Table 21.4). The first step is risk assessment. Individuals should be screened for contraindications to exercise participation, including recent myocardial infarction or electrocardiogram changes suggestive of myocardial infarction, uncontrolled arrhythmia, unstable angina, third-degree heart block, severe symptomatic aortic stenosis, suspected or known aortic dissection, or acute progressive heart failure. In addition, uncontrolled hypertension with a systolic blood pressure >200 mm Hg or diastolic blood pressure >120 mm Hg is a relative contraindication to exercise participation. Because adverse effects of exercise are more common with vigorous exercise, especially if undertaken by sedentary individuals, the second step is to start exercising at moderate intensity and for short duration. The net effect of regular physical activity is a lower risk of mortality from cardiovascular disease.

APPROACH TO PHYSICAL ACTIVITY PROMOTION IN THE CHRONIC KIDNEY DISEASE POPULATION

As a result of the growing body of literature on the benefits of physical activity among members of the general population as well as among persons with CKD, K/DOQI Clinical Practice Guidelines for Cardiovascular Disease in Dialysis Patients included a series of recommendations about physical activity (see Table 21.3). Key elements of these recommendations include

TABLE 21.4   Minimizing Risk of Exercise Participation

Proper screening	Rule out contraindications
	• Recent myocardial infarction or electrocardiogram changes consistent with myocardial infarction
	• Unstable angina
	• Uncontrolled arrhythmia
	• Third-degree heart block
	• Acute progressive heart failure
	• Elevated blood pressure
	• Any acute condition that would make exercise participation high risk
	• Inability to walk or unstable gait
Proper equipment	Comfortable, stable footwear
	Loose-fitting clothing
Exercise considerations	Begin at low intensity and short duration
	Encourage stretching before and after exercise
	Progress gradually according to perceived exertion
	Avoid excessively vigorous activity
	Include 5 min of warm up before and cool down after any session that is of at least moderate intensity
Evaluate frequently	• Provide encouragement, reinforcement
	• Monitor for problems
	• Reinitiate after intercurrent illnesses

a statement that assessment and counseling about physical activity should be done by nephrologists or dialysis unit staff. These guidelines specifically recommend a target of 30 minutes of moderate activity on most days, and stress that patients should be started at low levels and gradually progressed to the recommended levels. Unfortunately, however, a survey of nephrologists showed that most nephrologists are not counseling patients to become more active, and a major reason cited by nephrologists for not counseling was a lack of confidence in their ability to discuss this topic. Although the guidelines provide specific targets, they do not address implementation, something nephrologists urgently need.

Reasons for the lack of focus on the mechanics of exercise prescription include the facts that exercise was only one part of a large set of guidelines on cardiovascular disease and that there are no data specific to CKD populations on how to increase physical activity levels. Therefore, strategies for increasing physical activity among patients with CKD, as for many other aspects of their care, must be extrapolated from information available in persons without kidney disease. Nephrologists have several options available to increase physical activity participation among their patients. First, simply asking patients about their level of physical activity lets them know that this is an important aspect of their medical care. Second, nephrologists can educate patients about the potential benefits of exercise to further reinforce its role in their care. Third, nephrologists can provide written information about exercise and its benefits. A detailed exercise guide specifically designed for patients on dialysis is available at no cost online through Life Options, a program of research-based education and outreach that aims to improve quality of life among patients with kidney disease. This booklet contains information about the benefits of regular exercise as well as specific information about how to get started on an exercise program. Physicians can refer patients to this website, or they can download the booklet and provide it to patients directly. In addition, there are a multitude of Internet-based sources of exercise information directed at the general public or older individuals provided by organizations such as the Centers for Disease Control and Prevention, the U.S. Department of Agriculture, the American College of Sports Medicine, Harvard School of Public Health, and many others. These resources are valuable for patients who are healthy except for kidney disease, but some patients may need additional help or support. Patients who are unable to walk or who have difficulty walking can be referred to physical therapists for evaluation and for recommendations on how to increase strength and physical activity, which should be covered by Medicare. Patients who have known or suspected cardiac disease or congestive heart failure can be referred for cardiac rehabilitation, a large component of which is geared toward beginning an exercise program.

Finally, nephrologists can discuss the specifics of exercise with patients (Fig. 21.1) or can provide opportunities for physical activity participation during dialysis sessions for patients receiving in-center hemodialysis. The latter strategy has been shown to be beneficial and in some cases to improve the efficiency of dialysis and reduce adverse effects such as hypotensive episodes and cramping. Several authors have advocated exercise during dialysis because of better adherence, because it does not require additional time commitments from the patients, and because it can reverse the forced

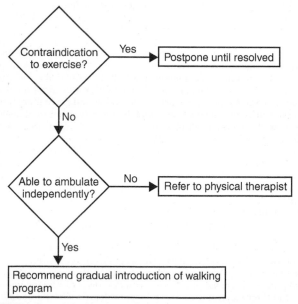

FIGURE 21.1 General algorithm for starting aerobic exercise program.

inactivity of dialysis that does not include exercise. However, although there are many programs in Canada and elsewhere that have successfully incorporated in-center exercise, in the United States, the dialysis provider system does not lend itself easily to incorporating such activity during the dialysis treatment. Dialysis staff are often less than enthusiastic about supporting dialysis unit-based exercise programs, citing concerns about lack of time, patient safety (the difficulty of maneuvering around exercise equipment in the case of an emergency), and staff safety (the possibility of injury when moving bulky exercise equipment to allow patient participation). These barriers are not trivial in any circumstance, but they become effectively insurmountable in the absence of strong physician and unit leadership support of exercise, as well as a designated individual to manage the prescription and monitoring of exercise. Unfortunately, very few units in the United States currently have the resources to provide an on-site exercise program, but this should not preclude encouragement of exercise outside the dialysis setting. In addition, because patients on home dialysis (peritoneal dialysis or other hemodialysis modality), those with CKD not requiring dialysis, and those who have received kidney transplants are also in need of exercise counseling, nephrologists should develop a mechanism to provide specific information to patients about how to become more physically active as part of their lifestyle.

The most important guiding principle when recommending that patients increase their level of physical activity is to encourage patients to start slowly and gradually increase the intensity and duration of their activity (see Table 21.4). A major barrier to exercise counseling by physicians and to beginning an exercise program for patients is the notion that exercise must be vigorous to be beneficial. Newer research has shown that while more may be better, "even a little is good," and this concept should be heavily emphasized when discussing physical activity with patients with CKD. The idea of "no pain, no gain" should be abandoned, and patients should be advised to start at a level that can be accomplished *without* pain. Although the target is 30 minutes of moderate exercise on most days of the week, it is important to recognize that many patients will need to start with a much shorter duration of activity and that "moderate exercise" should be defined relative to the individual's level of fitness rather than in absolute terms. Thus, rather than advising patients to walk at a certain speed (a difficult recommendation to follow in any case), patients should be advised to walk at a speed that they perceive as "somewhat hard" to "hard" but not "very hard." The example of walking will be used throughout this section, but bicycling or other activity can be prescribed following similar principles. Walking, however, has several advantages: it is generally safe; there is no need for special equipment; it can be done anywhere; intensity can be varied; and it can be tracked by time, distance, or number of steps. In addition, there is specific evidence for the benefit of walking through the Nurses' Health Study, the Harvard Alumni Health Study, the National Health Interview Survey, the Women's Health Initiative, among others.

A key component of a successful exercise program is monitoring, and this is where nephrologists or dialysis unit staff could make exercise a part of the patient care plan even without instituting a unit-based program. If patients were routinely asked about the time spent in physical activity and the intensity of the activity, progression to the recommended levels could be facilitated. The first goal is usually to increase the duration of exercise to at least 20 minutes per session, and preferably 30 minutes. This can be done gradually, with an increase of 1 to 2 minutes per week as tolerated. Then patients can be encouraged to increase the intensity of the activity. In the case of walking, this can be accomplished by increasing speed, adding uphill segments to the route, or by carrying hand weights and/or wearing ankle weights. Most patients should not be encouraged to increase the velocity to the point of jogging because this may increase the chances of injury. All patients should be advised of the target perceived level of exertion and should be told that exertion should not be so strenuous that they cannot talk during exercise.

In addition to walking or other aerobic activity, physical activity guidelines also state that to promote and maintain health and physical independence, older adults will benefit from performing activities that maintain or increase muscular strength and endurance for a minimum of 2 days each week. These activities include a progressive weight training program, weight-bearing calisthenics, and similar resistance exercises that use major muscle groups. The general principle of starting low and increasing gradually applies here as well. The starting weight should be one that can be lifted at least 10 to 15 times for each exercise at a level of exertion that is moderate. However, it may be more difficult for nephrologists to discuss the specifics of and monitor the safety of resistance training than walking programs, so the option of a physical therapy referral for detailed instructions should be utilized liberally, and physicians can reinforce progress by asking periodically and re-referring as needed for progress assessments and updated recommendations.

Finally, physical activity guidelines for older individuals also state that to maintain the flexibility necessary for regular physical activity and daily life, older adults should perform activities that maintain or increase flexibility on at least 2 days each week for at least 10 minutes each day. To reduce risk of injury from falls, community-dwelling older adults with substantial risk of falls (e.g., with frequent falls or mobility problems) should perform exercises that maintain or improve balance. Physical therapists are well equipped to provide balance and flexibility exercise recommendations to patients with CKD, and these can be incorporated into an overall exercise plan. Stretching exercises should be performed before and after aerobic exercise to warm up and cool down the muscles while also maintaining mobility.

Unfortunately, increasing physical activity and improving fitness are often not one-time endeavors. Patients with CKD suffer from many comorbid conditions and become ill or require hospitalization frequently, which must be taken into account when discussing physical activity with patients. Fitness declines rapidly during periods of bed rest, and it can be discouraging for patients to experience health-related setbacks. Physicians can help by acknowledging that it is not unexpected for there to be losses in ability to exercise associated with these events and by encouraging patients to repeat the process of initiating physical activity during recovery. Patients should find a new comfortable level, which may well be lower than previously tolerated activity, and should build gradually from there.

In general, it cannot be emphasized enough that physician involvement increases the chances that patients will increase and sustain their level of physical activity. When asked about their experience with physical activity, dialysis patients have reported that lack of encouragement from their healthcare team was a barrier to exercise participation. Patients often receive subtle or not-so-subtle messages from their physicians that they are not capable of being active. Asking about and encouraging physical activity should be part of our routine care for these patients.

Internet Resources

American Heart Association Recommendations for Physical Activity in Adults. http://www.heart.org/HEARTORG/HealthyLiving/PhysicalActivity/FitnessBasics/American-Heart-Association-Recommendations-for-Physical-Activity-in-Adults_UCM_307976_Article.jsp#.WAI4lpMrKHp. Accessed May 10, 2017.
Centers for Disease Control and Prevention. http://www.cdc.gov/nccdphp/dnpa/physical/. Accessed May 10, 2017.

Harvard School of Public Health. http://www.hsph.harvard.edu/nutritionsource /staying-active/. Accessed May 10, 2017.

Life Options. http://lifeoptions.org/catalog/catalog.php?prod-Cat=booklets:%20Exercise:%20A%20Guide%20for%20People%20on%20Dialysis. Accessed May 10, 2017.

National Institute on Aging. https://www.nia.nih.gov/health/publication/exercise-physical-activity/introduction. Accessed May 10, 2017.

National Kidney Foundation. K/DOQI Clinical Practice Guidelines for Cardiovascular Disease in Dialysis Patients. http://kidneyfoundation.cachefly.net/professionals /KDOQI/guidelines_cvd/index.htm . Accessed May 10, 2017.

Office of Disease Prevention and Health Promotion. Physical Activity Guidelines. https://health.gov/paguidelines/. Accessed May 10, 2017.

U.S. Department of Agriculture. Dietary Guidelines for Americans 2015–2020. 8th Ed. https://health.gov/dietaryguidelines/2015/resources/2015-2020_Dietary_ Guidelines.pdf. Accessed May 10, 2017.

Suggested Readings

Carlson SA, Hootman JM, Powell KE, et al. Self-reported injury and physical activity levels: United States 2000 to 2002. *Ann Epidemiol* 2006;16:712–719.

Cheema B, Abas H, Smith B, et al. Progressive exercise for anabolism in kidney disease (PEAK): a randomized, controlled trial of resistance training during hemodialysis. *J Am Soc Nephrol* 2007;18:1594–1601.

Fried LP, Tangen CM, Walston J, et al; Cardiovascular Health Study Collaborative Research Group. Frailty in older adults: evidence for a phenotype. *J Gerontol A Biol Sci Med Sci* 2001;56A:M146–M156.

Johansen KL. Exercise in the ESRD population. *J Am Soc Nephrol* 2007;18:1845–1854.

Johansen KL, Chertow GM, Kutner, NG, et al. Low level of self-reported physical activity in ambulatory patients new to dialysis. *Kidney Int* 2010;78:1164–1170.

Johansen KL, Painter PL, Sakkas GK, et al. Effects of resistance exercise training and nandrolone decanoate on body composition and muscle function among patients who receive hemodialysis: a randomized, controlled trial. *J Am Soc Nephrol* 2006;17:2307–2314.

National Institute on Aging. *Your Everyday Guide from the National Institute on Aging at NIH: Exercise & Physical Activity*. NIH Publication No. 15-4258. Bethesda, MD: U.S. Department of Health and Human Services, Public Health Service, National Institutes of Health, National Institute on Aging; 2015 .

National Kidney Foundation. K/DOQI Clinical Practice Guidelines for Cardiovascular Disease in Dialysis Patients. *Am J Kidney Dis* 2005;45(Suppl 3):S1–S154.

Nelson ME, Rejeski WJ, Blair SN, et al. Physical activity and public health in older adults: recommendation from the American College of Sports Medicine and the American Heart Association. *Circulation* 2007;116:1094–1105.

Office of the U.S. Surgeon General. *Physical activity and health: A report of the Surgeon General.* Washington, DC: U.S. Department of Health and Human Services, National Center for Chronic Disease Prevention and Health Promotion; 1996.

Shlipak MG, Stehman-Breen C, Fried LF, et al. The presence of frailty in elderly persons with chronic renal insufficiency. *Am J Kidney Dis* 2004;43:861–867.

U.S. Department of Health and Human Services. *2008 Physical Activity Guidelines for Americans.* Washington, DC: U.S. Department of Health and Human Services; 2008.

U.S. Department of Health and Human Services and U.S. Department of Agriculture. *Dietary Guidelines for Americans, 2015.* Washington, DC: U.S. Department of Health and Human Services and U.S. Department of Agriculture; 2015.

22 The Renal Dietitian in the Clinic—Medical Nutrition Therapy

Linda W. Moore

The complexity of nutritional needs of patients with chronic kidney disease (CKD) is reported throughout the literature and in the many chapters of this handbook. Nutrient requirements and metabolism change as kidney disease progresses. Thus, determining what, when, and how to implement medical nutrition therapy (MNT) requires knowledge of the level of kidney function, the specific nutrient needs, and the individual's nutrition history and medical history. Dietitians are uniquely skilled at determining and implementing nutritional recommendations, helping people understand how to make the necessary dietary changes, and monitoring the outcomes resulting from the dietary changes. The process is iterative, requiring multiple interactions to achieve success, and adjustments are likely necessary over time.

Another factor to be considered in providing nutritional care to non-dialysis patients with CKD is access to the renal dietitian. Nephrologists, dietitians, and patients may seek opportunities to partner in the provision of the much-needed nutritional care for nondialysis kidney diseases and find it difficult to find these services outside the confines of dialysis centers where the services of dietitians are federally mandated for dialysis patients.

This chapter will review some methods dietitians use in providing nutrition care to patients with nondialysis CKD and discuss some potential linkages to specialty care partnerships for both dietitians and physicians.

EXAMPLE TECHNIQUES USED BY DIETITIANS IN CKD-MNT

Prescribing dietary changes is common for people with hypertension, diabetes, or kidney diseases. For hypertension, primary prevention and intervention strategies involve a dietary component for weight loss, the reduction of dietary sodium intake, and an increase in dietary potassium intake. The treatment of diabetes includes fundamental dietary changes: energy and carbohydrate restrictions account for the main dietary alterations in treating diabetes. Finally, in the treatment of CKD, dietary modifications such as low-protein diets are used to slow the progression to kidney failure in people with advanced kidney disease. It is unknown whether instituting dietary changes for treating hypertension, diabetes, or kidney disease directly contributes to nutritional status changes. However, some studies have demonstrated that prescribed alterations in nutrient intake result in the unintentional reduction in macronutrient or micronutrient intake unless careful attention is provided.

Dietitians consider the patient's nutrition history and nutrition knowledge when implementing dietary intake recommendations. It is not practical to expect a patient to consume a low-sodium diet by only providing a list of foods high in sodium to avoid or even a list of foods low in sodium to include in their diet. Whereas the patient may attempt to follow the general recommendation, they are at risk for excluding vital nutrients by doing so. For illustration, a brief presentation of three cases where a renal dietitian provided CKD-MNT demonstrates the reality of what is required to assist patients through the web of a renal diet.

Example 1

A recently widowed 75-year-old gentleman was referred to the dietitian for uncontrolled diabetes and blood pressure. His nutrition history revealed that he was only eating processed and canned meats, eggs, bread, canned beans, and usually one meal per day from a fast-food restaurant. Nutrient analysis indicated dietary protein intake of 123 g per day (1.5 g per kg standardized body weight [SBW]) in ~2,500 kcal (31 kcal per kg SBW). His blood pressure was 140/89 mm Hg on three blood pressure medications. Body mass index (BMI) was 30.5 kg per m^2 (119% of SBW). Laboratory results included HbgA1c of 7.3%, blood urea nitrogen (BUN) of 43 mg per dL, a serum creatinine of 1.7, estimated glomerular filtration rate (eGFR) of 39 mL/min/1.73 m^2, and potassium of 5.3 mEq per L. His primary care physician did not mention kidney function in the referral. This patient would not have known what to do with the lists of foods allowed and not allowed. He had a food and nutrition-related knowledge deficit but was interested in learning what to do to improve his health. His nutrition education began with meal timing, owing to concern regarding his diabetes. Initial instructions were for avoiding salt, caution about high-potassium foods, and education on the process of food diaries. His physician was contacted to recommend a nephrology referral in light of his kidney function and potassium. Over the ensuing weeks, the patient and dietitian discussed how to include fruits and vegetables with his meals and continued to teach lower sodium choices. At each encounter, they also discussed his diabetes, and methods for monitoring his glucose, while communicating with his physician's office regarding his status.

Example 2

The patient was referred to the renal dietitian by a nephrologist. The patient was a 72-year-old well-nourished male employed full time, who had Stage 3 CKD (BUN 19 mg per dL, serum creatinine 1.3 mg per dL, eGFR range 45 to 57 mL/min/1.73 m^2), serum potassium 4.1 mEq per L, hemoglobin 16.6 g per dL, 25OHD3 19 ng per mL, and urine protein 7.4 g. His blood pressure was 174/90 mm Hg (on a β-blocker), BMI was 29.7 kg per m^2 (158% of SBW). His nephrologist requested MNT for CKD. His diet prescription was 0.6 to 0.8 g protein per kg body per day plus 6 to 8 g protein for proteinuria, 30 kcal/kg/d, and 2 g sodium, 800 mg phosphorus. He was prescribed a vitamin D supplement (to be rechecked in 8 weeks). The diet education was initiated with a manual on food groups and how to choose appropriate foods from each group to cover his prescription. He was also provided with a 7-day menu consisting of three meals each day that fit his diet prescription and was coded to his manual on food groups. He was instructed to work through this list for 4 weeks, noting any pitfalls and providing general comments, but the emphasis was placed on consuming everything on the menu. He met again with the renal dietitian and adjustments were made to the 7-day menu regarding items that did not work for him. His blood pressure on follow-up was 150/84 mm Hg, BMI was 29 kg per m^2, and serum creatinine was stable. The patient subsequently relocated to another state for his work and was lost to follow-up.

Example 3

A nephrologist referred a 72-year-old moderately nourished female with new-onset type 2 diabetes and Stage 4 CKD with a diet prescription that read "low protein (1 g per kg ideal body weight per day), to maintain blood pressure ≤ 130/80 mm Hg, HgbA1c ≤ 7.0, and a low phosphorus intake." The patient's blood pressure was 181/82 mm Hg (on a β-blocker and a calcium channel blocker), BMI was 17.8 kg per m^2 (82% of SBW). Her BUN was 33 mg per dL, serum creatinine 2.2 mg per dL (eGFR 22 mL/min/1.73 m^2), she had 1$^+$ protein in her urine, serum potassium was 3.8 mEq per L, glucose was

164 mg per dL, and serum albumin was 3.7 g per dL. Her ferritin was 60 ng per mL, and hemoglobin was 9.3 g per dL. The patient was also taking ferrous sulfate, B complex vitamins, vitamin E, and lecithin. An oral sulfonylurea was used for diabetes control. A diet for 0.8 to 1 g protein per kg SBW per day, 2 g sodium, 700 mg phosphorus was planned, but the sodium and phosphorus components were deferred to a later visit. She was provided with a manual on food groups and educated on how to choose appropriate foods from each group to cover her prescription. She indicated that she liked cooking and wanted to develop her own menu. She returned to the dietitian the following week with a food diary showing 1.2 g protein and 26 kcal per kg SBW per day, 3 g sodium and 1 g phosphorus per day. She was checking her blood glucose level 4 times a day but at ~2 hours postprandial; all but 1 time per day glucose levels were <100 mg per dL. The patient was provided more detail on how to divide carbohydrates throughout the day, retrained on protein sources, and instructed to return in 2 weeks with another diary. On return, her protein intake slightly improved to 1.1 g per kg of protein and 27 kcal per kg of SBW per day; her carbohydrate distribution and glucose monitoring improved. The 2 g sodium and 700 mg phosphorus restrictions were implemented after providing an additional handout on the phosphorus content of foods. She returned to the renal dietitian's office 1 month later with a diary indicating 0.9 g protein and 28 kcal per kg SBW per day, 1,700 mg sodium, and 730 mg of phosphorus. Her self-monitoring blood glucose remained in the desired range, and her weight was stable. The renal dietitian spent 3 hours with the patient throughout these visits and requested that the nephrologist refer the patient again if her condition changed.

The dietitian approaches nutrition care by implementing a nutrition assessment and determining the nutritional diagnosis, following with a nutrition intervention and nutrition evaluation and monitoring (Fig. 22.1). This method is somewhat standardized across dietetics practice. As in the cases described above, patients with CKD demonstrate multiple comorbidities, each of which alters the nutritional approach. These patients also showed some of the patient-centered nuances encountered by the dietitian: food and nutrition knowledge deficits, varying degrees of nutritional status, and levels of readiness or willingness to learn, as well as abilities for implementing change. The type of visit, the goals for the session, and whether the payer dictates the number of visits allowed usually determines the length and frequency of CKD-MNT visits (Table 22.1). For example, the initial visit is usually longer than follow-up visits (Table 22.1). Some insurance companies will indicate the number of visits allowed during the precertification process. However, the amount of time between visits is determined by the needs of the patient. A more complex diet for a patient having difficulty assimilating the information may require a shorter time between the first few visits, while a longer time between the later visits may be preferable.

The unique nutrient needs of these patients are best provided through physician-dietitian or registered dietitian/nutritionist (MD-RDN) partnerships, as has been recognized in dialysis facilities for decades. Gaining access to renal dietitians before dialysis presents a challenge to many patients and physicians. Building these partnerships may help patients who face a challenging future.

DIETITIANS PRACTICE IN PRIMARY CARE CLINICS, NEPHROLOGY CLINICS, OR PRIVATE PRACTICE

In the United States, dietitians are approved providers of MNT for patients with Stage 4 CKD and some of Stage 3 CKD (GFR < 50 mL/min/1.73 m^2) as well as patients who have diabetes. Thus, in these categories, the dietitian may provide fee-for-service. Some private insurance companies still do not

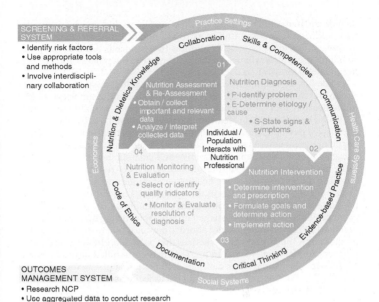

FIGURE 22.1 The nutrition care process (From Academy of Nutrition and Dietetics. Nutrition Terminology Reference Manual (eNCPT): Dietetics Language for Nutrition Care. http://ncpt.webauthor.com. Accessed July, 2017; reprinted with permission).

TABLE 22.1 Current Recommendations for Timing and Frequency of CKD-MNT Encounters

Encounter	Academy of Nutrition and Dietetics, Recommended Hours	Centers for Medicare & Medicaid Services, Covered Benefit, Allowed Hours
Year 1		3[*]
Month 1	0.75–1.5[†]	
Month 2	0.25–1.5 per encounter	
Month 3	every 1–3 months or	
Month 4	more if nutrient intake	
Month 5	is inadequate, protein–	
Month 6	energy malnutrition, or	
Month 7	intercurrent illness that	
Month 8	would further compromise	
Month 9	nutrition status	
Month 10		
Month 11		
Month 12		
Year 2 and beyond		2 per year[‡]

[*]Number of hours may be achieved over multiple visits. However, the first visit is usually an hour or longer to accommodate the time to perform initial nutrition assessment.
[†]Patients should receive MNT from a dietitian at least 12 months before initiation of dialysis.
[‡]Number of hours may be achieved over multiple visits. However, usually 2–3 visits per year beyond year one will suffice for follow-up within the hours allowed. If the patient's condition changes, however, more hours may be needed along with a new referral form outlining the changes and new diet prescription.
CKD, chronic kidney disease; MNT, medical nutrition therapy.

include the benefit of dietitians for their customers, but may be persuaded with additional documentation as to the need. Thus, precertification is necessary. Fee-for-service MNT requires that service is billed to the payer, so billing specialists will need to become aware of the process and codes to use in billing for MNT by dietitian providers.

Fee-for-service may be waning across U.S. healthcare systems, however. According to the current U.S. Secretary of Health and Human Services, 85% of Medicare fee-for-service payments should be tied to quality or value in 2016, and by 2018, 50% of Medicare payments should be delivered through alternative payment models. Accountable care organizations and bundled payment arrangements are examples of some alternative payment models being explored. Dietitians are effective and cost-efficient providers, especially in the primary care setting where a significant return on investment has been demonstrated. Fewer hospital admissions and reduced physician visits have shown cost savings in these contexts. Less time with physicians per patient could also lead to increased availability for the physician to see more patients. Many physicians would welcome having dietitians in their practice but perceive they cannot afford to pay the dietitian. By reducing hospitalizations, the primary care practices that participate in these alternative payment models may realize an increase in their bundled payment, which could help offset some of the dietitian cost. For patients who have diabetes or CKD, the dietitian provider can still bill as fee-for-service and thus cover that part of the dietitian cost.

Dietitians Transitioning from Dialysis to Nondialysis CKD-MNT Providers or General Dietitians Seeking to Include MNT for CKD in Their Scope

The Academy of Nutrition and Dietetics, together with the Council on Renal Nutrition of the National Kidney Foundation, has published a consensus statement on the standards of practice (SOP) and standards of professional performance (SOPP) of dietitians working in nephrology settings. This report delineates the elements of nutrition care practice in nephrology nutrition and identifies the level of practice (competent, proficient, or expert) that would be required for each indicator. Dietitians may use the SOP and SOPP to assess their own individual competence and determine areas that may need to be strengthened.

In addition to the SOP and SOPP for dietitians in nephrology nutrition, the Academy of Nutrition and Dietetics offers a tool for self-assessment of competence in a dietetics practice area. The *Scope of Practice Decision Tool* is an online, interactive tool intended to aid dietetics practitioners in determining if a function is within their scope and offers advice on a process for increasing proficiency in the area. For dietitians transitioning from being a dialysis dietitian to seeing patients in a nondialysis CKD clinic or primary care group, using the *Scope of Practice Decision Tool* may be a useful exercise to complete prior to the transition.

Likewise, for dietitians who do not practice in a dialysis setting but wish to develop skills for CKD-MNT, the *Scope of Practice Decision Tool* could be useful to detect areas that should be strengthened. A dietitian without the certified specialist in renal nutrition (CSR) credential (see below) or without dialysis experience will require a higher level of proficiency when working with patients with CKD, especially due to the increased prevalence of patients with comorbidities such as diabetes and cardiovascular disease.

A number of organizations have training materials for dietitians who wish to provide CKD-MNT for patients not on dialysis (Table 22.2), including the Academy of Nutrition and Dietetics, such as the Chronic Kidney Disease Toolkit (http://www.eatrightstore.org/) and the National Kidney Foundation Council on Renal Nutrition (http://www.kidney.org). The National Institute

TABLE 22.2	Summary of Resources Available for Self-Assessment and Training on CKD-MNT
Resource	**Description**
AND "Scope of Practice Decision Tool"	An online, interactive tool to assist dietitians in self-assessment of preparedness for an activity. If the activity is outside the dietitian's scope, then it should be deferred until training in that area can be satisfied.
AND "Chronic Kidney Disease Toolkit"	A comprehensive package of materials produced from evidence-based guidelines. Materials include the MNT protocol, forms for implementation of the protocol, as well as data collection tools for monitoring quality. Covers Stages 1–5 CKD including kidney transplantation for adults.
AND "eMentoring and Mentoring Resources"	A program to connect dietitians with a matched mentor or mentee based on goals, communication style, and availability. This program could be used, by mutual agreement, for nonrenal dietitians entering the renal field who wish to gain insight from experienced renal dietitians. Additionally, the Entrepreneurs Dietetic Practice Group have a specific mentoring program for dietitians entering the private practice role.
NIDDK, NKDEP "CKD Nutrition Management Training Program"	A series of online modules to be used by dietitians and dietetics educators in preparing to provide MNT for patients with CKD. The five training modules include case studies and tests the participant's knowledge of the stages of CKD and appropriate CKD-MNT.
NKF Council on Renal Nutrition "Pocket Guide to Nutritional Assessment of the Patient with Chronic Kidney Disease"	A complete manual on nutrition assessment, this guide covers the diet and nutrient recommendations for the stages of CKD and renal replacement therapy types, including transplantation. The guide also provides lists of vitamins and nutrition supplements commonly used in this target population.
NKF Council on Renal Nutrition and AND Renal Dietitians DPG joint project "A Clinical Guide to Nutrition Care in Kidney Disease"	A guide that covers the spectrum of nutrition care for kidney disease in children and adults at any stage of CKD or renal replacement therapy type. The guide is written for new renal dietitians, dietitians working in nondialysis settings and dialysis settings, and can be used by educators and students.
ISRNM and Abbott Nutrition project "Total Nutrition Therapy: Renal, A Hands-on Renal Nutrition Course for Healthcare Professionals"	A global clinical course for nephrologists and allied health professionals in renal disease. The program focuses on protein–energy wasting and identification of risks for malnutrition at the stages of CKD, as well as methods for monitoring and managing nutrition therapy to improve outcomes.

AND, Academy of Nutrition and Dietetics; CKD, chronic kidney disease; DPG, Dietetics Practice Group; ISRNM, International Society of Renal Nutrition and Metabolism; MNT, medical nutrition therapy; NIDDK, National Institute of Diabetes and Digestive and Kidney Diseases; NKDEP, National Kidney Disease Education Program ; NKF, National Kidney Foundation.

of Diabetes and Digestive and Kidney Diseases developed a National Kidney Disease Education Program on CKD (Table 22.2). Other training options for dietitians who do not have experience in CKD-MNT include attending a workshop such as the one provided at the Spring Clinical Meeting of the National Kidney Foundation (http://www.kidney.org/spring-clinical). The workshop is entitled "Foundations of Nutrition Practice for Kidney Disease" and "Advanced Practice in Renal Nutrition," which represent both an entry level and an advanced level component for dietitians in CKD. The *Journal of Renal Nutrition* also offers Continuing Professional Education in CKD topics, which is another resource for dietitians new to CKD practice (http://www.jrnjournal.org).

Dietitians should be cautious of embarking on CKD-MNT without self-assessment of their skills in this area. Utilizing the tools mentioned (Table 22.2) could provide a method for self-assessment as well as training to qualify for providing CKD-MNT prior to taking on that role. Once a thorough review of the tools, toolkits, and guides mentioned are completed, it might be beneficial for a new CKD-MNT provider to find a dietitian experienced in CKD-MNT to arrange for mentorship and practice a few cases together. Additionally, the dietitian should maintain an open forum with the referring physician and, if the referring physician is the primary care doctor, reaching out to the patient's nephrologist is essential for assuring success of the CKD-MNT.

What are additional skills that dietitians need to be able to work in an integrated primary care or nephrology clinic environment or what do the practices need from the dietitian? Dietitians must be familiar with what is going on in their state or region and evaluate how they can provide value before embarking on practicing in these settings, especially any statutory requirements of the state in which they practice. Some of the unique skills needed are (1) motivational interviewing, ability to engage patients in their care, (2) knowledge of how to measure quality, and (3) understand quality improvement (plan-do-study-act cycles), especially those of interest to the primary care or nephrology clinic practice.

Another tool available to dietitians is the Academy of Nutrition and Dietetics Health Informatics Infrastructure tool (ANDHII; https://www.andhii.org). Dietitians can use ANDHII to build a nutrition outcomes database using the terminology unique to MNT in a de-identified, Health Insurance Portability and Accountability Act (HIPAA)-compliant venue. Once the data are entered, ANDHII will also create the progress note for the encounter that can be printed or pasted into the clinic's electronic health record. The tool can be used as a dietetics outcomes registry or repository as well as a database for nutrition research.

A Physician Referral Is Required for CKD-MNT

If the dietitian has access to the patient's electronic health record, the amount of information required on a referral form is minimal: patient name, medical record number, date of birth, the medical diagnosis for MNT (preferably the stage of CKD), the referral request, and physical activity limitations, if any. The referral request may be written as a specific diet order, a diet concordant with a named guideline, or in some states where the dietitian is approved to write the diet order, the physician may simply write "CKD-MNT" to indicate the purpose of the referral. Without access to the patient's electronic health record, however, the referring physician will need to supply qualifying laboratory data (e.g., >3 months confirmed abnormality of kidney function or structure, medications, insurance information, and progress notes) in addition to the above. Likewise, if the physician determines that the patient needs additional MNT during the course of a year because of changes from the initial diagnosis, another referral will be required with documentation as to the changes and a revised diet prescription, as appropriate.

NEPHROLOGISTS NEED ACCESS TO QUALIFIED DIETITIANS

Finding Qualified Dietitians to Provide CKD-MNT for Your Patients

More than 600 dietitians in the United States are board CSR, a certification offered by the Commission on Dietetic Registration, the credentialing agency for the Academy of Nutrition and Dietetics. To qualify for board certification, the registered dietitian must have maintained registration with the Commission for at least 2 years and have 2,000 hours of documentable practice experience in kidney disease within the previous 5 years, and pass the Commission's rigorous examination. A dietitian who holds the CSR works directly with patients who have kidney disease, and the board certification is testament to their knowledge of the various settings and nutritional requirements associated with the stages of kidney disease. Dietitians who hold the CSR might also work in education, research, or management in kidney diseases. Recertification is required every 5 years.

Another credential offered by the Commission that might be useful in the management of patients with CKD is the Advanced Practice Certification in Clinical Nutrition (RDN-AP or RD-AP). To qualify for this certification, the dietitian must have held the RDN or RD for 4 years and have 8,000 documented hours of clinical nutrition practice during the previous 15 years with 800 of these from the past 2 years. A graduate degree or demonstrated leadership and peer-reviewed publication activity or Board Certification in a specialty is also required. Finally, the dietitian must pass a rigorous examination administered by the Commission. The dietitians with AP provide direct clinical nutrition care to patients. The Advanced Practitioner often functions autonomously in their area of practice.

Nephrologists and clinic managers or hiring personnel may also choose to use the Academy's SOP and SOPP for dietitians in nephrology nutrition to determine the level of practice of the dietitian they may be interviewing. The patient with kidney disease and multiple comorbidities likely needs a "proficient" or "expert" MNT practitioner in most cases. A dietitian with the CSR or AP would be able to fill that role. Without one or both of these credentials, the interviewer may turn to the SOP and SOPP for guidance on assessing the skill level.

Supporting CKD-MNT in the Nephrology Clinic

As mentioned above, several payment methods are available for dietitians to work in nondialysis CKD settings. Combining a fee-for-service system for patients who have diabetes or qualifying CKD (GFR <50 mL/min/1.73 m^2) with other methods such as incident-to-MD when a patient does not have the qualifying condition would be a way to pay for having access to on-site dietitians in a nephrology practice. Good record keeping will be necessary for assuring there is no cross-over between incident-to-MD and fee-for-service provider encounters, however.

Another consideration for how to include dietitians in a nephrology practice is The Joint Commission Accredited Chronic Kidney Disease (ACKD) program. The Joint Commission ACKD program (https://www.joint commission.org/certification/chronic_kidney_disease.aspx) is a certificate of distinction for CKD centers. A center with this certificate provides care to all the stages of CKD utilizing a cohesive clinical team within a culture of excellence, and ACKD programs improve patient care quality by emphasizing practice guidelines. The ACKD would include patient access to dietitians as well as other healthcare professionals.

CONCLUSION

Patients with CKD have complex nutritional needs relating to the metabolism of nutrients as well as finessing the implementation of the nutrient recommendations. Dietitians are uniquely skilled at helping patients achieve nutritional goals, but finding the right physician–dietitian partnership is often challenging. Utilizing practice guidelines and SOP may assist in selecting partners. Incorporating new programmatic approaches to interdisciplinary care in primary practice or specialty practice may help physicians to build partnerships with dietitians that will benefit their patients and their practice.

Suggested Readings

Academy Quality Management Committee and Scope of Practice Subcommittee of the Quality Management Committee. Academy scope of practice decision tool: a self-assessment guide. *J Acad Nutr Diet* 2013;113(Suppl 6):S10.

Burwell SM. Setting value-based payment goals – HHS efforts to improve U.S. health care. *N Engl J Med* 2015;372:897–899.

Goldstein DJ, LaPierre AF. Nutrition and kidney disease. In: Gilbert SJ, Weiner DE, Gipson DS, et al, eds. *National Kidney Foundation's Primer on Kidney Diseases.* 6th ed. 2009;467–475.

Johns TS, Yee J, Smith-Jules T, et al. Interdisciplinary care clinics in chronic kidney disease. *BMC Nephrol* 2015;16:161.

Johnson R. The Lewin Group — what does it tell us, and why does it matter? *J Am Diet Assoc* 1999;99:426–427.

Kent PS, McCarthy MP, Burrowes JD, et al. Academy of Nutrition and Dietetics and National Kidney Foundation: revised 2014 standards of practice and standards of professional performance for registered dietitian nutritionists (competent, proficient, and expert) in nephrology nutrition. *J Acad Nutr Diet* 2014;114(9):1448–1457. e45.

Moore LW, Byham-Gray L, Parrott JS, et al. The mean dietary protein intake at different stages of chronic kidney disease is higher than current guidelines. *Kidney Int* 2012;83(4):724–732.

Mueller C, Rogers D, Brody RA, et al. Report from the Advanced-Level Clinical Practice Audit Task Force of the Commission on Dietetic Registration: results of the 2013 advanced-level clinical practice audit. *J Acad Nutr Diet* 2015;115(4):624–634.

Price JA, Kent S, Cox SA, et al. Using Academy standards of excellence in nutrition and dietetics for organization self-assessment and quality improvement. *J Acad Nutr Diet* 2014;114:1277–1292.

Soman SS, Yee J, Ho K. Quality improvement initiatives in kidney disease. In: Skorecki K, Chertow GM, Marsden PA, et al., eds. *Brenner & Rector's the Kidney.* 10th ed. Elsevier Saunders, Philadelphia. 2016:2620–2626. e4.

Wolf AM, Siadity M, Yaeger B, et al. Effects of lifestyle intervention on health care costs: The ICAN Project. *J Am Diet Assoc* 2007;107(8):1365–1373.

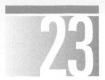

23

Nutritional Support in Acute Kidney Injury

Edward D. Siew and Kathleen D. Liu

Acute kidney injury (AKI), previously termed acute renal failure, results in a complex array of metabolic derangements due to the underlying precipitant, the systemic response to illness, the kidney injury itself, and therapies used to treat the AKI. These perturbations, including systemic inflammation and oxidative stress, and associated imbalances in electrolyte, acid–base, and volume status can contribute to profound alterations in macro- and micronutrient metabolism (Fig. 23.1). Not surprisingly, the extent of these abnormalities and the processes that drive them are important predictors of outcome in this growing population.

In the absence of specific therapies for AKI, providing nutritional and metabolic support is essential, but challenging. In addition to the fundamental question of how well patients with AKI can successfully incorporate macro- and micro nutrients, the added complexity of impaired excretion and the effects of renal replacement therapy (RRT) raise critical questions about its timing, route, amount, and safety. This chapter provides an overview of the metabolic and nutritional abnormalities in AKI and reviews the debates and current recommendations surrounding nutritional support in this growing population.

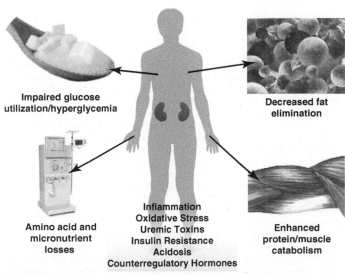

Impaired glucose utilization/hyperglycemia

Decreased fat elimination

Amino acid and micronutrient losses

**Inflammation
Oxidative Stress
Uremic Toxins
Insulin Resistance
Acidosis
Counterregulatory Hormones**

Enhanced protein/muscle catabolism

FIGURE 23.1 Metabolic and Nutritional Disorders Associated with AKI

DEFINITIONS AND EPIDEMIOLOGY

A variety of terms have been applied to describe impaired nutritional status in acute and chronic kidney disease (CKD), including "uremic wasting," "renal cachexia," and "protein–energy malnutrition." The complexity of these derangements extends beyond a lack of substrate and often involves impaired utilization and frank catabolism. In 2008, the International Society of Renal Nutrition and Metabolism proposed the term "protein–energy wasting" (PEW) to provide a consensus definition that characterized the generic loss of lean body mass and fuel reserves in patients with kidney disease (see Chapter 2). These criteria remain to be validated in both community-acquired and hospital-acquired AKI.

Components of the PEW syndrome have been observed in patients with AKI throughout the literature. Several studies have found evidence for PEW, as assessed by the Subjective Global Assessment or biochemical markers hypoalbuminemia ($<$3.5 g per dL) or hypocholesterolemia (150 mg per dL), in up to 42% in early AKI. Although not studied specifically in AKI, patients admitted to general medical services also often develop PEW during the course of hospitalization. These parameters are potent predictors of in-hospital mortality. A longitudinal study of prealbumin levels in 161 patients with AKI requiring renal consultation observed that low serum prealbumin ($<$11 mg per dL) independently predicted in-hospital mortality after adjustment for illness severity, stage of AKI, and AKI treatment. Furthermore, every 5 mg per dL increase in the prealbumin level was associated with an additional 29% decrease in-hospital mortality (hazard ratio [HR] 0.71; 95% confidence interval [CI] 0.52 to 0.96). Whether prealbumin and other plasma nutritional markers reflect recent nutritional status or are governed by the extent of underlying inflammation and illness severity has not been elucidated. Moreover, whether treatment and/or prevention of PEW impacts outcomes in AKI also remains poorly addressed.

METABOLIC AND NUTRITIONAL DERANGEMENTS IN ACUTE KIDNEY INJURY

Carbohydrate Metabolism

The kidney plays an important role in glucose metabolism. Isotopic dilution studies have demonstrated that the renal cortex is responsible for between 15% and 30% of total body gluconeogenesis whereas the medulla accounts for up to 20% of systemic glucose utilization. As kidney function declines, diminished clearance of insulin coupled with decreased glucose utilization in skeletal muscle likely contribute to the insulin resistance observed in uremia. This altered insulin sensitivity appears to be primarily a postreceptor defect of PI3K-Akt signaling, which is also subject to influence from inflammation, oxidative stress, and the accumulation of "uremic toxins." The kidney is also an important site of insulin degradation. In humans, less than 1% of the filtered insulin is freely excreted in the urine with the catabolism occurring primarily via peritubular uptake. The kidney also catabolizes the insulin precursor proinsulin and C-peptide, with the kidney accounting for most of the proinsulin catabolism.

Hyperglycemia, along with other aspects of insulin resistance, is common in critical illness and an important risk factor for death and morbidity. Up to 75% of intensive care unit (ICU) patients may have detectable insulin resistance on admission as assessed by Homeostasis Model Assessment with approximately two-thirds exhibiting overt hyperglycemia (serum glucose $>$126 mg per dL). Traditionally, insulin resistance and hyperglycemia were considered to be a part of an overall adaptive response to increase substrate and energy availability during physiologic stress. However, these responses, known as the 'diabetes of injury' are unregulated, maladaptive, and may contribute to organ dysfunction, infection, polyneuropathy of critical illness, and mortality. Some evidence suggests that intracellular accumulation of glucose has toxic effects on cellular function via enhanced generation of free radicals (oxidative stress) from increased uncoupling of oxidative phosphorylation and deleterious effects on mitochondrial ultrastructure and function. It is also known that hyperglycemia hampers the immune system, largely through the impairment of neutrophil and macrophage function. Increased hepatic gluconeogenesis and glycogenolysis and decreased insulin-driven peripheral utilization are the main effectors of this phenomenon, although excessive counterregulatory hormones, including glucagon, epi- and nor-epinephrine, cortisol, and growth hormone, also contribute. Acute illness often induces a generalized inflammatory response with the release of potent inflammatory mediators into the systemic circulation. Many of these mediators are known to be involved in both the pathogenesis of AKI and insulin resistance. Tumor necrosis factor α (TNF-α) has been associated with the development of insulin resistance in patients with renal impairment and those undergoing acute stress. In addition to secretion by macrophages, TNF-α is also found in skeletal muscle where the levels are known to inversely correlate with glucose disposal. Although the mechanism remains to be fully elucidated, a recent study demonstrated that infusion in humans induces directly suppresses phosphorylation of Akt substrate 160 leading to dysfunction of GLUT4 translocation and glucose uptake. Interleukin-6 (IL-6) is another proinflammatory cytokine that has been shown to inhibit insulin receptor tyrosine phosphorylation and downstream signaling in hepatocytes as well as in skeletal muscle in animal models. Elevated levels of IL-6 appear to predict insulin resistance in patients during acute stress such as cardiac surgery and have also been associated with the development of AKI.

The high prevalence of AKI in acutely ill patients and the known impairments of glucose metabolism resulting from loss of kidney function place patients with AKI at extraordinarily high risk for insulin resistance. A large multicenter observational study of critically ill patients with established AKI demonstrated that hyperglycemia and insulin resistance are common and independently associated with poor outcome. In this study, insulin resistance, defined by hyperglycemia in the setting of hyperinsulinemia, was associated with increased mortality rates. Moreover, glucose levels over a period of 5 weeks were significantly higher in nonsurvivors compared to survivors, and insulin levels were higher in those who died, independent of demographics and severity of illness.

Protein Metabolism

The normal adaptive response to protein malnutrition is to reduce the degradation of protein and essential amino acids. However, in patients with AKI and other acute illness, enhanced protein catabolism is often evident and reflected by excess amino acid release from the skeletal muscle and negative nitrogen balance. Protein catabolic rates of 1.4 to 1.8 g/kg/d have been reported in severe AKI, particularly among those receiving RRT. Amino acid transport into the skeletal muscle for protein synthesis may also be impaired, partly because of hepatic extraction to support gluconeogenesis and the synthesis of acute phase proteins. Negative nitrogen balance is associated with poor prognosis in patients with AKI and may also have adverse consequences on endothelial and immune function.

The mechanisms driving enhanced protein catabolism in AKI have not been well characterized, but may be related to increased activation of the ubiquitin-proteasome pathway (UPP) system. Potential contributing factors include inflammation, oxidative stress, hormone imbalances, and metabolic acidosis. Experimental infusion studies with TNF-α have demonstrated an enhanced proteolysis of muscle protein as well as a reduction in protein synthesis. Elevated IL-1 levels also appear to enhance muscle protein breakdown in animal models which may improve with pharmacologic blockade. IL-6 has been demonstrated to be associated with accelerated muscle atrophy which may be through direct upregulation of the UPP system and attenuated by IL-6 receptor antibody. Elegant studies in models of acute uremia and in patients on chronic dialysis have demonstrated that acidosis is associated with accelerated skeletal muscle and total body protein degradation, respectively, and improves with correction of the acidosis. Although often overshadowed by its effects on carbohydrate metabolism, insulin also has critical protein-anabolic affects. The earliest observations of patients with uncontrolled type 1 diabetes mellitus were characterized by markedly net negative nitrogen balance, hyperaminoacidemia, and lean tissue atrophy. However, these effects seem to also extend to insulin-resistant phenotypes and insulin-deficient states. Studies in insulin-resistant animal models have demonstrated increased protein degradation in skeletal muscle via enhanced activation of caspase-3 and the UPP system. Dialysis patients with diabetes or insulin resistance (without diabetes) exhibit increase in skeletal muscle protein breakdown compared to nondiabetic counterparts, and that diabetes predicts loss of lean body mass over time.

Lastly, RRT itself can impact protein balance. For example, chronic hemodialysis patients have demonstrated markedly enhanced whole-body and skeletal muscle protein catabolism during dialysis, likely through the induction of inflammation and oxidative stress. RRT can also itself remove significant amounts of amino acids and proteins. For example, a standard run of intermittent hemodialysis can result in as high as 8 to 10 g of amino acid loss into the dialysate, with an even greater capacity for loss during continuous renal replacement therapy (CRRT). Depending on the modality and pretreatment plasma protein concentrations, protein losses from CRRT have generally been reported to be between 1 and 15 g per day, although losses as high as 20 to 30 g per day have been observed. Although heavily influenced by flow and filtration rates, convective clearance of amino acids may exceed that of dialysis by up to 30%. These findings have direct implications for nutritional support because a significant amount of amino acids received during supplementation may be lost during treatment.

Lipid Metabolism

Several studies suggest that lipid metabolism is profoundly altered in the setting of AKI. In particular, the triglyceride content of lipoproteins is increased, whereas cholesterol content is decreased. This is true for both low-density lipoprotein (LDL) and high-density lipoprotein (HDL). The major cause of impairment in lipid metabolism appears to be inhibition of lipolytic enzyme function, including peripheral lipoprotein lipase and hepatic triglyceride lipase. These abnormalities can be exacerbated by acidosis or if heparin is administered as an anticoagulant for dialysis therapy. As a result of diminished lipolytic function, fat elimination is impaired. For example, if lipid is administered intravenously as part of parenteral nutrition (PN), clearance of fat emulsion is reduced by as much as 50%. This includes clearance of both long- and medium-chain triglycerides.

PROVIDING NUTRITION

Although AKI patients have proven to be especially susceptible to PEW and its complications, several challenges confront the provision of nutritional support to this population. It is well known, for example, that AKI patients are especially prone to fluid and solute overload from aggressive resuscitation, diminished clearance, and third spacing. Not only can this hinder accurate assessment of nutritional status, but can also heighten concerns over the potential consequences of overfeeding, including worsening azotemia, hyperglycemia, volume status, hypercapnia, electrolyte abnormalities, lipid toxicity, and increased infections. These concerns, however, must be reconciled with observations that targeted goals of supplementation are often unmet in the ICU and associated with adverse clinical outcomes. Unfortunately, the provision of nutritional support in AKI remains hindered by a paucity of adequate randomized controlled trials targeting clinical outcomes. In addition, the heterogeneity in type, timing, and severity of AKI as well as the varying co-morbidity burden of these patients makes a uniform set of recommendations for all AKI patients impossible. However, consensus guidelines, based largely on expert opinion, are available for patients with AKI from various nutritional societies, including the 2009 European Society for Clinical Nutrition and Metabolism (ESPEN) and the 2016 American Society for Parenteral and Enteral Nutrition (ASPEN)/Society of Critical Care Medicine (SCCM) (Table 23.1).

Route

Traditional teaching promotes enteral nutrition (EN) as the preferred route of supplementation in the acutely ill patients with purported benefits being maintenance of intestinal mucosa to minimize bacterial translocation, less infectious risk, and lower cost. Although systemic reviews of the trials have failed to demonstrate a clear mortality benefit with EN compared to PN, earlier studies suggested that infectious complications may be reduced, possibly because of a higher incidence of hyperglycemia and the need for central access with PN. While the relative benefits have not been well studied in AKI, additional considerations for the volume of infusion of PN and potentially the need for additional central access may be required. In one study of 182 patients with AKI, the feasibility and tolerance of EN was examined. Side effects were observed more commonly in patients with AKI than those with normal kidney function, but EN remained well tolerated overall.

ESPEN, ASPEN, and the Critical Care Group of Canada have historically supported the primary use of EN and do not recommend the routine exclusive

TABLE 23.1	Macronutrient Guidelines from Major Nutritional Societies for Patients with AKI		
Guidelines	**Energy**	**Protein**	**Comments**
ESPEN Guidelines 2006	20–30 kcal/kg/d Carbohydrate: 3–5 (max 7) g/kg/d Fat: 0.8–1.2 (max 1.5) g/kg/d	Conservative: 0.6–0.8 g/kg/d Extracorporeal therapy: 1.0–1.5 g/kg/d CRRT: up to maximum of 1.7 g/kg/d	Adapt to individual needs in cases of underweight/ obesity
SCCM/ASPEN 2016	25–30 kcal/kg/d	1.2–2.0 g/kg/d Up to 2.5 g/kg/d on RRT	Protein should not be restricted as a means to avoid/ delay initiating dialysis therapy

AKI, acute kidney injury; ASPEN, American Society for Parenteral and Enteral Nutrition; CRRT, continuous renal replacement therapy; ESPEN, European Society of Parenteral and Enteral Nutrition; RRT, renal replacement therapy; SCCM, Society of Critical Care Medicine.

use of PN in patients with functioning gastrointestinal tracts. However, a more recent pragmatic trial (CALORIES Trial) randomized 2,388 patients to EN versus PN for initiation of nutrition therapy among patients who were anticipated to be in the ICU for more than 3 days. Target energy replacement was 25 kcal per kg actual body weight within 48 to 72 hours of ICU admission. The amount of protein and caloric intake and adherence rates were similar in both groups; however, targets were not met for the majority of patients. No difference in the primary outcome of 30-day mortality (33.1% PN vs. 34.2% EN, $p = 0.57$) was observed. The mean number of infectious complications were also similar in both groups (0.22 vs. 0.21, $p = 0.72$). Adverse events differed between groups with patients receiving EN experiencing more vomiting and hypoglycemia, whereas patients receiving PN tending to have more frequent elevation of liver enzymes. Notably, most patients did not have malnutrition defined on the basis of body mass index and weight loss, and the protocol duration was 5 days. While providing some support that the negative impact of PN on clinical outcomes in modern-day practice may be overstated, these findings remain to be validated.

Timing

The optimal timing to initiate nutritional therapy in patients with AKI is not well-established, but has been addressed by recent trials in the critically ill patients (Table 23.2). The Early versus Late Parenteral Nutrition in Critically Ill Adults (EPaNIC) study randomized 4,640 critically ill patients already receiving EN to early initiation of PN within 48 hours of ICU admission versus initiation after Day 7. The amount of PN was titrated to meet caloric requirements in combination with EN to reach caloric goals. The primary endpoint of the number of ICU days differed between the two groups, with patients in the late initiation group experiencing a median 1 day shorter stay than the early-initiation group and a 6.3% relative increase in the likelihood of being discharged from the ICU earlier and alive. Modest reductions in infectious complications (26.2% vs. 22.8%, $p = 0.008$), mean cost ($1,600), and a median reduction of 3 days in the duration of RRT ($p = 0.008$) were also observed in the late-initiation group; however, no difference in mortality at 90 days were noted. In the EDEN randomized trial, 1,000 adults with acute lung injury (ALI) requiring mechanical ventilation were randomized within 48 hours of ALI to trophic or full enteral feeding during the first 6 days. Patients were excluded if there was a contraindication to enteral feeding, including high-dose vasopressors. Eligible patients were randomized to initial trophic feeding (EN at 10 mL per hour, or 10 to 20 kcal per hour) compared to the full-feeding group, which was initiated at 25 mL per hour and rapidly titrated to a target of 25 to 30 kcal/kg/d of nonprotein calories and 1.2 to 1.6 g/kg/d of protein. No difference in the primary outcome of ventilator-free days nor in other important secondary outcomes including 60-day mortality and infectious complications were observed, although the early full-feeding group experienced higher rates of vomiting, high gastric residuals, and insulin requirements. A similar study (PermiT) was recently performed in 895 general ICU patients randomized within 48 hours of ICU admission to permissive underfeeding (40% to 60% of caloric requirements until Day 14 or initiation of oral feeding) or standard feeding targeting 70% to 100% of caloric requirements with enteral feeds. During the intervention period, the average caloric intake was 46% of daily requirements in the underfeeding group versus 71% in the full-feeding group. Protein intake did not significantly differ between the groups. No difference in 90-day mortality was observed between the groups (27.2% in the underfeeding vs. 28.9% in the full-feeding group, $p = 0.58$) or in days of mechanical ventilation or hypoglycemia. Post hoc analysis suggested that incident RRT was required less frequently in the permissive underfeeding group (7.1% vs. 11.4%, $p = 0.04$) generating an interesting hypothesis about whether caloric

TABLE
23.2

Summary of Recent Clinical Trials of Nutrition in the Critically Ill Patients

Study Name/Journal/ Date/Author	Topic	Size	Setting	Intervention	Outcomes
CALORIES, NEJM 2014, Harvey	Route	2,400	Critically ill adults in the United Kingdom with unplanned admission to the ICU	EN vs. PN within 36 hr of admission and used exclusively for 5 d. Energy target = 25 kcal/kg/d within 48–72 hr	1. No difference in 30-d mortality. 2. No differences in infectious complications or mortality at 90 d. Less hypoglycemia and vomiting in PN group. Trend toward more elevation of liver enzymes in the PN group. Caloric intake similar in both the groups but target not commonly achieved.
EPaNIC, NEJM 2011, Casaer	Timing (of PN)	4,640	Critically ill adults receiving EN	Early: Day 1 400 kcal (20% glucose), Day 2, 800 kcal, Day 3 PN+EN to meet caloric needs Late: 5% glucose initiated at the same volume as the early group for hydration with PN on day 8 if insufficient calories	1. Length of ICU stay. Late initiation group had a relative 6.3% increase in the likelihood of being discharged alive earlier from the ICU, $p = 0.04$. 2. Late initiation group with relatively lower risk of mechanical ventilation >2 d and a median reduction of 3 d of RRT, and lower cost.
OMEGA, JAMA 2011, Rice	Supplements	272	Critically ill adults with acute lung injury in the United States	n-3 fatty acids, γ-linolenic acid, and antioxidants until the earliest of 21 d, 48 hr of unassisted breathing, or extubation.	1. No difference in ventilator-free days to study day 28. Stopped early for futility.
NEJM 2013, Heyland	Supplements	1,223	Critically ill adults in Canada	2 × 2 factorial: glutamine (0.35 g/kg/d IV per IBW) Antioxidants (500 μg selenium, 20 mg zinc + 10 mg β-carotene, 500 mg vitamin E, 1,500 mg vitamin C)	1. Trend toward increasing mortality at 28 d among glutamine (32.4% vs. 27.2%, $p = 0.05$). 2. No difference in mortality at 28 d in antioxidant arms (30.8% vs. 28.8%, $p = 0.48$).

EN, enteral nutrition; IBW, ideal body weight; ICU, intensive care unit; IV, intravenous; PN, parenteral nutrition; RRT, renal replacement therapy.

restriction might be renoprotective as has been demonstrated in animal studies, although further research is needed.

In summary, these recent studies suggest that early enteral support is generally well tolerated in those without contraindication (e.g., anatomic, ongoing active resuscitation); however, there may be little difference in clinical outcomes such as death or time on the ventilator between early full versus early trophic feeds in critically ill patients. Further, PN, in the short term, has a comparable safety profile to EN in the overall ICU population, although the risk of infectious complications increases over time and is higher in patients admitted with a diagnosis of sepsis. PN can be considered as an adjunct if enteral goals are not being met, although it does remain more costly and may lack some non-nutritional benefits to the gut.

Amount
Energy Requirements
Observational studies using indirect calorimetry suggest that resting energy expenditure in AKI appears to be principally determined by the acute illness associated with AKI rather than by the renal impairment itself. One study found an approximate 30% relative increase in resting energy expenditure in patients with sepsis-related AKI compared to healthy controls. However, when patients with "isolated" AKI including causes such as drug-induced interstitial nephritis or glomerulonephritis were examined, there was no similar increase in energy expenditure relative to these same controls. Another study comparing indirect calorimetry versus estimating equations in stable mechanically ventilated patients could not demonstrate a marked increase in energy expenditure between those with and without kidney injury. Based on these observations, ESPEN has recently recommended an energy intake of 20 to 30 kcal/kg/d (nonprotein calories) depending on the estimated requirement. More recently, the 2016 ASPEN/SCCM guidelines recommend a 25 to 30 kcal/kg/d target using standard enteral formulations. However, specialty formulations lower in certain electrolytes can be used if electrolyte abnormalities develop.

Protein Requirement
As previously discussed, AKI and the need for RRT markedly enhance protein catabolism with normalized protein catabolic rates of between 1.4 and 1.8 g/kg/d. Optimal dosing of protein in AKI as well as the appropriate target for nitrogen balance remains to be determined. An early observation of 40 patients on continuous venovenous hemofiltration estimated that between 1.5 and 1.8 g/kg/d of protein would be needed to achieve nitrogen balance. A subsequent nonrandomized study of AKI patients on CRRT compared a higher dose of dietary protein supplementation (2.5 g/kg/d) to a group of patients receiving standard of care (1.2 g/kg/d) with both receiving equal amount of calories. Patients receiving the higher dose of protein were more likely to achieve a positive nitrogen balance at any time during follow-up (53.6% vs. 36.7%, $p < 0.05$) and trended toward having less overall negative nitrogen balance but required more CRRT due to azotemia. Scheinkestel et al. performed a study randomizing patients to 2.0 g/kg/d or an escalating regimen of 1.5, 2.0, and 2.5 g/kg/d of protein supplementation with energy requirements estimated by Schonfield equation or indirect calorimety. Nitrogen balance was more likely to be positive with doses of greater than 2 g/kg/d associated with improved outcome after adjustment for age, sex, and severity of illness. A subsequent study examined the effect of varying energy intakes on achieving positive nitrogen balance using a crossover design in a small group of patients with acute renal failure. Comparing nutrition providing 30 versus 40 kcal/kg/d using a fixed protein dose (approximately 1.5 g/kg/d), the higher energy regimen did not

improve nitrogen balance and was associated with increased fluid administration, serum triglyceride and glucose levels, and insulin requirement. Based
on the above data, ESPEN recommends protein dosing based on the expected
degree of catabolism with 0.6 to 0.8 g/kg/d for conservative therapy, 1 to
1.5 g/kg/d for extracorporeal treatment, and a maximum of 1.7 g/kg/d in "hypercatabolism." More recent ASPEN/SCCM guidelines recommend a standard
enteral formulation targeting protein intake of 1.2 to 2 g per kg actual body
weight per day and up to a maximum of 2.5 g/kg/d among those receiving RRT.
Clearly, further adequately powered, well-designed trials with clinical endpoints
and safety monitoring are required to make more specific recommendations.

Lipids

Impaired lipolysis characterizes the main lipid abnormality of AKI, resulting
in hypertriglyceridemia, elevated very-low-density lipoprotein and LDL levels,
and diminished HDL levels. Consequently, it has been recommended that
supplementation remains between 0.8 and 1.2 g/kg/d and that total caloric
intake from fat calories not exceed 25% to 35%. This goal can usually be met with
10% to 30% lipid formulations. The impact of lipid-based medications such as
propofol should be considered into calculations. The advantages of intravenous
lipids include their high specific energy content, a low osmolality, provision of
essential fatty acids to prevent deficiency syndromes, a lower rate of hepatic
lipid accumulation, a lower risk of inducing hyperglycemia, and reduced carbon
dioxide production (especially relevant in patients with respiratory failure).

Parenteral lipid emulsions usually contain long-chain triglycerides that
are mostly derived from soybean oil, but fat emulsions containing a various
mixture of long- and medium-chain triglycerides (coconut oil) and/or olive
oil and/or fish oil are available. Whether a lower content of polyunsaturated
fatty acids yields the proposed advantages and a reduction in proinflammatory side effects is unknown. The benefits of medium-chain triglycerides in
PN formulations compared to long-chain triglycerides also remain unclear
and are not widely available. Frequent monitoring of triglyceride levels
and liver function is also recommended, especially when PN is employed
with adjustments made as necessary to avoid problems associated with
hypertriglyceridemia.

Micronutrients and Other Additives

The use of key additives to EN to modulate inflammatory or immune response,
including glutamine, arginine, and ω-3 fatty acids, has garnered interest in
recent years. Glutamine is a nonessential amino acid abundantly synthesized
in skeletal muscle that has often been regarded as "conditionally essential"
during catabolic illness. Observations of increased utilization by immune cells
and that low levels associated with poor outcomes have led to the hypothesis
that supplementation may be beneficial. Similarly, oxidative stress is involved
both in the pathogenesis of AKI and as a common finding in patients with
AKI. The applicability of the so-called "immunonutrition," or more recently,
"pharmaconutrition," in critically ill patients has been examined in several
small studies largely failing to demonstrate significant mortality benefit. In
addition to being underpowered, many of these early studies suffered from
heterogeneity in the patient populations, and formulations applied may be
contributing to the lack of a demonstrable effect. Even less is known about
their role in AKI; however, significant losses of glutamine (3.5 to 3.6 g per
day) have been demonstrated in patients on CRRT, suggesting the need for
supplementation although dose and safety remain undetermined.

A more recent trial randomized 1,223 mechanically ventilated patients
with two or more organ failures in a 2 × 2 factorial design to treatment with
glutamine versus no glutamine and antioxidants versus no antioxidants,

the latter containing selenium, zinc, β-carotene, and vitamins E and C. Supplements were started within 24 hours of ICU admission and provided enterally and intravenously. Median time to starting nutrition was within 24 hours of the first organ failure. In all, 80% of patients received EN only, and <10% received any PN. There were no differences in the type or amount of calories or protein received in each study arm. The primary outcome of the study was 28-day mortality, and there was a trend toward higher mortality among those receiving glutamine compared with those who did not (32.4% vs. 28.2%, $p = 0.05$), with no significant differences in mortality between those receiving antioxidant supplements and those who did not. No interaction was observed in patients receiving both. Among secondary outcomes, in-hospital mortality and 6-month mortality were higher among patients receiving glutamine compared to those who did not as well as longer length of ICU stay. Supplementation with glutamine (enterally or parenterally) is currently NOT recommended for routine use in critically ill patients; however, some interest remains in the use of these formulations in specific subpopulations with specific pathologies, including traumatic brain injury and trauma.

Other antioxidants have been evaluated in the ICU setting, albeit not specifically for AKI. N-acetyl-cysteine (NAC), a thiol-containing antioxidant, has minimal toxicity and is routinely used for the treatment of fulminant hepatic failure caused by acetaminophen (and more recently, other types of fulminant hepatic failure). Several small trials evaluating the use of NAC therapy in critically ill patients have been performed with somewhat mixed results. Although PN enriched with anti-inflammatory fish oils and antioxidants was shown in a small trial in patients with acute respiratory distress syndrome to improve clinical outcomes, there was no benefit in the larger OMEGA clinical trial, which was stopped for futility. In a single-center randomized clinical trial, patients receiving methylene blue (an inhibitor of the nitric oxide pathway) had improved oxygen delivery, reduced body temperature, and reduced requirements for pressor support. In animal models of ischemic AKI, edaravone (a free-radical scavenger) and mesna (a thiol-containing antioxidant) have demonstrated renoprotective effects and thus may be suitable for clinical trials in patients with AKI. However, the lack of compelling evidence for immunomodulatory nutrition regimens has made them difficult to recommend for routine use in the critically ill patients or in AKI patients.

Alterations in the metabolism of vitamins and trace elements in AKI patients have not been well studied. In patients receiving CRRT, losses of water-soluble vitamins in effluent have been reported although limited data exist to support specific recommendations for replacement. For example, vitamin C losses have been reported during CRRT, but concerns over the possibility of secondary oxalosis led the ESPEN in 2009 to recommend replacement not exceed between 30 and 50 mg per day, recognizing that greater amounts may be needed in some patients on CRRT. Similarly, vitamin A is known to accumulate in renal impairment as a result of diminished clearance of retinol-binding protein and retinol which are also poorly dialyzed. As a result, a careful weighing of the risk/potential benefit of significant supplementation in patients with AKI should be considered. If replacement is deemed necessary, a conservative approach with close monitoring for signs and symptoms of vitamin A toxicity is reasonable, the latter being recommended in the most recent ESPEN guidelines. Folate losses have also been reported in one study to be about 265 μg per day. Thiamine (vitamin B_1), vitamin B_6, selenium, zinc, and copper losses have also been reported in patients undergoing CRRT with suggestions for replacement at doses greater than the recommended dietary allowance.

Lastly, as electrolyte requirements will vary among a heterogeneous AKI population and can change quickly (particularly in patients receiving RRT), there are also currently no "standard" recommendations for electrolytes. Although special formulations lower in potassium and phosphorous may be of benefit in some patients, replacement and decision-making needing to be evaluated on an individual and day-to-day basis. Conversely, patients on CRRT may need phosphorus supplementation after 3 to 5 days.

Insulin

Given the adverse impact that hyperglycemia and insulin resistance have on clinical outcomes, the optimal level of glycemic control in critically ill patients has been a subject of great interest. One early study of intensive insulin therapy designed to maintain blood glucose at or below 110 mg per dL was shown to reduce morbidity and mortality in a surgical ICU. Although mortality data in a subsequent study from a medical ICU at the same institution were equivocal, subgroup analysis suggested that benefit might be derived in those staying in the ICU for greater than 3 days. The effect of intensive insulin therapy in patients with established AKI remains to be determined; however, intensive insulin therapy has been postulated to have a role in the prevention of AKI. The potential mechanism of benefit is unclear, but may be related to a decrease in cellular glucotoxicity or another metabolic effect of insulin such as reduction in protein catabolism or improvements in dyslipidemia. However, there is a significant risk of life-threatening hypoglycemia with intensive insulin therapy, and two subsequent trials in mixed ICU populations were terminated early because of increased hypoglycemia without apparent clinical benefit. The largest study in this field, the multinational prospective randomized Normoglycemia in Intensive Care Evaluation – Survival Using Glucose Algorithm Regulation (NICE-SUGAR) Study, confirmed these earlier signals regarding the potential harm of overly tight glucose control by randomizing 6,104 critically ill patients anticipated to remain in the ICU for more than 3 days to tight (81 to 108 mg per dL) or moderate (144 to 180 mg per dL) glycemic control using a uniform standardized intravenous insulin administration protocol. Intensive glucose control was associated with a higher rate of death at 90 days (27.5% vs. 24.9%, $p = 0.02$) and a greater incidence of severe hypoglycemia (blood glucose level $\leq$40) (6.8% vs. 0.5%, $p < 0.001$). Of note, no differences in the need for or days of RRT were observed between the groups despite similar renal function at study entry.

Based on these results, the target blood glucose of 140- or 150 to 180 mg per dL for general ICU populations has been recommended. As the attendant risk of hypoglycemia may be even more severe in patients with AKI because of impaired insulin metabolism by the kidney, attention to potential contributions from nephrologic care to both hypoglycemia and hyperglycemia is warranted. For example, awareness of how changes in delivery/dose of RRT may impact glucose levels in patients receiving insulin therapy as well as the glucose content of dialysate/replacement fluids, PN, and medications are paramount to reducing risk.

CONCLUSION

In conclusion, AKI is a complex disease associated with a wide array of metabolic derangements resulting from loss of renal homeostatic function, the byproducts of injury, and the impact of RRT. Inflammation, oxidative stress, and insulin resistance can have profound implications for the utilization and catabolism of key substrates, ultimately hindering the ability of afflicted patients to promote cellular recovery. Although adequately designed and powered studies examining the optimal approach to metabolic and nutritional support in patients with AKI are lacking, nutritional risk is high in this patient population and independently predicts morbidity and mortality. Consequently, frequent ascertainment of the nutritional and metabolic demands of patients is warranted with an individualized therapeutic approach coupling the best-available evidence and guidelines for patients with comparable illness severity with vigilant monitoring for complications.

Suggested Readings

Arabi YM, Aldawood AS, Haddad SH, et al. Permissive underfeeding or standard enteral feeding in critically ill adults. *N Engl J Med* 2015;372:2398–2408.

Basi S, Pupim LB, Simmons EM, et al. Insulin resistance in critically ill patients with acute renal failure. *Am J Physiol Renal Physiol* 2005;289:F259–F264.

Berger MM, Shenkin A, Revelly JP, et al. Copper, selenium, zinc, and thiamine balances during continuous venovenous hemodiafiltration in critically ill patients. *Am J Clin Nutr* 2004;80:410–416.

Cano NJ, Aparicio M, Brunori G, et al. ESPEN guidelines on parenteral nutrition: adult renal failure. *Clin Nutr* 2009;28:401–414.

Casaer MP, Mesotten D, Hermans G, et al. Early versus late parenteral nutrition in critically ill adults. *N Engl J Med* 2011;365:506–517.

Fiaccadori E, Lombardi M, Leonardi S, et al. Prevalence and clinical outcome associated with preexisting malnutrition in acute renal failure: a prospective cohort study. *J Am Soc Nephrol* 1999;10:581–593.

Fiaccadori E, Maggiore U, Giacosa R, et al. Enteral nutrition in patients with acute renal failure. *Kidney Int* 2004;65:999–1008.

Fiaccadori E, Maggiore U, Rotelli C, et al. Effects of different energy intakes on nitrogen balance in patients with acute renal failure: a pilot study. *Nephrol Dial Transplant* 2005;20:1976–1980.

Finfer S, Chittock DR, Su SY, et al. Intensive versus conventional glucose control in critically ill patients. *N Engl J Med* 2009;360:1283–1297.

Harvey SE, Parrott F, Harrison DA, et al. Trial of the route of early nutritional support in critically ill adults. *N Engl J Med* 2014;371:1673–1684.

Heyland D, Muscedere J, Wischmeyer PE, et al. A randomized trial of glutamine and antioxidants in critically ill patients. *N Engl J Med* 2013;368:1489–1497.

Himmelfarb J, McMonagle E, Freedman S, et al. Oxidative stress is increased in critically ill patients with acute renal failure. *J Am Soc Nephrol* 2004;15:2449–2456.

Klein CJ, Moser-Veillon PB, Schweitzer A, et al. Magnesium, calcium, zinc, and nitrogen loss in trauma patients during continuous renal replacement therapy. *JPEN J Parenter Enteral Nutr* 2002;26:77–92; discussion 92–73.

Macias WL, Alaka KJ, Murphy MH, et al. Impact of the nutritional regimen on protein catabolism and nitrogen balance in patients with acute renal failure. *JPEN J Parenter Enteral Nutr* 1996;20:56–62.

National Heart, Lung, and Blood Institute Acute Respiratory Distress Syndrome (ARDS) Clinical Trials Network, Rice TW, Wheeler AP, Thompson BT, et al. Initial trophic vs full enteral feeding in patients with acute lung injury: the EDEN randomized trial. *JAMA* 2012;307:795–803.

Scheinkestel CD, Adams F, Mahony L, et al. Impact of increasing parenteral protein loads on amino acid levels and balance in critically ill anuric patients on continuous renal replacement therapy. *Nutrition* 2003;19:733–740.

Schetz M, Vanhorebeek I, Wouters PJ, et al. Tight blood glucose control is renoprotective in critically ill patients. *J Am Soc Nephrol* 2008;19:571–578.

Simmons EM, Himmelfarb J, Sezer MT, et al. Plasma cytokine levels predict mortality in patients with acute renal failure. *Kidney Int* 2004;65:1357–1365.

Taylor BE, McClave SA, Martindale RG, et al. Guidelines for the provision and assessment of nutrition support therapy in the adult critically ill patient: Society of Critical Care Medicine (SCCM) and American Society for Parenteral and Enteral Nutrition (A.S.P.E.N.). *Crit Care Med* 2016;44:390–438.

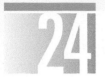

Nutrition in Pediatric Kidney Disease

Vimal Chadha, Rosanne J. Woloschuk, and Bradley A. Warady

The nutritional management of children with chronic kidney disease (CKD) poses several unique challenges that must be addressed if target outcomes such as normal growth and bone health are to be achieved. This is particularly important for those children with CKD from early infancy in whom optimal nutrition plays a very essential role in growth during this stage of life. Clinical experience also suggests that inadequate nutrition may contribute to an impaired neurodevelopmental outcome in the youngest patients with CKD. Most importantly, physical manifestations of poor growth, such as short stature and low body mass index (BMI), have been associated with an increased risk of mortality in children with CKD. Dietary restrictions in children, therefore, should be limited as much as possible with a goal of enhancing nutrient intake while always taking the severity of CKD and the clinical implications of dietary management into consideration.

ASSESSMENT OF NUTRITIONAL STATUS

Assessment of the nutritional status of children with CKD requires the evaluation of multiple indices because there is no single measure that by itself can accurately reflect a patient's nutritional status. A variety of physical measurements and anthropometric data plotted on appropriate growth charts, along with an evaluation of the dietary intake, are required to provide a comprehensive picture. The recommended frequency of the nutritional evaluation depends on both the age of the child and the severity of CKD, as recommended in the Kidney Disease Outcomes Quality Initiative (KDOQI) pediatric nutrition guidelines (Table 24.1).

Evaluation of Nutrient Intake

Dietary recall and food intake records kept in a diary are the two most common methods used for estimating nutrient intake. The dietary recall (usually obtained for the previous 24 hours) is a simple, rapid method of obtaining a crude assessment of dietary intake. Because it relies on the patient's (or their parents) memory, the responses may not always be valid. However, the advantages of the recall method are that respondents usually will not be able to modify their eating behavior in anticipation of this dietary evaluation. The most important limitation of the 24-hour recall method is its poor ability to capture the day-to-day variability in dietary intake. Children may be even more susceptible to this limitation than adults because they tend to exhibit more day-to-day variability. Therefore, it may be useful to obtain three 24-hour recalls to more completely evaluate the food intake pattern.

A dietary diary is a prospective written report of food eaten during a specified length of time, including a weekend day. A food intake diary provides a more reliable estimate of an individual's nutrient intake than do single-day records. Although dietary diaries have been shown to give unbiased estimates of energy intake in normal weight children younger than 10 years of age,

TABLE
24.1

Recommended Parameters and Frequency of Nutritional Assessment for Children with CKD Stages 2 to 5 and 5D

| | Minimum Interval in months | | | | | | | | | |
| Measure | Age 0 to <1 yr | | | Age 1-3 yr | | | Age >3 yr | | | |
	CKD 2-3	CKD 4-5	CKD 5D	CKD 2-3	CKD 4-5	CKD 5D	CKD 2	CKD 3	CKD 4-5	CKD 5D
Dietary intake	0.5-3	0.5-3	0.5-2	1-3	1-3	1-3	6-12	6	3-4	3-4
Height or length-for-age percentile or SDS	0.5-1.5	0.5-1.5	0.5-1	1-3	1-2	1	3-6	3-6	1-3	1-3
Height or length velocity-for-age percentile or SDS	0.5-2	0.5-2	0.5-1	1-6	1-3	1-2	6	6	6	6
Estimated dry weight and weight-for-age percentile or SDS	0.5-1.5	0.5-1.5	0.25-1	1-3	1-2	0.5-1	3-6	3-6	1-3	1-3
BMI-for-height-age percentile or SDS	0.5-1.5	0.5-1.5	0.5-1	1-3	1-2	1	3-6	3-6	1-3	1-3
Head circumference-for-age percentile or SDS	0.5-1.5	0.5-1.5	0.5-1	1-3	1-2	1-2	N/A	N/A	N/A	N/A
nPCR	N/A	N/A	N/A	N/A	N/A	N/A	N/A	N/A	N/A	1*

BMI, body mass index; CKD, chronic kidney disease; HD, hemodialysis; N/A, not applicable; nPCR, normalized protein catabolic rate; SDS, standard deviation score.
*Only applies to adolescents receiving HD.

underreporting is common in adolescents. Accordingly, 24-hour recalls may be better suited to the adolescent population.

Physical Measurements (Anthropometry)

The evaluation of anthropometric parameters is a fundamental component of the nutritional assessment in pediatrics, and must be accurately measured using calibrated equipment according to standardized techniques. Recumbent length, height, weight, and head circumference are measured directly, and BMI is calculated as weight (in kg) divided by height (in meters) squared; reference values are available for children older than 2 years of age. It is important to note that serial measurements are necessary for the assessment of growth.

Once measured, weight, length/height, head circumference, and BMI should be plotted on the appropriate growth chart, specific for the patient's age and sex. For premature infants, the growth parameters should be plotted after correcting for their gestational age until they are 2 years old. In 2000, the Center for Disease Control (CDC) published revised North American growth reference charts for infants and children up to 20 years of age and in 2006, the World Health Organization (WHO) released new growth standards for children from birth to 5 years of age. The WHO growth *standards* are distinguished from the CDC *reference* charts in that the WHO *standards* are based on the outcomes of children growing under ideal conditions (nonsmoking mothers, lived in areas of high-socioeconomic status, and received regular pediatric health care), with a subset of the children breastfed for at least 4 months, in contrast to the general population.

Because the WHO Child Growth *Standards* represent ideal growth and ideal growth should be the goal for children with CKD as well, the WHO Child Growth *Standards* should be used as the reference for children from birth to 2 years of age. Thereafter, the differences between the CDC reference curves and the WHO Child Growth *Standards* are minimal. For this reason and because the switch is made from length to height measurement at 2 years, transition from the WHO Child Growth *Standards* to the CDC reference curves should be made at this age.

Normalized Protein Catabolic Rate

In adolescent patients undergoing maintenance hemodialysis (HD), the normalized protein nitrogen appearance (nPNA), also known as normalized protein catabolic rate (nPCR), should be determined. The PCR is the amount of protein that is catabolized in excess of the amount that is synthesized and in a person in steady state, the PCR is a reflection of the dietary protein intake (DPI). It is dependent upon the urea generation rate (G) during the interdialytic period, and it can be calculated simultaneously during formal Kt/V estimations by urea kinetic modeling. Recent pediatric data have demonstrated that a nPCR <1 g/kg/d of protein predicted a sustained weight loss of at least 2% per month for 3 consecutive months in adolescent and young adult–aged HD patients. In younger patients, the nPCR was not effective in predicting weight loss.

Serum Albumin

Many studies have shown that hypoalbuminemia present at the time of dialysis initiation, as well as during the course of chronic dialysis, is a strong independent predictor of patient morbidity and mortality. However, despite its clinical utility, serum albumin levels may be insensitive to short-term changes in nutritional status, do not necessarily correlate with changes in other nutritional parameters, and can be influenced by non-nutritional factors such as infection/inflammation, hydration status, peritoneal or urinary albumin losses, and acidemia. Therefore, while hypoalbuminemia remains an important component of the general evaluation of patients with CKD, its value as an exclusive marker of nutritional status is questionable.

NUTRITIONAL REQUIREMENTS

Energy Requirements

A number of studies have shown that the majority of pediatric patients with CKD exhibit an inadequate dietary energy intake, and the energy intake progressively decreases with worsening kidney function. However, there is no evidence that the energy requirements for children with CKD should be any different than those for healthy children. In turn, the energy requirements for children with CKD should be 100% of the estimated energy requirement (EER) for chronologic age (Table 24.2), and then adjusted for the individual physical activity level and gender. It is important to note that the calculated energy requirements are estimates only, and some children will require more or less for normal growth; therefore, all dietary prescriptions should be individualized. In fact, because prevention and treatment of obesity in children with CKD is also important, it is imperative to recognize that energy requirements for overweight or obese children are lower and can be estimated by using equations specific for children heavier than a healthy weight.

Energy requirements for pediatric patients who receive maintenance HD or peritoneal dialysis (PD) are similar to those of predialysis patients with CKD. In children receiving PD, variable glucose absorption takes place from the dialysis fluid depending on the PD modality, the dialysate glucose concentration, and the peritoneal membrane solute transport capacity, with the mean energy intake derived from peritoneal glucose absorption in one study found to be 9 kcal/kg/d. Because many children who receive chronic PD are underweight, the prescribed dietary energy intake in them should exclude the estimated calorie absorption from the dialysate because failure to do so may compromise the nutritional quality of the diet. However, some children and particularly infants receiving PD therapy, gain weight at a faster rate than normal; in these cases, the calorie contribution from dialysate should be taken into account when estimating energy requirements.

Protein Requirements

It has been postulated that a high-protein diet results in glomerular hyper-filtration, which may result in kidney injury. In addition, there is a nearly

Age	EER (kcal/d) = Total Energy Expenditure + Energy Deposition
0–3 mo	EER = [89 × weight (kg) – 100] + 175
4–6 mo	EER = [89 × weight (kg) – 100] + 56
7–12 mo	EER = [89 × weight (kg) – 100] + 22
13–35 mo	EER = [89 × weight (kg) – 100] + 20
3–8 yr boys	EER = 88.5 – 61.9 × age (y) + PA × [26.7 *x* weight (kg) + 903 × height (m)] + 20
Girls	EER = 135.3 – 30.8 × age (y) + PA × [10 *x* weight (kg) + 934 × height (m)] + 20
9–18 yr boys	EER = 88.5 – 61.9 × age (y) + PA × [26.7 × weight (kg) + 903 × height (m)] + 25
Girls	EER = 135.3 – 30.8 × age (y) + PA × [10 × weight (kg) + 934 × height (m)] + 25

TABLE 24.2 Equations to Estimate Energy Requirements for Children at Healthy Weights

EER, estimated energy requirement; PA, physical activity.

linear relationship between protein and phosphorus intake that results in the frequent association between a high-protein diet, hyperphosphatemia, and the associated risks of cardiovascular disease (CVD). On the other hand, low-protein diets reduce the generation of nitrogenous wastes and inorganic ions, both of which might be responsible for many of the clinical and metabolic disturbances characteristic of uremia. In children, however, there is concern about the potential harmful effects of severe dietary protein restriction, particularly as it pertains to the growth of infants and young children with CKD. To that end, the largest randomized pediatric trial designed to study the impact of dietary protein restriction investigated nearly 200 children with CKD Stages 3 and 4 and found that there was no evidence for a nephroprotective effect of modest dietary protein restriction, and that the DPI can be safely restricted to 0.8 to 1.1 g/kg/d in children with CKD without compromising growth.

Although the spontaneous DPI is reduced in progressive CKD in a manner similar to that of energy intake, the DPI typically remains far in excess of the average requirements, ranging from 150% to 200% of the recommended daily allowance. Current KDOQI Pediatric Nutrition guidelines recommend maintaining the DPI at 100% to 140% of the dietary reference intakes (DRI) for ideal body weight in children with CKD Stage 3 and at 100% to 120% of the DRI in children with CKD Stages 4 and 5 (Table 24.3). These dietary protein recommendations refer to the needs of a stable child and assume that the energy intake is adequate (i.e., meets 100% of EER). Protein requirements may be increased in patients with proteinuria and during recovery from intercurrent illness and may be adjusted to height age instead of chronologic age if evidence of protein deficiency exists.

Protein requirements for children receiving maintenance dialysis therapy are higher than those of children predialysis because of protein/nitrogen losses associated with the dialysis procedure. In those receiving PD, daily peritoneal protein losses decrease with age across childhood from an average of 0.28 g per kg in the first year of life to less than 0.1 g per kg in adolescents (Table 24.3). Patients with high peritoneal membrane transport characteristics tend to have low serum albumin levels, likely because of increased peritoneal protein losses; these patients may have slightly greater protein requirements.

Amino acid and protein losses during HD vary according to dialyzer membrane characteristics and reuse. Whereas losses have not been quantified

TABLE 24.3   Recommended Dietary Protein Intake in Children with CKD Stages 3 to 5 and 5D

Age	DRI (g/kg/d)	Recommended for CKD Stage 3 (g/kg/d) (100%–140% DRI)	Recommended for CKD Stages 4 and 5 (g/kg/d) (100%–120% DRI)	Recommended for HD (g/kg/d)*	Recommended for PD (g/kg/d)†
0–6 mo	1.5	1.5–2.1	1.5–1.8	1.6	1.8
7–12 mo	1.2	1.2–1.7	1.2–1.5	1.3	1.5
1–3 yr	1.05	1.05–1.5	1.05–1.25	1.15	1.3
4–13 yr	0.95	0.95–1.35	0.95–1.15	1.05	1.1
14–18 yr	0.85	0.85–1.2	0.85–1.05	0.95	1.0

CKD, chronic kidney disease; DRI, dietary reference intakes; HD, hemodialysis; PD, peritoneal dialysis.
*DRI + 0.1 g/kg/d to compensate for dialysis losses.
†DRI + 0.15 – 0.3 g/kg/d depending on patient age to compensate for peritoneal losses.

in children, an average of 8 to 10 g of amino acids and less than 1 to 3 g of protein are lost per HD session in adults. On the basis of three HD sessions per week for a 70 kg adult, this equates to 0.08 g/kg/d. Assuming that dialytic amino acid losses are linearly related to urea kinetics, children can be expected to have similar or slightly higher amino acid losses than adults, and an added DPI of 0.1 g/kg/d should be appropriate to compensate for pediatric HD losses.

The most convincing argument for limiting DPI in dialyzed children is derived from the solid evidence for a key etiologic role of dietary phosphorus load in the pathogenesis of secondary hyperparathyroidism and dialysis-associated calcifying arteriopathy. Hence, it appears most appropriate to limit protein intake and associated phosphorus intake in children on dialysis to the safe levels known to ensure adequate growth and nutrition in healthy children. Apart from the quantity of protein intake, the source of protein is also important. It is advised that at least 50% of the total protein intake consist of protein of high biologic value such as the protein from milk, eggs, meat, fish, and poultry. Attention should also be paid to the ratio of the phosphorus to the protein content of the foods with preference given to foods with a low phosphorus to protein content ratio.

Lipid Management

Dyslipidemia is a frequently recognized complication of CKD in children, occurs relatively early in the course of CKD (i.e., CKD Stage 3), and increases in prevalence with decreasing kidney function. The dyslipidemia seen in children with CKD has complex underlying metabolic alterations and is characterized by increased levels of serum triglycerides (TG) in combination with high levels of very-low-density lipoprotein and intermediate-density lipoproteins, low levels of HDL particles, and normal or modestly increased levels of total and low-density lipoprotein (LDL) cholesterol. This pattern of dyslipidemia has been labeled "atherogenic."

The optimal management of dyslipidemia in children with CKD is not clearly defined. Treatment of malnutrition related to impaired kidney function is essential and should supersede any potential rise in lipid levels that might result from it. In children with hypercholesterolemia, less than 25% to 30% of calories should come from dietary fat, of which ≤7% should be from saturated fatty acids; the daily cholesterol intake should be <200 mg. For those patients with serum triglyceride >150 mg per dL, therapeutic lifestyle changes are recommended along with a low-fat diet and a low intake of simple carbohydrates. The child should be encouraged to ingest complex carbohydrates in lieu of simple sugars and concentrated sweets and to use unsaturated fats such as oils and margarines from corn, safflower and soy. Plant stanol esters in the form of dietary supplements reduce intestinal cholesterol absorption and may provide a safe and effective means of reducing serum cholesterol.

A high intake of n-3 polyunsaturated fatty acids (omega-3 fatty acids, docosahexanoic acid and eicosapentanoic acid) are associated with decreasing TG levels and a decreased risk of heart disease, whereas dietary fiber, particularly naturally occurring viscous fiber or mineral- and electrolyte-free powdered forms of fiber (e.g., Unifiber, Benefiber), may help reduce total and LDL cholesterol levels; high intakes have been associated with reduced rates of CVD.

BONE MINERAL METABOLISM

Calcium

Adequate dietary calcium intake during childhood is necessary for skeletal development and acquisition of optimal peak bone mass. The current recommendation is that patients with CKD should achieve a calcium intake of 100% of the DRI (Table 24.4). Infants and young children usually meet the DRI for calcium with the consumption of adequate volumes of breast milk formula. Unfortunately, the largest source of dietary calcium for most persons are dairy products which are also rich in phosphorus; in turn, phosphorus restriction universally leads to a decreased calcium intake. In these situations, calcium supplementation may be required. The target calcium intake can be achieved through the use of calcium-containing phosphate binders or supplemental calcium salts such as carbonate (40% elemental calcium), acetate (25% elemental calcium), and gluconate (9% elemental calcium). When used for calcium supplementation alone, ingesting these products between meals maximizes calcium absorption. Chloride and citrate salts of calcium should be avoided because the former may lead to acidosis in patients with CKD and the latter may enhance aluminum absorption.

On the other hand, excessive calcium intake in conjunction with activated vitamin D analogs can lead to hypercalcemia, adynamic bone disease, and systemic calcification. Accordingly, the KDOQI guidelines recommend that the combined elemental calcium intake from nutritional sources and phosphate binders should not exceed 2 times the DRI for age, except for ages 9 to 18 years (both genders) where 2 times the DRI (2,600 mg) exceeds the tolerable upper intake level of 2,500 mg.

Phosphorus

In an effort to prevent/control CKD-associated bone disease and CVD, serum phosphorus concentrations above the normal reference range for age should be avoided in patients with advanced CKD/end stage renal disease (ESRD). Dietary phosphorus restriction decreases parathyroid hormone (PTH) levels and increases $1,25(OH)_2D$, whereas dietary phosphorus intakes approximately twice the DRI for age aggravate hyperparathyroidism despite little or no change in serum phosphorus levels (likely the result of elevated fibroblast growth factor-23 levels and enhanced phosphorus excretion). It is important to note that the higher physiologic serum concentrations of calcium and phosphorus that are observed in healthy infants and young children presumably reflect the increased requirements for these minerals by the rapidly growing skeleton. As such, rickets caused by phosphorus deficiency can occur in preterm infants whose diet provides insufficient quantities of phosphorus; hence, subnormal serum phosphorus values are equally important to avoid. Recently published recommendations suggest that in children with CKD whose serum PTH concentration exceeds the target range, but whose

Age	DRI	Upper Limit (for Healthy Children)	Upper Limit for CKD Stages 2–5, 5D (Dietary + Phosphate Binders*)
0–6 mo	210	ND	≤420
7–12 mo	270	ND	≤540
1–3 yr	500	2,500	≤1,000
4–8 yr	800	2,500	≤1,600
9–18 yr	1,300	2,500	≤2,500

Recommended Calcium Intake for Children with CKD Stages 2 to 5 and 5D

CKD, chronic kidney disease; DRI, dietary reference intakes; ND, not determined.
*Determined as 200% of the DRI, to a maximum of 2,500 mg elemental calcium.

Recommended Maximum Oral and/or Enteral Phosphorus (mg per day) Intake for Children with CKD

Age	DRI (mg/d)	High PTH and Normal Phosphorus*	High PTH and High Phosphorus†
0–6 mo	100	≤100	≤80
7–12 mo	275	≤275	≤220
1–3 yr	460	≤460	≤370
4–8 yr	500	≤500	≤400
9–18 yr	1,250	≤1,250	≤1,000

CKD, chronic kidney disease; DRI, dietary reference intakes; PTH, parathyroid hormone.
*≤100% of the DRI.
†≤80% of the DRI.

serum phosphorus concentration remains normal, the dietary phosphorus intake should be restricted to 100% of the DRI; in contrast, the intake should be restricted to 80% of the DRI when the serum phosphorus concentration exceeds the normal reference range for age (Table 24.5).

It is important to note that an overly strict dietary phosphorus restriction is not only often impractical, but extremely low-phosphorus diets are typically unpalatable. While young infants are characteristically managed with a low-phosphorus containing milk formula such as Similac PM 60/40 (Abbott Nutrition), or Renastart (Vitaflo Nutrition), or by pretreatment of breastmilk/infant formula with sevelamer carbonate (Renvela), some infants may require phosphorus supplementation in the form of sodium phosphate (Neutra-Phos) because of their higher physiologic needs, as mentioned previously. Most other patients with CKD/ESRD require oral intestinal phosphate binders to control hyperphosphatemia. Whereas food labels rarely state the phosphorus content, foods rich in phosphorus such as chocolates, nuts, dried beans, and the many foods and fluids that contain phosphorus-based food additives (e.g., cola soft drinks) should be avoided; nondairy creamers and certain frozen nondairy desserts may be used in place of milk and ice cream.

Vitamin D
Recent clinical evidence suggests a high prevalence (typically 80% to 90%) of nutritional vitamin D insufficiency in both children and adults with CKD. Ali et al. reported a 20% to 75% prevalence of vitamin D deficiency (25(OH)D <15 ng per mL) in children with CKD Stages 1 to 5, with higher prevalence rates in Hispanics and African-Americans, likely because of increased melanin content of their skin. This insufficiency may aggravate secondary hyperparathyroidism in patients with CKD because the availability of 25(OH)$_2$D becomes a rate-limiting step for the synthesis of 1,25(OH)$_2$D. Accordingly, the latest KDOQI Pediatric Nutrition Guidelines suggest checking serum 25(OH)$_2$D levels once per year in children with CKD Stages 2 to 5 and 5D. If the serum level of 25(OH)$_2$D is <30 ng per mL, supplementation with vitamin D$_2$ (ergocalciferol) or vitamin D$_3$ (cholecalciferol) is suggested, with the specific dosing regimen dependent on the severity of the deficiency (Table 24.6).

ELECTROLYTES
Sodium
Sodium requirements in children with CKD are dependent on the underlying kidney disease and the degree of renal insufficiency. Children who have CKD

Recommended Supplementation for Vitamin D Deficiency/ Insufficiency in Children with CKD

Serum 25(OH)D (ng/mL)	Definition	Ergocaliferol (Vitamin D₂) or Cholecalciferol (Vitamin D₃) Dosing	Duration (mo)
<5	Severe vitamin D deficiency	8,000 IU/d orally or enterally × 4 wk or (50,000 IU/wk × 4 wk); then 4,000 IU/d or (50,000 IU twice per mo for 2 mo) × 2 mo	3
5–15	Mild vitamin D deficiency	4,000 IU/d orally or enterally × 12 wk or (50,000 IU every other wk, for 12 wk)	3
16–30	Vitamin D insufficiency	2,000 IU daily or (50,000 IU every 4 wk)	3

CKD, chronic kidney disease.

as a result of obstructive uropathy (i.e., posterior urethral valves) or renal dysplasia are most often polyuric and may experience substantial urinary sodium losses despite advanced degrees of CKD. Sodium depletion adversely affects growth and nitrogen retention, and its intake supports the normal expansion of the extracellular fluid volume needed for muscle development and mineralization of bone. In turn, infants and children with polyuric salt-wasting forms of CKD who do not have their sodium and water losses corrected may experience vomiting, constipation, and significant growth retardation associated with chronic intravascular volume depletion and a negative sodium balance. It should be emphasized that normal serum sodium levels do not rule out sodium depletion and the need for supplementation. Sodium supplementation can be given as chloride or bicarbonate depending upon the patient's acid–base status.

In contrast, children with CKD resulting from a primary glomerular disease, or those who are oliguric or anuric, typically require a sodium and fluid restriction to minimize fluid gain, edema formation, and hypertension. These patients should be advised to avoid processed foods and snacks from fast-food restaurants because the majority (75%) of sodium in the diet comes from salt added during food processing.

Infants receiving PD are predisposed to substantial sodium losses, even when anuric. High ultrafiltration requirements per kilogram of body weight result in removal of significant amounts of sodium chloride during dialysis. These losses are not adequately replaced through the low-sodium content of breast milk or standard commercial infant formulas, and infants on PD are, therefore, at risk for developing hyponatremia and hypotension that can result in cerebral edema and blindness. Sodium supplementation (2 to 10 mEq/kg/d) should be individualized based on clinical symptoms, including hypotension, hyponatremia, and/or abnormal serum chloride levels.

Potassium

Potassium homeostasis in children with CKD is usually unaffected until the glomerular filtration rate (GFR) falls to <10% of normal. However, children with renal dysplasia, postobstructive kidney damage, severe reflux nephropathy, and renal insufficiency secondary to interstitial nephritis often demonstrate renal tubular resistance to aldosterone and may manifest hyperkalemia, even when their GFR is relatively well preserved. The hyperkalemia experienced by these children is exacerbated by volume contraction (and can be particularly common in salt losers), and the majority of patients respond to salt and water

Nutrient Content per 100 kcal

Formula (kcal/oz)	Volume (mL)	Protein (g)	Sodium (mg)	Potassium (mg)	Calcium (mg)	Phosphorus (mg)
Human milk (20)	150	1.3	25	83	53	21
Similac PM 60/40 (20)	150	2.2	24	80	56	28
Renastart (30)	100	1.6	50	23	22	19
Suplena (54)	56	2.5	44	63	59	40
Nepro (54)	56	4.5	59	59	59	40
Renalcal (60)	50	1.7	3	4	3	5
Cow's milk (19)	158	5.2	92	216	205	190

Conversion mg to mEq: sodium 23 mg = 1 mEq, potassium 39 mg = 1 mEq.

repletion. Moderate-to-severe hyperkalemia may require treatment with a potassium binder such as sodium polystyrene sulfonate (Kayexalate). In the case of infants and young children being fed milk formula, the potassium content of the formula can be reduced by pretreating it with kayexalate or an alternative formula with a lower potassium concentration can be used (Table 24.7). If constipated, the patient should be treated aggressively because significant quantities of potassium are eliminated through the gastrointestinal route in patients with CKD. In patients who are persistently hyperkalemic, dietary potassium intake should be limited, and foods rich in potassium to be minimized/avoided should include chocolates, potatoes (all forms), bananas, avocado, green leafy vegetables, dried fruits, concentrated tomato preparations, and orange juice. Altering the methods of food preparation, such as soaking vegetables before cooking, helps decrease the potassium content.

In children undergoing HD, dietary potassium intake should be distributed throughout the day, as high serum concentrations of potassium can develop when a large quantity of potassium is ingested at one time, regardless of the total daily dietary content. On the other hand, some patients receiving PD may become hypokalemic because of potassium losses in the dialysate and will require potassium supplementation.

VITAMINS AND MICRONUTRIENTS

The vitamin and mineral needs of pediatric patients with CKD are not clearly defined (other than for vitamin D), and the limited data that is available is derived from patients undergoing maintenance dialysis. Children with CKD are prone to develop vitamin deficiencies because of anorexia and dietary restrictions, while they are also at risk for developing toxic levels of vitamins when the renal clearance is significantly impaired. All of the water-soluble vitamins except pyridoxine are eliminated by the kidneys, and their clearance in patients with CKD is not known. However, most water-soluble vitamins are lost during maintenance dialysis and, in turn, dialysis patients are routinely provided special vitamin formulations that do not contain vitamins A and D, such as Nephronex (LLorens Pharmaceuticals) and Nephro-Vite (R&D Laboratories, Inc., Marina Del Rey, CA).

Based on the limited data, the current KDOQI Pediatric Nutrition Guidelines recommend the intake of at least 100% of the DRI for thiamin (B$_1$), riboflavin (B$_2$), niacin (B$_3$), pantothenic acid (B$_5$), pyridoxine (B$_6$), biotin (B$_8$), cobalamin (B$_{12}$), ascorbic acid (C), retinol (A), α-tocopherol (E), vitamin K, folic acid, copper, and zinc for children with CKD Stages 2 to 5, and those receiving maintenance dialysis. The guidelines suggest supplementation of vitamins and trace elements if dietary intake alone does not meet 100% of the DRI or if clinical evidence of a deficiency, possibly confirmed by low blood levels of the vitamin or trace element, is present. As most infant milk formulas, including Similac PM 60/40, are fortified with both water-soluble and fat-soluble vitamins, the majority of infants with CKD (and not yet on dialysis) receive the DRI for all vitamins (including vitamin A) by dietary intake alone and likely do not require vitamin supplementation. For children not receiving formula, supplementation with vitamin A is not recommended unless the dietary intake is very low, because of the risk for developing vitamin A toxicity.

STRATEGIES FOR ACHIEVING NUTRITION GOALS

Once the individualized quantity of various dietary components has been determined, the next step is to develop a nutrition plan that can meet these needs. This can be particularly challenging in pediatrics and requires the input of the family because many of the foods that are desirable in patients with CKD are not ones commonly liked/eaten by children, especially if their appetite is already suppressed. Because cultural food preferences often play an important role in the family's ability to adhere to dietary changes, dietary recommendations should also be tailored to help families modify, but not eliminate cultural food preferences. The nutrition plan should be modified as necessary according to changes in the child's nutritional status, kidney function, dialytic therapy, medication regimen, and psychosocial situation.

Ideally, the dietitian will establish a positive rapport with both the child and the primary caretakers in order to enhance compliance with the recommended nutritional regimen. In the case of infants, the parents or primary caretaker who is responsible for feeding the child have the greatest interaction with the dietician; in contrast, adolescents should receive the majority of information directly because they often eat independently. It is noteworthy that the two most vulnerable groups of patients in terms of the risk for malnutrition are infants and adolescents. While infants are at special risk because of the frequent occurrence of anorexia and emesis, many adolescents have poor eating habits.

Energy and Protein

Infants with CKD can initially be fed breast milk. The most commonly used milk formula in the United States for infants with moderate to severe CKD is Similac PM 60/40 (Abbott Nutrition), a product whose protein, sodium, potassium, calcium, and phosphorus content closely resembles breast milk (Table 24.7). If hyperkalemia and/or hyperphosphatemia exist, the Similac PM 60/40 can be mixed with renal-specific formulas such as Renastart (Vitaflo, USA) or Renalcal (Nestle) to decrease the concentration of potassium and phosphorus. The potassium and phosphorus concentration of the formula can also be decreased by treating the formula with a potassium resin sodium polystyrene sulfonate (Kayexalate) or sevelamer carbonate (Renvela), respectively. The liquid formulation of sodium polystyrene sulfonate should be avoided because of a recent report of aluminum contamination associated with its use.

Infants with CKD or receiving dialysis who are prescribed a fluid restriction may require a greater caloric density of their milk formula than the standard 20 kcal per oz. It is important to recognize that concentrating the milk formula will also increase the protein and electrolyte/mineral content; thus, this approach should be used cautiously. Instead, the provision of extra calories can be achieved by adding carbohydrate and/or fat modules to the formula with a glucose polymer such as SolCarb (Solace Nutrition) or in the form of corn oil. However, the use of corn and other oils as additives is not common because they do not mix well with formula and can obstruct feeding tubes. Microlipid (Nestle Nutrition), a 50% fat emulsion from safflower oil with 4.5 kcal per mL and Duocal (Nutricia North America), a fat and carbohydrate combo modular with 5 kcal per g of powder (59% calories from carbohydrate and 41% from fat), are additional commercially available products for energy supplementation. The latter is not approved for infants younger than 1 year. The quantity of both carbohydrate and fat modules can gradually be increased to raise the caloric density of the formula to as much as 60 kcal per oz. It is advisable to wait at least 24 hours following each 2- to 4-kcal per oz incremental increase in concentration to enhance patient tolerance.

To help meet the energy needs of older children, calorie-dense (1.8 kcal per mL) preparations such as Nepro and Suplena (Abbott Nutrition) have been formulated specifically for renal patients. Suplena has a lower protein content than Nepro (2.5 g vs. 4.5 g per 100 kcal), and is thus preferable for predialysis patients. Dilution of these preparations to half to two-third strength may improve acceptance and tolerance in young children. In children beyond infancy, common foods that have a high-caloric content, but a relatively low mineral and protein content are often more readily accepted than high-calorie carbohydrate supplements. Powdered fruit drinks, frozen fruit flavored desserts, candy, jelly, honey, and other concentrated sweets can be used for this purpose. However, the altered taste acuity associated with uremia may limit the acceptability of these foods. In addition, one may need to avoid high-carbohydrate foods in the presence of hypertriglyceridemia. Under these circumstances, unsaturated fats may be the preferred choice of high-calorie food sources. Children and adolescents should also be encouraged to use margarine on popcorn, bread, vegetables, rice, and noodles for added calories.

In contrast to energy intake, the protein requirements of older children and adolescents with CKD are usually met by voluntary, unsupplemented consumption. If the protein intake is insufficient owing to concomitant phosphorus restriction in the patient with severe CKD/ESRD, the protein module, Beneprotein (Nestle Nutrition), a whey protein concentrate, can be provided. One gram of Beneprotein is equivalent to 0.86 g protein. Whey protein powder can also be added to food items for older children.

Nutritional therapy, irrespective of the route of administration or caloric density of the formula, should provide a balance of calories from carbohydrate and unsaturated fats within the physiologic ranges recommended as the acceptable macronutrient distribution ranges (AMDRs) of the DRI. The recommended AMDRs for children older than 4 years are 45% to 65% from carbohydrate, 25% to 35% from fat (polyunsaturated/saturated ratio of 1), and 10% to 30% from protein; children younger than 3 years need a somewhat lower proportion of protein (5% to 20%) and a greater proportion of fat (30% to 40%) in their diets to meet energy needs. An adequate amount of nonprotein calories should be provided for protein-sparing effects. It should, however, be noted that during the advanced stages of uremia, the protein-sparing effect of added fat calories may be inferior to the effect of added concentrated carbohydrate calories.

Enteral Nutritional Support

Enteral feeding should be considered if nutritional intake by the oral route is suboptimal. The use of enteral support has resulted in maintenance or improvement of standard deviation scores for weight and/or height in infants and young children with moderate to severe CKD and those undergoing maintenance dialysis. In fact, many clinicians have advocated for early enteral feeding at the first sign of growth failure during infancy.

Nasogastric (NG) tubes, gastrostomy tubes/buttons, and gastrojeju-nostomy tubes have been used to provide supplemental enteral feedings, which can be given as an intermittent bolus or more commonly by continuous infusion during the night. Continuous overnight feeds are generally preferred to allow time during the day for regular oral intake. Historically, the NG tube has been used most frequently in infants and young children because it is easily inserted and is generally well tolerated. However, this route of therapy is often complicated by recurrent emesis and the need for frequent tube replacement, in addition to the risk of pulmonary aspiration, nasoseptal erosion, and psychologic distress of the caretaker because of the cosmetic appearance. Persistent emesis can be addressed by slowing the rate of formula delivery and by the addition of antiemetic agents such as metoclopramide or domperidol. Additionally, whey-predominant formulas can be beneficial because they have been shown to stimulate gastric emptying.

The gastrostomy tube or button has been used as the enteral route of choice by many clinicians, and has the cosmetic advantage of being hidden beneath clothing. Once placed, it can be used within several days. Many, but not all clinicians recommend that the patient should be investigated for gastroesophageal reflux prior to undertaking gastrostomy placement so that a Nissen fundoplication can be created at the same time, if required. Potential complications of gastrostomy tubes/buttons include exit-site infection, leakage, obstruction, gastrocutaneous fistula, and peritonitis in patients receiving PD. To decrease the risk of peritonitis, the gastrostomy should be placed either before or simultaneously during PD catheter placement, in the latter case accompanied by antibiotic and antifungal prophylaxis. In addition, it may be better to avoid combining gastrostomy placement and PD catheter placement in a severely malnourished patient until the nutritional status and general immune status of the patient can be improved by other means, such as with NG feeds.

A common and serious complication of using any form of enteral tube feeding is a prolonged and potentially difficult transition from tube to oral feeding. Regular non-nutritive sucking and repetitive oral stimulation are recommended for all tube-fed infants. A multidisciplinary feeding team consisting of a dietitian, occupational therapist, and behavioral psychologist can help facilitate the transition from tube to oral feeding.

Alternative Routes of Nutritional Support

The substitution of amino acids for dextrose in the PD fluid and the provision of parenteral nutrition during HD sessions (intradialytic parenteral nutrition) are two additional aggressive approaches to nutritional supplementation that have had limited pediatric application.

Suggested Readings

Ali FN, Arquelles LM, Langman CB, et al. Vitamin D deficiency in children with chronic kidney disease: uncovering an epidemic. *Pediatrics* 2009; 123:791–796.

Brewer ED. Growth of small children managed with chronic peritoneal dialysis and nasogastric tube feedings: 203-month experience in 14 patients. *Adv Perit Dial* 1990;6:269–272.

Chadha V, Warady BA. Nutritional management of the child with kidney disease. In: Kopple JD, Massry SG, Kalantar-Zadeh K, eds. *Nutritional Management of Renal Disease*. 3rd ed. Amsterdam: Elsevier Inc; 2013:581–603.

Dibas B, Warady BA. Vitamin D status of children receiving chronic dialysis. *Pediatr Nephrol* 2012;27:1967–1973.

Expert Panel on Integrated Guidelines for Cardiovascular Health and Risk Reduction in Children and Adolescents: Summary Report. *Pediatrics* 2011;128(suppl 5): S213–S256.

Food and Nutrition Board: Dietary reference intakes for energy, carbohydrate, fiber, fat, fatty acids, cholesterol, protein, and amino acids (macronutrients). *Food and Nutrition Board.* Washington, DC: National Academies; 2002.

Kari JA, Gonzalez C, Ledermann SE, et al. Outcome and growth of infants with severe chronic renal failure. *Kidney Int* 2000;57:1681–1687.

National Kidney Foundation. KDOQI clinical practice guideline for nutrition in children with CKD: 2008 update. *Am J Kidney Dis* 2009;53(suppl 2):S1–S124.

Parekh RS, Flynn JT, Smoyer WE, et al. Improved growth in young children with severe chronic renal insufficiency who use specified nutritional therapy. *J Am Soc Nephrol* 2001;12:2418–2426.

Rees L, Azocar M, Borzych D, et al. Growth in very young children undergoing chronic peritoneal dialysis. *J Am Soc Nephrol* 2011;22:2303–2312.

Rees L, Brandt ML. Tube feeding in children with chronic kidney disease: technical and practical issues. *Pediatr Nephrol* 2010;25:699–704.

Rees L, Jones H. Nutritional management and growth in children with chronic kidney disease. *Pediatr Nephrol* 2013;28:527–536.

Saland JM, Ginsberg H, Fisher EA. Dyslipidemia in pediatric renal disease: epidemiology, pathophysiology, and management. *Curr Opin Pediatr* 2002;14:197–204.

Srivaths PR, Wong C, Goldstein SL. Nutrition aspects in children receiving maintenance hemodialysis: impact on outcome. *Pediatr Nephrol* 2009; 24:951–957.

Strologo LD, Principato F, Sinibaldi D, et al. Feeding dysfunction in infants with severe chronic renal failure after long-term nasogastric tube feeding. *Pediatr Nephrol* 1997;11:84–86.

Taylor JM, Oladitan L, Carlson S, et al. Renal formulas pretreated with medications alters the nutrient profile. *Pediatr Nephrol* 2015;30:1815–1823.

Warady BA, Kriley M, Alon U, et al. Vitamin status of infants receiving long-term peritoneal dialysis. *Pediatr Nephrol* 1994;8:354–356.

Warady BA, Weis L, Johnson L. Nasogastric tube feeding in infants on peritoneal dialysis. *Perit Dial Int* 1996;16:S521–S525.

Watson AR, Coleman JE, Warady BA. When and how to use nasogastric and gastrostomy feeding for nutritional support in infants and children on CAPD/CCPD. In: Fine RN, Alexander SR, Warady BA, eds. *CAPD/CCPD in Children.* Boston, MA: Kluwer Academic; 1998:281–300.

Wong CS, Gipson DS, Gillen DL, et al. Anthropometric measures and risk of death in children with end-stage renal disease. *Am J Kidney Dis* 2000;36:811–819.

World Health Organization. *WHO Child Growth Standards: Length/Height-for-Age, Weight-for-Age, Weight-for-Length, Weight-for-Height and Body Mass Index-for-Age. Methods and Development.* Geneva Switzerland: World Health Organization; 2006:332.

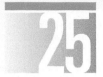

Sample Menus for Chronic Kidney Disease Patients

Jane H. Greene

MEAL PLANNING

No matter what stage of kidney disease, planning meals to meet nutritional requirements, prevent malnutrition, and maintain acceptable blood chemistries, blood pressure, and fluid status is a daunting task for any patient.

Most renal dietitians use the *average* calorie, protein, sodium, potassium, and phosphorus content for the food groups lists developed by the Renal Dietitians dietetic practice group of the American Dietetic Association when calculating a meal plan for a patient with chronic kidney disease (CKD). Steps involved to calculate a meal plan for any patient are as follows:

- Determine the nutrition prescription.
- Determine the amount of high-biologic value (HBV) protein needed.
- Determine the number of meat and milk choices needed to supply the HBV protein.
- Distribute the remainder of protein between starch, milk substitute, fruit, and vegetable choices.
- Provide for the remainder of caloric requirements with fat and high-calorie choices (foods high in carbohydrates that contain only a trace of protein and minimal electrolytes).
- Total each nutrient and adjust the diet to meet the previously established nutrition prescription.

The following sample menus and meal planning suggestions are a starting point for the health care team to assist patients and their caregivers. Each example is based on the nutritional requirements of a 70-kg patient, adapted from the Kidney Disease Outcomes Quality Initiative guidelines for the nutrition prescription.

Chronic Kidney Disease Stages 3 and 4
Nutrition Prescription: 0.6 g protein per kg body weight (42 g) and 30 calories per kg (2,100 calories) <2,400 mg sodium, 800 mg phosphorus, <2,400 mg potassium.

Goals/Outcomes: prevent malnutrition, slow progression of kidney disease, decrease nitrogenous waste products, and prevent symptoms of uremia.

American Diet

Breakfast	½ cup almond milk, 1 cup fruit loops cereal, 1 medium powdered sugar donut, 1 cup apple juice, 1 cup coffee with cream and sugar
Lunch	Chicken salad on croissant (2 oz cooked chicken, 1 tsp mayonnaise, ¼ tsp dried tarragon, and 2 tsp chopped celery), wedge of iceberg lettuce with 1 tsp Catalina dressing, poached pear with 1 tsp brown sugar, ¼ tsp nutmeg, and 12 oz lemon-lime soda

Dinner	2 oz fish and 2 hushpuppies fried in ¼ cup vegetable oil, ½ cup green beans seasoned with onion, ½ cup coleslaw with 1 tsp mayonnaise, and 12 oz lemonade
Snacks	Fruit-flavored Popsicle and 8 oz cranberry juice cocktail

Nutritional Analysis: 2,140 calories, 42.5 g protein, 1,979 mg sodium, 803 mg phosphorus, and 1,535 mg potassium.

Dietary Reference Intake
The diet for CKD contains less than the dietary reference intake for several water-soluble vitamins because of the restriction of high-protein and high-potassium foods. Supplementation of particular vitamins and/or minerals may be required in some patients.

Chronic Kidney Disease Stage 5: Dialysis
Nutrition Prescription: 1.2 g protein per kg body weight (84 g protein) and 35 calories per kg (2,450 calories) <2,400 mg sodium, <1,200 mg phosphorus, and <2,400 mg potassium with 1,000 mL fluid restriction.

Goals/Outcomes: adequate protein and calorie intake to maintain nutritional status, interdialytic fluid weight gains within acceptable range, laboratory values within acceptable range, blood pressure within appropriate limits, and level of functional ability maintained.

American Diet

Breakfast	½ cup fresh blueberries, 1 cup frosted corn flakes, 4 oz 2% milk, 1 scrambled egg, 1 toaster muffin, and 6 oz brewed coffee with half and half and sugar
Lunch	2 slices white bread, ½ cup low sodium, water-packed tuna, 1 tsp mayonnaise with 2 tsp sweet pickle relish and ¼ tsp celery seed and lettuce leaf, ½ cup carrot sticks, ½ cup sweetened applesauce, 10 vanilla wafers, and 8 oz lemon-flavored drink mix with sugar
Dinner	4 oz braised chuck roast, ½ cup parsley buttered noodles, ½ cup frozen French-style green beans, 1½ to 2 cups tossed salad: Bibb lettuce, red and yellow bell pepper strips, sliced cucumbers, 2 tsp Catalina dressing, dinner roll with 2 tsp unsalted tub margarine, ½ cup fruit sorbet, and 8 oz iced tea with sugar
Snack	2 Fruit roll-ups

Nutritional Analysis: 900 mL fluid, 2,330 calories, 82 g protein, 2,519 mg sodium, 1,100 mg phosphorus, and 2,267 mg potassium.
Dialysis patients may be tired and not interested in cooking on the days they receive their hemodialysis treatment. Offering ideas for quick meals at home and nutritional supplements could prevent a trip to the drive-thru window for a high-sodium fastfood meal on the way home.

Dietary Reference Intake
The diet for hemodialysis patients contains less than the daily recommended intake for several water-soluble vitamins because of the restriction of foods high in potassium and phosphorus, dialysate losses, and decreased intestinal absorption. Again, supplementation of particular vitamins and/or minerals may be required in some patients.

Kidney Transplant—Maintenance Needs
Nutrition Prescription: 1 g protein per kg body weight (70 g protein) and 25 to 30 calories per kg body weight (1,750 to 2,100 calories or adequate to

maintain desirable weight), fat <30% total calories (70 g total fat for 2,100 calories) with <300 mg cholesterol per day. Restrict or supplement vitamins and minerals as needed to meet recommended daily intake.

Goals/Outcomes: achieve or maintain desirable weight, maintain acceptable blood glucose levels, maintain serum cholesterol levels <200 mg per dL, maintain normal blood pressure, maintain optimal bone density, minimize side effects of medications, and maintain healthy lifestyle.

American Diet

Breakfast	¾ cup oatmeal, ½ cup blueberries, 8 oz skim milk, 1 slice whole-grain toast, 2 tsp tub margarine, 2 tsp jelly, and 4 oz orange juice, coffee, or tea
Lunch	3 oz turkey breast, 2 slices whole-grain bread, lettuce, tomato, mustard, 1 cup carrot sticks, salad of ½ cup chopped apple, 2 tsp diced celery and 2 tsp chopped walnuts blended with 1 to 2 tsp light mayonnaise, and iced tea
Dinner	3 oz flank steak, steamed broccoli with lemon, small baked potato, 2 tsp tub margarine, 1 slice Italian bread, ½ cup sliced strawberries, and 1 slice angel food cake, iced tea

Nutritional Analysis: approx. 1,776 calories, 74 g protein.

Asian Indian

The staple food of western and northern India is wheat, whereas in eastern and southern India rice is more common. Chicken, fish and mutton are the main meats consumed in India. Beef is generally not eaten by Hindus (the predominant religion), and pork is not consumed by Muslims. Different religions observe dietary laws that could impact eating patterns, especially related to fasting and feasting.

Chronic Kidney Disease Stages 3 and 4

Breakfast	1 paratha with 2 tsp margarine/ghee, ½ cup cereal, ½ cup milk, $^1/_3$ small papaya, and coffee/masala tea
Lunch	1 chapati with margarine/ghee, ½ cup chicken curry, ½ cup rice, ½ cup carrots, and1 apple, coffee/tea
Dinner	1 chapati with margarine/ghee, ½ cup mutton curry, ½ cup cabbage, ½ cup raita, and coffee/tea

Chronic Kidney Disease Stages 3 and 4: Vegetarian

Breakfast	1 paratha with 2 tsp margarine/ghee, ½ cup cereal, ½ cup milk, $^1/_3$ small papaya, coffee/masala tea
Lunch	1 chapati with margarine/ghee, ½ cup mung dhal, ½ cup carrots, 1 apple, and coffee/tea
Dinner	1 chapati with margarine/ghee, ¾ cup dhal with vegetables, and ½ cup raita, coffee/tea

Nutritional Analysis: approx. 2,170 calories, 46 g protein, 1,692 mg sodium, 1,722 mg potassium, and 766 mg phosphorus.

Chronic Kidney Disease Stage 5: Dialysis

Breakfast	2 parathas with margarine/ghee, 1 egg, 1 cup cereal, ½ cup milk, ½ cup mango, and 6 oz coffee/masala tea

| Lunch | 2 chapati with margarine/ghee, 1 cup chicken curry, 1 cup rice, ½ cup carrots, ½ cup peas, 1 apple, and 8 oz coffee/tea |
| Dinner | 2 chapati with margarine/ghee, 1 cup mutton curry, 1 cup rice, ½ cup cabbage, ½ cup raita, and 8 oz coffee/tea |

Chronic Kidney Disease Stage 5: Vegetarian/Dialysis

Breakfast	2 paratha with margarine/ghee, 1 egg, ½ cup milk, ½ cup mango, and 6 oz coffee/masala tea
Lunch	2 chapati with margarine/ghee, ¾ cup mung dhal, ½ cup carrots, ½ cup peas, 1 apple, and 8 oz coffee/tea
Dinner	2 chapati with margarine/ghee, 1 cup dhal with vegetables, ½ cup rice, 1 tangerine, ½ cup raita, and 8 oz coffee/tea

Nutritional Analysis: approx. 3,000 calories, 88 g protein, 2,800 mg sodium, 2,550 mg potassium, and 1,340 mg phosphorus.

Kidney Transplant

Breakfast	1 paratha with margarine/ghee, ½ cup cereal, 2 eggs, 1 banana, 1 cup milk, and coffee/masala tea
Lunch	1 chapati with margarine or ghee, 1 cup fish curry, ½ cup rice, ½ cup cabbage, ½ cup carrots, ½ cup grapes, and coffee/tea
Dinner	1 chapati with margarine or ghee, 1 cup chicken curry, ½ cup rice, ½ cup mixed vegetables, and coffee/tea

Nutritional Analysis: approx. 2,400 calories and 92 g protein.

Vegetarian Kidney Transplant

Breakfast	1 paratha with margarine or ghee, ½ cup cereal, 2 eggs, 1 banana, 1 cup milk, and coffee/masala tea
Lunch	1 chapati with margarine or ghee, 1 cup dhal, ½ cup rice, ½ cup carrots, 1 apple, and coffee/tea
Dinner	1 chapati with margarine or ghee, 1 cup mung dhal, ½ cup rice, ½ cup mixed vegetables, 2 tsp chutney, ½ cup raita, and coffee/tea

Nutritional Analysis: approx. 2,400 calories and 85 g protein.

Mexican

The traditional diet of Mexico is high in carbohydrates with corn, beans, and rice eaten in some form at almost every meal. The diet is usually composed of three meals with lunch as the largest meal and may include an afternoon snack. Diet restrictions needed for kidney disease can require major changes in the Mexican diet because of the high sodium, potassium, and phosphorus content of the foods usually eaten by this culture.

Chronic Kidney Disease Stages 3 and 4

Breakfast	1 sweet roll, 1 cup café con leche (coffee with milk), and 1 fried egg
Lunch	2 oz grilled chicken, ½ cup Spanish rice with chili peppers, ½ cup corn, 2 small corn tortillas, 1 small apple, and 12 oz lemon-lime soda
Dinner	6 oz bowl lentil soup, ½ cup buttered rice, ½ cup mustard greens, 2 small corn tortillas, ½ cup mango, and 12 oz iced tea

Nutritional Analysis: approx. 1,800 calories, 47 g protein, 1,050 mg sodium, 2,000 mg potassium, and 810 mg phosphorus.

Chronic Kidney Disease Stage 5: Dialysis

Breakfast	1 sweet roll, 1 cup café con leche (coffee with milk), 2 fried eggs, and ½ cup oatmeal.
Lunch	4 oz grilled chicken, ½ cup Spanish rice with chili peppers, ½ cup corn, 2 small corn tortillas, and 12 oz lemon-lime soda
Dinner	1 cup chili con carne, 2 small corn tortillas, 1 small apple, and 12 oz lemon-lime soda

Nutritional Analysis: approx. 1,960 calories, 82 g protein, 2,007 mg sodium, 2,138 mg potassium, and 1,365 mg phosphorus.

Kidney Transplant

Breakfast	1 cup oatmeal, 1 cup milk, 1 cup café con leche (coffee with milk), and 1 cup papaya
Lunch	4 oz grilled chicken, ½ cup Spanish rice with chili peppers, 1.2 cup corn, 2 small corn tortillas, and 12 oz soda (colas acceptable)
Dinner	1 cup chili con carne, 2 small corn tortillas, 1 small apple, and 12 oz soda (colas acceptable)

Nutritional Analysis: 1,810 calories and 72 g protein.

Suggested Readings

Fox M. Global food practices, cultural competency, and dietetics. *J Acad Nutr Diet* 2015;115:342–348.

Fox M. Global food practices, cultural competency, and dietetics: Part 2. *J Acad Nutr Diet* 2015;115:499–504.

Fox M. Global food practices, cultural competency, and dietetics: Part 3. *J Acad Nutr Diet* 2015;115:701–705.

SUBJECT INDEX

Page numbers followed by *f* or *t* indicate material in figures or tables, respectively.